Benefits of exercise

Benefits of exercise: the evidence

P. H. Fentem, N. B. Turnbull *and* E. J. Bassey

Manchester University Press
Manchester and New York
Distributed exclusively in the USA and Canada by St. Martin's Press

Published by Manchester University Press
Oxford Road, Manchester M13 9PL, UK
and Room 400, 175 Fifth Avenue,
New York, NY 10010, USA

Distributed exclusively in the USA and Canada
by St. Martin's Press, Inc.,
175 Fifth Avenue, New York, NY 10010, USA

British Library cataloguing in publication data
   Fentem, P.H. *(Peter H.)*
   Benefits of exercise : the evidence.
   1. Man. Health. Role of physical fitness.
   Bibliographies
   I. Title II. Turnbull, N.B. III. Bassey, E.J. (E.
   Joan)
   016.6137

   ISBN 0-7190-2430-7

Library of Congress cataloguing in publication data
Fentem, P. H. (Peter H.)
   Benefits of exercise: the evidence/P. H. Fentem, N.B. Turnbull,
E. J. Bassey.
      p. cm.
   ISBN 0–7190–2430–7: $90.00 (est.)
    1. Exercise—Health aspects—Bibliography. I. Turnbull, N. B.
II. Bassey, E. J. (E. Joan) III. Title.
   Z6663. E9F46   1989
   [QP301]
   016.6137'1—dc20   89–31595

   ISBN 0 7190 2430 7 *hardback*

Typeset in Great Britain
by Megaron, Cardiff, Wales
Printed in Great Britain by
Billing and Sons Ltd., Worcester

Contents

Acknowledgements

We are grateful to the Sports Council and the Health Education Authority who provided a research grant to support the work which lead to the publication of 'The New Case for Exercise' and the assembly of this bibliography. The encouragement and advice which the authors received from Professor Jerry Morris, Mr Michael Collins and members of the Fitness and Health Advisory Group is gratefully acknowledged.

We are greatly indebted for their help to colleagues both in Nottingham and elsewhere who are too numerous to mention individually. As physiologists we have had to range far outside our own research areas in order to produce this book. We have therefore been glad to rely when necessary on the expertise of others, for instance, in establishing the validity of methodologies, in interpretating results and identifying up to date sources of information.

Special thanks are due to Mrs Avrille Blecher for unstinting hard work in entering and sorting references during the assembling of the bibliography.

We hope that those authors whose work would have enhanced the bibliography, but whom we have failed to include, will accept our apologies.

Introduction

This is a selected bibliography of the evidence that exercise is of benefit to health. The evidence has been drawn from the scientific and medical literature published world-wide during the last 15 years. It covers a range of disciplines and deals with the mechanisms for improvement in physical capabilities, and the prevention and amelioration of disease through exercise. It also considers the hazards of exercise and the deleterious effects of lack of activity. It is the result of a search commissioned in 1986 by the Sports' Council and the Health Education Council. The findings of the search have been published as 'The New Case for Exercise', 1988. The outcome of a previous search was published by the Sports' Council in 1978 as 'The Case for Exercise'.

The searches were instigated because of widespread interest in the potential health benefits of exercise and national concern about the prevalence of inactivity-related disability. Of particular interest was the possibility that exercise might have an important role in preventing disease, notably coronary heart disease, and in maintaining physical capabilities, especially in the elderly and handicapped. In addition there was concern about the hazards of exercise, particularly in those with a health problem. This leads to a need to define the balance of benefit and risk.

The published literature contains strong evidence that suitable exercise is of benefit in many chronic diseases and disorders and it also improves positive health. For example, exercise has preventive effects on the development of coronary heart disease and osteoporosis, ameliorating effects on arthritis and respiratory diseases and curative effects on hypertension and mild late-onset diabetes. Improvements in positive health are apparent in an ability to work harder and longer with less fatigue than previously. The range of activities in which a person of any age can participate comfortably is thus widened and the incapacitating effects of disability or old age minimized. The evidence fully justifies encouraging participation of all age groups in physical exercise as part of a national health education programme.

The bibliography

The bibliography is divided by physiological function into eight major sections. These are further divided into sub-sections, prefaced by a brief summary. References are allocated to one sub-section only and given a unique reference number, the first three digits of which identify the section and sub-section. Because of the large amount of material within Cardiovascular Function, Primary Prevention has been further sub-divided, e.g. 231.4, 'Lipids'. Each reference has been given keywords which are not constrained by sub-section and are detailed below under organization of material.

The scope of the search

The search was concentrated on material published between 1978 and 1988, although earlier references, some from the previous search, were included if more recent work on the subject was not available or if they were of special interest.

This is not a comprehensive bibliography, many papers have been omitted and the selection inevitably reflects the judgement of the authors. Our aim was to list within a single volume the best evidence available concerning the effects of exercise on health. Its breadth therefore precludes an exhaustive listing. Our searches have been thorough and we feel that this approach enhances the usefulness of the book. For those embarking upon an in-depth review of a topic within the bibliography, it should serve as a useful starting point.

The search concentrated on identifying original research papers which reported controlled studies in humans, using validated methods, appropriate statistics and ample numbers of subjects. Priority was given to papers in which the initial exercise capacity of the subjects was defined. A few animal studies have been included where the nature of the intervention made human studies impossible.

The quality of the references varies somewhat between sections. Where evidence was scarce the quality is poorer than in sections where much evidence was available and choices could be made. If possible, papers which used different approaches were chosen. For example, references using epidemiological and intervention methods and prospective and retrospective assessment were included in preference to several papers using the same method. Papers by a number of different authors and from different countries were favoured over a number by the same author. If several papers were similar in content and quality the more recent were included. Unbiased reviews and books were accepted, but letters, case reports, unreferenced papers and papers published in obscure journals or written in a language other than English were rejected,

unless information on the topic was scarce.

The following aspects were addressed:-

1) The mechanisms by which exercise changes function or capacity
2) The scale of health benefits of exercise
3) The prescription which leads to a definable positive benefit
4) Details of any hazard or deterioration of exercise
5) The role of exercise in preventing disease
6) The role of exercise in ameliorating the effects of disease

Exercise included contrived exercise training programmes, leisure activity, occupational activity, and customary daily activity.

References which investigated the effects of lack of physical activity in a controlled manner were included, but sports or activities which did not involve physical effort were not. References in which exercise was used acutely as a provocative test rather than chronically as a training intervention were not included except where they seemed essential as background material or for explaining mechanisms.

In the summaries which head each sub-section, unless otherwise specified, exercise is taken to mean rhythmic activity of a moderate nature using large muscle groups at an intensity a little greater than that to which the individual is accustomed, sustained for at least 20 minutes and repeated at least three times a week.

Sources of information

The search has been helped by reference to Medline from 1980 – 1986, Current Contents, Citation Indices, Index Medicus and Physical Fitness/Sports Medicine (U.S.President's Council on Physical Fitness and Sport). Searches have been made of the relevant journals in the Nottingham University Libraries (Medical School and the Science Libraries) and the Pilkington Library, Loughborough University of

Technology. Consultation with appropriate colleagues in Nottingham and elsewhere (see acknowledgements) has both widened and focused the scope of our search.

Organization of material

Indices. The section and sub-sections are listed in the table of contents by number and heading. There is a complete author index with a list of reference numbers after each name and two indices of keywords (see below).

Reference numbers. Within the sub-sections the references are listed alphabetically by first author and each reference has a unique number. The first digit indicates its section and the second two digits indicate its sub-section. The last two digits are unique within sub-section, and are appear in order of entry. For example, reference 210/25 is in section CARDIOVASCULAR FUNCTION (2), sub-section Cardiac performance'(10), and is the 25th entry listed in that sub-section.

Keywords are listed in alphabetical order after each reference. There are two categories of keywords, global which are used throughout the bibliography and specific which operate within sub-section. The 'Alphabetical Index of Keywords' contains all the keywords both global and specific.

Global keywords include section and sub-section headings as well as items which allow retrieval from perspectives other than physiological function such as male/female, children/adult/elderly. They are defined in the 'Grouped Index of Global Keywords'.

Specific keywords allow retrieval in addition to the global keywords within sub-section. They are listed and defined at the beginning of each sub-section and pertain to relevant measurements, diseases and conditions. They are only used within that sub-section.

Cross-referencing. As references are allocated to one sub-section only, according to the major topic of the paper, references containing material relevant to another section or sub-section will have the appropriate section heading as a keyword in capital letters but no specific keywords from the other section. For instance, a study primarily about changes in lipid levels in diabetics will be in the sub-section CARBOHYDRATE TOLERANCE, however, if changes in blood lipids were measured, the global keyword LIPIDS would appear, but not the specific keyword 'Apoproteins'. Similarly, to find any papers about 'Osteoporosis' *outside* the BONES section, the search must be on the global keyword BONES, because there will be no entries carrying the specific keyword 'Osteoporosis'.

KEYWORDS are listed in the appendix

Summary of evidence: exercise ameliorates, prevents or reverses poor physical capability arising from low levels of customary activity

THE PROBLEM

Inactivity related disability was suspected to be widespread and to prejudice the quality of life especially in the elderly. Improvements in maximal performance, aerobic capacity and adaptation to exercise are well known in athletic individuals. Are they also available to the sedentary, old or disabled? Exercise implies rhythmic activity using large muscle groups at an intensity a little greater than that to which the individual is accustomed and sustained for 20 minutes 3 times a week.

SCOPE

This section contains references dealing primarily with changes produced by exercise in physical capability assessed as maximal oxygen uptake (measured or predicted), maximal or functional performance, maximal working capacity, or submaximal response to a standard level of exercise. There is a large literature, this section therefore contains a representative selection not a comprehensive listing. It contains references on the intensity and amount of exercise needed for effective improvement in physical capabilities, and on the effects of inactivity as well as exercise. It contains studies of all age groups, of the sedentary and the athletic, and includes studies of those who are physically handicapped.

METHODOLOGICAL DIFFICULTIES

Directly measured maximal oxygen uptake, maximal working capacity or performance require highly motivated and completely healthy subjects, consequently the information is selective. Objective criteria for maximal effort are only available for maximal oxygen uptake which reaches a plateau during exercise at a maximal work rate. The other studies rely on sub-maximal measurements of the relation between heart rate and oxygen uptake or work rate. The prediction of maximal oxygen uptake for an individual from such submaximal data carries an error of $\pm$ 15% or more depending on the data from which it has been predicted. The problem is exacerbated in older people because an age-related reduction in maximal heart rate is applied which carries a large standard deviation. In addition baseline data consisting of measurements on a single occasion are not usually satisfactory because of the effect of mild anxiety on heart rate. The intensity of the exercise must be related to the initial physical condition of the subject, otherwise it will not produce the overload upon which improvements depend. Useful epidemiological evidence on levels of customary activity or functional capabilities is scarce.

EVIDENCE

Despite these difficulties it is clear that improvements in these physical capabilities are available to almost anyone. The magnitude of the improvement in maximal oxygen uptake varies between 10% and 50% and it is due to various improvements in both cardiovascular and muscle function. The evidence for this improved adaptation to exercise is in sections 120, 140, 210. Maximal work capacity is also increased, stamina is improved, effort tolerance increased and fatigue diminished. This amounts to an improvement in positive health and in the quality of life which is especially important for those handicapped by disease or disability and in the elderly. Their physical safety margins for maintaining an independent lifestyle may be small and should therefore be optimized.

110/1   **Abrams, M.**   (1978)
Beyond Three Score years and ten – a first report on a survey of the elderly
Age Concern Research Publication.
Elderly, Review

110/2   **Adams, F.H.**   (1973)
Factors affecting working capacity of children and adolescents. In: Physical Activity, Human Growth and Development (Ed.) Lawrence Rarick, G.
Academic Press
Children, GROWTH, Review

110/3   **Adams, M. & de Vries, H.A.**   (1973)
Physiological effects on an exercise training regimen upon women aged 52 to 79
J Gerontol **28**, 50-55
AEROBIC CAPACITY, BLOOD PRESSURE, Body composition, Elderly, Exercise programme, Female

110/4   **American College of Sports Medicine**   (1978)
Position Statement on: The recommended quantity and quality of exercise for developing and maintaining fitness in healthy adults
Med Sci Sports **10**, vii-x
Review

110/5   **Andersen, K.L., Ilmarinen, J., Rutenfranz, J., Ottmann, W., Berndt, I., Kylian, H. & Ruppel, M.**   (1984)
Leisure time sports activities and maximal aerobic power during late adolescence
Eur J Appl Physiol **52**, 431-436
AEROBIC CAPACITY, Body composition, Children, Leisure activity

110/6   **Andersen, K.L., Seliger, V., Rutenfranz, J. & Skrobak-Kaczynski, J.**   (1976)
Physical performance capacity of children in Norway. Part iv. The rate of growth in maximal aerobic power and the influence of improved physical education in a rural community – population parameters in a rural community
Eur J Appl Physiol **35**, 49-58
AEROBIC CAPACITY, Children, Longitudinal

110/7   **Anderson, L.B., Henckel, P. & Saltin, B.**   (1987)
Maximal oxygen uptake in Danish adolescents 16-19 years of age
Eur J Appl Physiol **56**, 74-82
AEROBIC CAPACITY, Body composition, Children

110/8   **Aniansson, A., Grimby, G., Rundgren, A., Svanborg, A. & Orlander, J.**   (1980)
Physical training in old men
Age and Ageing **9**, 186-187
AEROBIC CAPACITY, Elderly, Exercise programme, Intervention, Male, MUSCLE METABOLISM, MUSCLE STRENGTH

110/9   **Aniansson, A., Rundgren A. & Sperling L.**   (1980)
Evaluation of functional capacities in activities of daily living in 70-year-old men and women
Scand J Rehabil Med **12**, 145-154
Customary activity, Elderly

110/10   Asayama, K., Nakamura, Y.,
Ogata, H., Hatada, K., Okuma, H. &
Deguchi, Y.   (1985)
Physical fitness of paraplegics in full
wheelchair marathon racing
Paraplegia **23**, 277-287
*Adult, Handicap, Leisure activity,
Marathon*

110/11   Asmussen, E., Fruensgaard, K., &
Norgaard, S.   (1975)
A follow-up longitudinal study of
selected physiologic functions in former
physical education students – after forty
years
J Am Geriatr Soc **23**, 442-450
*Adult, AEROBIC CAPACITY, BLOOD
PRESSURE, Longitudinal, MUSCLE
STRENGTH, RESPIRATORY
FUNCTION*

110/12   Åstrand, P-O.   (1976)
Quantification of exercise capability and
evaluation of physical capacity in man
Prog Cardiovasc Dis **19**, 51-67
Review

110/13   Åstrand, P-O.   (1987)
Exercise physiology and its role in disease
prevention and in rehabilitation
Arch Phys Med Rehabil **68**, 305-309
Adult, Review

110/14   Åstrand, P-O. & Rodahl,
K.   (1986)
Textbook of work physiology
McGraw Hill
Review

110/15   Badenhop, D.J., Cleary, P.A.,
Schaal, S.F., Fox, E.L. & Bartels,
R.L.   (1983)
Physiological adjustments to higher or
lower intensity exercise in elders
Med Sci Sports Exerc **15**, 496-502
*AEROBIC CAPACITY, Elderly,
Female, Male, Exercise programme,
Intervention,*

110/16   Bailey, D.A., Shephard, R.J.,
Mirwald, R.L. & McBride, G.A.   (1974)
A current view of Canadian cardio-
respiratory fitness
Can Med Ass J **111**, 25-30
*Adult, AEROBIC CAPACITY,
Comparative*

110/17   Bale, P.   (1981)
Pre- and post-adolescent physiological
response to exercise
Br J Sports Med **15**, 246-249
*AEROBIC CAPACITY, BLOOD
PRESSURE, Children, Longitudinal*

110/18   Bar-Or, O., Skinner, J.S., Buskirk,
E.R. & Borg, G.   (1972)
Physiological and perceptual indicators
of physical stress in 41 to 60 year old men
who vary in conditioning level and in
body fatness
Med Sci Sports **4**, 96-100
*Adult, Body composition, Comparative,
Male, PERCEIVED EXERTION*

110/20   Bassey, E.J.   (1978)
Age, inactivity and some physiological
responses to exercise
Gerontology **24**, 66-77
*AEROBIC CAPACITY, Elderly,
Female, Inactivity, Male, Review*

110/21   Bassey, E.J.   (1985)
Benefits of exercise in the elderly. In:
Recent advances in geriatric medicine
(Ed.) Isaacs, B.
Churchill Livingstone, London 91-112
Elderly, Review

110/19   Bassey, E.J.   (1976)
The relations between age, inactivity and
the physiological response to exercise
PhD Thesis, University of Nottingham
Elderly, Review

110/22   Bassey, E.J., Patrick, J.M., Irving, J.M., Blecher, A. & Fentem, P.H.   (1983)
An unsupervised aerobics physical training programme in middle-aged factory workers: feasibility, validation and response
Eur J Appl Physiol **52**, 120-125
Adult, Customary activity, Exercise programme, Female, Intervention, Male

110/23   Beasley, C.R.   (1982)
Effects of a jogging program on cardiovascular fitness and work performance of mentally retarded adults
Am J Ment Defic **86**, 609-613
Adult, Exercise programme, Handicap, Intervention

110/24   Bengtsson, C., Vedin, J.A., Grimby, G. & Tibblin, G.   (1978)
Maximal work performance test in middle-aged women; results from a population study
Scand J clin Lab Invest **38**, 181-188
Acute exercise, Adult, BLOOD PRESSURE, Female, PERCEIVED EXERTION

110/25   Boileau, R.A.   (1984)
Advances in Pediatric Sport Sciences
Human Kinetics Publishers, Champaign, Illinois **1**,
Review

110/26   Borms, J.   (1986)
The child and exercise: an overview
J Sports Sci **4**, 3-20
Children, Review

110/27   Bouchard, C., Lesage, R., Lortie, G., Simoneau, J-A, Hamel, P., Boulay, M.R., Pérusse, L., Theriault, G. & Leblanc, C.   (1986)
Aerobic performance in brothers, dizygotic and monozygotic twins
Med Sci Sports Exerc **18**, 639-646
AEROBIC CAPACITY, Body composition, Comparative

110/28   Brown, M. & Gordon, W.A.   (1987)
Impact of impairment on activity patterns of children
Arch Phys Med Rehabil **68**, 828-832
Children, Customary activity, Handicap

110/29   Bundschuh, E.L. & Cureton, K.J.   (1982)
Effect of bicycle ergometer conditioning on the physical work capacity of mentally retarded adolescents
Am Correct Ther J **36**, 159-163
Children, Exercise programme, Handicap, Intervention

110/30   Buskirk, E.R. & Hodgson, J.L.   (1987)
Age and aerobic power: the rate of change in men and women
Fed Proc **46**, 1824-1829
AEROBIC CAPACITY, Review

110/31   Clausen, J.P.   (1977)
Effect of physical training on cardiovascular adjustments to exercise in man
Physiol Rev **57**, 779-815
Review

110/32   Clausen, J.P., Trap-Jensen, J. & Lassen, N.A.   (1970)
The effects of training on the heart rate during arm and leg exercise
Scand J clin Lab Invest **26**, 295-301
Adult, Exercise programme, Intervention, Male

110/33   Collis, M.L.   (1973)
The effects of a sustained training programme of breath-hold swimming on selected physiological parameters and swimming performance
Br J Sports Med **7**, 182-184
Athlete, Intervention, Leisure activity, RESPIRATORY FUNCTION, Vigorous

110/34   Conner, M.K., Smith, L.G., Fryer, A., Erickson, S., Fryer, S. & Drake, J.   (1986)
Future fit: a cardiovascular health education and fitness project in an after-school setting
J School Health **56**, 329-333
Children, Exercise programme, Intervention

110/35   Convertino, V.A., Goldwater, D.J. & Sandler, H.   (1986)
Bedrest-induced peak VO2 reduction associated with age, gender, and aerobic capacity
Aviat Space Environ Med **57**, 17-22
Adult, AEROBIC CAPACITY, Inactivity, Female, Male

110/36   Coutts, K.D. & Strogryn, J.L.   (1987)
Aerobic and anaerobic power of Canadian wheelchair track athletes
Med Sci Sports Exerc **19**, 62-65
Adult, AEROBIC CAPACITY, ANAEROBIC CAPACITY, Athlete, Handicap

110/37   Cowell, L.L., Squires, W.G. & Raven, P.B.   (1986)
Benefits of aerobic exercise for the paraplegic: a brief review
Med Sci Sports Exerc **18**, 501-508
Handicap, Review

110/38   Coyle, E.F., Martin, W.H., Bloomfield, S.A., Lowry, O.H.,& Holloszy, J.O.   (1985)
Effects of detraining on responses to submaximal exercise
J Appl Physiol **59**, 853-859
AEROBIC CAPACITY, Adult, CARDIAC PERFORMANCE, Inactivity, MUSCLE METABOLISM

110/39   Crockett, S.J.   (1987)
The family team approach to fitness: a proposal
Public Health Reports **102**, 546-551
Review

110/40   Cullinane, E.M., Sady, S.P., Vadeboncoeur, L., Burke, M. & Thompson, P.D.   (1986)
Cardiac size and VO2max do not decrease after short-term exercise cessation
Med Sci Sports Exerc **18**, 420-424
Adult, AEROBIC CAPACITY, Athlete, BLOOD PRESSURE, Body composition, CARDIAC PERFORMANCE, Inactivity, Intervention, Male

110/41   Cumming, G.R., Goulding, D. & Baggley, G.   (1971)
Working capacity of deaf and visually and mentally handicapped children
Arch Dis Child **46**, 490-494
AEROBIC CAPACITY, Children, Comparative, Handicap

110/42   Cunningham, D.A., Rechnitzer, P.A., Howard, J.H. & Donner, A.P.   (1987)
Exercise training of men at retirement: A clinical trial
J Gerontol **42**, 17-23
AEROBIC CAPACITY, Body composition, Elderly, Exercise programme, Intervention, JOINTS, LIPIDS, Male

110/43   Davies, C.T.M. & Knibbs, A.V.   (1971)
The training stimulus : the effects of intensity, duration and frequency of effort on maximum aerobic power output
Int Z Angew Physiol **29**, 299-305
Adult, AEROBIC CAPACITY, Comparative, Exercise programme, Intervention, Male

110/44   Davis, G.M., Shephard, R.J. & Leenen, F.H.   (1987)
Cardiac effects of short term arm crank training in paraplegics: echocardiographic evidence
Eur J Appl Physiol **56**, 90-96
Adult, CARDIAC PERFORMANCE, Exercise programme, Handicap, Intervention, Male

110/46   **de Vries, H.A.**   (1971)
Exercise intensity threshold for
improvement of cardiovascular-
respiratory function in older men
Geriatrics **26**, 94-101
*Elderly, Exercise programme,
Intervention, Male*

110/45   **de Vries, H.A.**   (1970)
Physiological effects of an exercise
training regimen upon men aged 52 to 88
J Gerontol **25**, 325-336
*AEROBIC CAPACITY, BLOOD
PRESSURE, Body composition, Elderly,
Exercise programme, Intervention, Male,
MUSCLE STRENGTH,
RESPIRATORY FUNCTION,*

110/47   **Dehn, M.M. & Bruce, R.A.**   (1972)
Longitudinal variations in maximal
oxygen uptake with age and activity
J Appl Physiol **33**, 805-807
*Adult, AEROBIC CAPACITY, Leisure
activity, Longitudinal, Male*

110/48   **Desplanches, D., Mayet, M.H.,
Sempore, B., Frutoso, J. & Flandrois,
R.**   (1987)
Effect of spontaneous recovery or
retraining after hindlimb suspension
J Appl Physiol **63**, 1739-1743
*AEROBIC CAPACITY, Animal,
Exercise programme, Intervention,
MUSCLE METABOLISM, MUSCLE
STRENGTH*

110/49   **Dobeln, W. & Eriksson,
B.O.**   (1972)
Physical training, maximal oxygen
uptake and dimensions of the oxygen
transporting organs in boys 11-13 years
of age
Acta Paediatr Scand **61**, 653-660
*AEROBIC CAPACITY, CARDIAC
PERFORMANCE, Children, Exercise
programme, GROWTH, Intervention,
Male*

110/50   **Dowdy, D.B., Cureton, K.J.,
DuVal, H.P. & Ouzts, H.G.**   (1985)
Effects of aerobic dance on physical work
capacity, cardiovascular function and
body composition of middle-aged women
Res Quart **56**, 227-233
*Adult, AEROBIC CAPACITY, BLOOD
PRESSURE, Body composition, Exercise
programme, Female, Intervention*

110/51   **Downey, A.M., Frank, G.C.,
Webber, L.S., Harsha, D.W., Virgilio,
S.J., Franklin, F.A. & Berenson,
G.S.**   (1987)
Implementation of Heart Smart: A
cardiovascular school health promotion
program
J School Health **57**, 98-104
*Children, Cohort, Exercise programme,
Leisure activity*

110/52   **Drinkwater, B.L. & Horvath,
S.M.**   (1972)
Detraining effects on young women
Med Sci Sports **4**, 91-95
*Adult, AEROBIC CAPACITY, Female,
Inactivity, Intervention*

110/53   **Edwards, M.A.**   (1974)
The effects of training at predetermined
heart rate levels for sedentary college
women
Med Sci Sports **6**, 14-19
*Adult, AEROBIC CAPACITY, Exercise
programme, Female, Intervention*

110/54   **Eisenman, P.A. & Golding,
L.A.**   (1975)
Comparison of effects of training on VO2
max in girls and young women
Med Sci Sports **7**, 136-138
*Adult, AEROBIC CAPACITY,
Comparative, Exercise programme,
Female, Intervention*

110/56   **Ekblom, B.**   (1986)
Factors determing maximal aerobic
power
Acta Physiol Scand (Suppl 556) **128**, 15-
19
AEROBIC CAPACITY, Adult, Review

110/55   **Ekblom, B.** (1969)
Effect of physical training on oxygen
transport system in man
Acta Physiol Scand (Suppl) **328**, 1-45
Review

110/57   **Eriksson, B.O.** (1975)
Girl swimmers then and later – a
longitudinal study of young girls
undergoing hard training
Lakartidningen **72**, 469-472
*AEROBIC CAPACITY, CARDIAC
PERFORMANCE, Children, Female,
GROWTH, Longitudinal, Swimming*

110/58   **Eriksson, B.O., Freychuss, U.,
Lundlin, A. & Thoren, C.A.R.** (1978)
Effect of physical training in former
female top athletes in swimming. In:
Children and Exercise IX (Eds) Berg, K
& Eriksson, B.O.
University Park Press, Baltimore
*AEROBIC CAPACITY, Body
composition, CARDIAC
PERFORMANCE, Children, Exercise
programme, Female, Intervention,
Swimming*

110/59   **Fahey, T.D., del Valle-Zuris, A.,
OehWen, G., Trieb, M & Seymour,
J.** (1979)
Pubertal stage differences in hormonal
and haematological responses to
maximal exercise in males
J Appl Physiol **46**, 823-827
*AEROBIC CAPACITY, Children,
Endocrine, GROWTH, Male*

110/60   **Farrally, M.R., Watkins, J. &
Ewing, B.G.** (1980)
The physical fitness of Scottish
schoolboys aged 13, 15 & 17 years
*Jordanhill College of Education, Glasgow,
Scotland.*
*Children, JOINTS, Male, MUSCLE
STRENGTH*

110/61   **Fentem, P.H., Bassey, E.J. &
Turnbull, N.B.** (1988)
The new case for exercise
*Sports Council & Health Education
Authority*
Review

110/62   **Fischer, A., Parizkova, J & Roth,
Z.** (1965)
The effect of systematic physical activity
on maximal performance and functional
capacity in senescent men
Int Z Angew Physiol **21**, 269-304
*AEROBIC CAPACITY, Body
composition, Comparative, Elderly,
Leisure activity*

110/63   **Gatch, W. & Byrd, R.** (1979)
Endurance training and cardiovascular
function in 9- and 10- year-old boys
Arch Phys Med Rehabil **60**, 574-577
*CARDIAC PERFORMANCE, Children,
Exercise programme, Intervention, Male*

110/64   **Gauthier, R., Massicote, D.,
Hermiston, R. & Macnab, R.** (1983)
The physical work capacity of Canadian
children, aged 7 to 17, in 1983. A
comparison with 1968
CAHPER J 4-9
Children, Longitudinal

110/65   **Getchell, L.H. & Moore,
J.C.** (1975)
Physical training; comparative responses
of middle-aged adults
Arch Phys Med Rehabil **56**, 251-254
*Adult, AEROBIC CAPACITY, Body
composition, Exercise programme,
Intervention*

110/66   **Gilliam, T.B. & Freedson,
P.S.** (1980)
Effects of a 12-week school physical
fitness program on peak VO2, body
composition and blood lipids in 7- to 9-
year old children
Int J Sports Med **1**, 73-78
*AEROBIC CAPACITY, Body
composition, Children, Exercise
programme, Intervention, LIPIDS*

110/67   Gilliam, T.B., Freedson, P.S., Greenen, D. & Shahraray, B.   (1981)
Physical activity patterns determined by heart rate monitoring in 6- to 7-year old children
Med Sci Sports Exerc **13**, 65-67
Children, Customary activity

110/68   Gleser, M.A.   (1973)
Effects of hypoxia and physical training on hemodynamic adjustments to one-legged exercise
J Appl Physiol **34**, 655-659
Adult, AEROBIC CAPACITY, CARDIAC PERFORMANCE, Exercise programme, Intervention, Male

110/69   Godin, G. & Shephard, R.J.   (1983)
Physical fitness promotion programmes: effectiveness in modifying exercise behaviour
Can J Appl Sport Sci **8**, 104-113
Review

110/70   Gore, I.Y.   (1972)
Physical activity and aging – a survey of Soviet literature
Gerontol Clin (Basel) **14**, 65-69
Elderly, Review

110/71   Goslin, B.R.   (1986)
Physical fitness of South African schoolchildren
J Sports Med Phys Fitness **26**, 128-136
AEROBIC CAPACITY, Body composition, Children, Comparative, Leisure activity, MUSCLE STRENGTH

110/72   Gossard, D., Haskell, W.L., Barr-Taylor, C., Mueller, J.K., Rogers, F., Chandler, M., Ahn, D.K., Miller, N.H. & DeBusk, R.F.   (1986)
Effects of low- and high-intensity home-based exercise training on functional capacity in healthy middle-aged men
Am J Cardiol **57**, 446-449
Adult, AEROBIC CAPACITY, Exercise programme, Intervention, Male

110/74   Grimby, G. & Saltin, B.   (1971)
Physiological effects of physical training
Scand J Rehabil Med **3**, 6-14
AEROBIC CAPACITY, CARDIAC PERFORMANCE, Exercise programme, Intervention, Male

110/73   Grimby, G. & Saltin, B.   (1966)
Physiological analysis of physically well-trained middle-aged and old athletes
Acta Med Scand **179**, 513-526
Adult, AEROBIC CAPACITY, CARDIAC PERFORMANCE, Comparative, Male, MUSCLE STRENGTH

110/75   Haber, P., Honiger, B., Klicpera, M. & Niederberger, M.   (1984)
Effects in elderly people 67-76 years of age of three-month endurance training on a bicycle ergometer
Eur Heart J (Suppl E) **5**, 37-39
AEROBIC CAPACITY, CARDIAC PERFORMANCE, Elderly, Exercise programme, Intervention

110/76   Hagberg, J.M   (1987)
Effect of training on the decline of VO2 max with aging
Fed Proc **46**, 1830-1833
Elderly, Review

110/77   Hartley, L.H., Grimby, G., Kilbom, A., Nilsson, N.J., Åstrand, I., Ekblom, B. & Saltin, B.   (1969)
Physical training in sedentary middle-aged and older men III. Cardiac output and gas exchange at sub-maximal and maximal exercise
Scand J clin Lab Invest **24**, 335-344
Adult, CARDIAC PERFORMANCE, Exercise programme, Intervention, Male

110/78   Hattin, H., Frase, M., Ward, G.R., & Shephard, R.J.   (1986)
Are deaf children unusually fit? A comparison of fitness between deaf and blind children
Adapt Phys Ed Quart **3**, 268-275
Children, Handicap

110/79   Heath, G.W., Hagberg, J.M.,
Ehsani, A.A. & Holloszy, J.O.   (1981)
A physiological comparison of young
and older endurance athletes
J Appl Physiol **51**, 634-640
Adult, AEROBIC CAPACITY, Athlete,
Comparative, Elderly, Leisure activity

110/80   Hickson, R.C. ,Bomze, H.A. &
Holloszy, J.O.   (1978)
Faster adjustment of O2 uptake to the
energy requirement of exercise in the
trained state
J Appl Physiol **44**, 877-881
Adult, AEROBIC CAPACITY, Exercise
programme, Intervention, Male

110/81   Hickson, R.C., Hagberg, J.M.,
Ehsani, A.A. & Holloszy, J.O.   (1981)
Time course of the adaptive responses of
aerobic power and heart rate to training
Med Sci Sports Exerc **13**, 17-20
Adult, AEROBIC CAPACITY, Exercise
programme, Intervention

110/82   Hickson, R.C., Kanakis, C. Jr.,
Davis, J.R., Moore, A.M., & Rich,
S.   (1982)
Reduced training duration effects on
aerobic power, endurance, and cardiac
growth
J Appl Physiol **53**, 225-229
Adult, AEROBIC CAPACITY,
CARDIAC PERFORMANCE, Exercise
programme, Inactivity, Intervention

110/83   Hoffman, M.D.   (1986)
Cardiorespiratory fitness and training in
quadriplegics and paraplegics
Sports Med **3**, 312-330
Adult, Exercise programme, Handicap,
Intervention

110/84   Hopkins, W.G., Gaeta, H., Thomas,
A.C. & Hill, P. McM.   (1987)
Physical fitness of blind and sighted
children
Eur J Appl Physiol **56**, 69-73
AEROBIC CAPACITY, Children,
Comparative, Customary activity,
Handicap

110/85   Houlsby, W.T.   (1986)
Functional aerobic capacity and body
size
Arch Dis Child **61**, 388-393
AEROBIC CAPACITY, Body
composition, Children, Cohort, Female,
Male

110/86   Huibregtse, W.H., Hartley, L.H.,
Jones, L.G., Doolittle, W.H. & Criblez,
T.L.   (1973)
Improvement of aerobic work capacity
following nonstrenuous exercise
Arch Environ Health **27**, 12-15
Adult, AEROBIC CAPACITY,
Intervention, Male, Occupational activity

110/87   Ilmarinen, J., Ilmarinen, R.,
Koskela, A., Korhonen, O., Fardy, P.,
Partanen, T. & Rutenfranz, J.   (1979)
Training effects of stair-climbing during
office hours on female employees
Ergonomics **22**, 507-516
Adult, AEROBIC CAPACITY, Body
composition, Female, PERCEIVED
EXERTION

110/88   Ilmarinen, J. & Rutenfranz,
J.   (1978)
Longitudinal studies of the changes in
habitual physical activity of
schoolchildren and working adolescents
In: Children and Exercise IX (Eds) Berg,
K. & Eriksson, B.O.
University Park Press, Baltimore
AEROBIC CAPACITY, Children,
Leisure activity, Longitudinal

110/89   Ilmarinen, J., Rutenfranz, J.,
Knauth, P., Ahrens, M., Kylian, H., Siuda,
A., Korallus, U.   (1978)
The effect of an on the job training
program – stairclimbing – on the physical
working capacity of employees
Eur J Appl Physiol **38**, 25-40
Adult, AEROBIC CAPACITY, Exercise
programme, Intervention, Male

110/90   **Ismail, A.H. & Montgomery, D.L** (1979)
The effect of a 4-month physical fitness programme on a young and an old group matched for physical fitness
Eur J Appl Physiol **40**, 137-144
Adult, AEROBIC CAPACITY, Body composition, BLOOD PRESSURE, Comparative, Exercise programme, Intervention, LIPIDS

110/91   **Johannessen, S., Holly, R.G., Lui, H. & Amsterdam, E.A.** (1986)
High frequency, moderate intensity training in sedentary middle-aged women
Phys Sports Med **14**, 99-102
Adult, AEROBIC CAPACITY, Body composition, Exercise programme, Female, Intervention

110/92   **Jones, N.L. & McCartney, N.** (1986)
Influence of muscle power on aerobic performance and the effects of training
Acta Med Scand (Suppl 711) **220**, 115-122
Adult, AEROBIC CAPACITY, Body composition, Exercise programme, Intervention

110/93   **Kasch, F.W.** (1973)
Physiological changes resulting from twenty-four months training in previously sedentary middle-aged males
Br J Sports Med **7**, 221.
Adult, AEROBIC CAPACITY, Exercise programme, Intervention, Male

110/94   **Kasch, F.W.& Kulberg, J.** (1981)
Physiological variables during 15 years of endurance exercise
J Sports Sci **3**, 59-62
Adult, AEROBIC CAPACITY, BLOOD PRESSURE, Longitudinal, Male

110/95   **Kasch, F.W. & Wallace, J.P.** (1976)
Physiological variables during 10 years of endurance exercise
Med Sci Sports **8**, 5-8
Adult, AEROBIC CAPACITY, Longitudinal, Male

110/96   **Kasch, F.W., Wallace, J.P. & Van Camp, S.P.** (1985)
Effects of 18 years of endurance exercise on the physical work capacity of older men
J Cardiac Rehabil **5**, 308-312
Adult, AEROBIC CAPACITY, Elderly, Longitudinal, Male

110/97   **Kemper, H.C.** (1986)
Longitudinal studies on the development of health and fitness and the interaction with physical activity of teenagers
Pediatrician **13**, 52-59
Children, Customary activity, Longitudinal

110/98   **Kemper, H.C.** (1987)
Longitudinal study of maximal aerobic power in teenagers
Ann Hum Biol **14**, 435-444
AEROBIC CAPACITY, Body composition, Children, GROWTH, Longitudinal

110/99   **Kemper, H.C.G., Verschuur, R., Ras, K.G.A., Snel, J., Splinter, P.G. & Tavecchio, L.W.C.** (1978)
Investigation into the effects of two extra physical education lessons per week during one school year upon physical development of 12- and 13-year-old boys
Med Sport **11**, 159-166
Children, Customary activity, GROWTH

110/100   **Kilbom, A.** (1971)
Physical training with sub-maximal intensities in women
Scand J clin Lab Invest **28**, 331-175
Adult, Customary activity, Female, Intervention, PERCEIVED EXERTION

110/101   **Kilbom, A. & Åstrand, I.**   (1971)
Physical training with submaximal
intensities in women. II. Effect on cardiac
output
Scand J clin Lab Invest **28**, 163-175
*Adult, AEROBIC CAPACITY, BLOOD
PRESSURE, CARDIAC
PERFORMANCE, Exercise programme,
Female*

110/102   **Kriska, A.M., Bayles, C., Cauley,
J.A., Laporte, R.E., Sandler, R.B. &
Pambianco, G.**   (1986)
A randomized exercise trial in older
women: increased activity over two years
and the factors associated with
compliance
Med Sci Sports Exerc **18**, 557-562
*Adult, BLOOD PRESSURE, Body
composition, Female*

110/103   **Lambert, C.A., Netherton, D.R.,
Finison, L.J., Hyde, J.N. & Spaight,
S.J.**   (1982)
Risk factors and life-style: a statewide
health interview survey
N Eng J Med **306**, 1048-1051
*Adult, Female, Leisure activity, Male,
Weight*

110/104   **Lampman, R.M.**   (1987)
Evaluating and prescribing exercise for
elderly patients
Geriatrics **42**, 63-76
Elderly, Review

110/105   **Lee, M., Ward, G.R. & Shephard,
R.J.**   (1985)
Physical capacities of sightless
adolescents
Dev Med Child Neurol **27**, 767-774
*AEROBIC CAPACITY, Body
composition, Children, Exercise
programme, Handicap, Intervention,
RESPIRATORY FUNCTION*

110/106   **Lesmes, G.R., Fox, E.L., Stevens,
C. & Otto, R.**   (1978)
Metabolic responses of females to high
intensity interval training of different
frequencies
Med Sci Sports **10**, 229-232
*Adult, AEROBIC CAPACITY,
Comparative, Exercise programme,
Female, Intervention*

110/107   **Lewis, S. F., Taylor, W.F.,
Graham, R. M., Pettinger, W. A., Schutte,
J.E. & Blomqvist, C.G.**   (1983)
Cardiovascular responses to exercise as
functions of absolute and relative
workload
J Appl Physiol **54**, 1314-1323
*Adult, AEROBIC CAPACITY, Body
composition, CARDIAC
PERFORMANCE, Male*

110/108   **Lewis, S.F., Thompson, P.,
Areskog, N., Vodak, P., Marconyak, M.,
DeBusk, R., Mellen, S. & Haskell,
W.**   (1980)
Transfer effects of endurance training to
exercise with untrained limbs
Eur J Appl Physiol **44**, 25 -34
*Adult, AEROBIC CAPACITY, Exercise
programme, Intervention, Male,
PERCEIVED EXERTION*

110/109   **Lo, P.-Y. & Dudley, G.A.**   (1987)
Endurance training reduces the
magnitude of exercise-induced
hyperammonemia in humans
J Appl Physiol **62**, 1227-1230
*Adult, AEROBIC CAPACITY, Female,
Intervention, Male*

110/110   **Lundgren-Lindquist, B.,
Aniansson, A. & Rundgren, A.**   (1983)
Functional capacities in 79-year-olds. III-
Walking performance and climbing
capacity
Scand J Rehabil Med **15**, 125-131
Elderly, Customary activity

110/111   **Lundgren-Lindquist, B. & Sperling, L.L.**   (1983).
Functional studies in 79-year-olds. II –
Upper extremity function
Scand J Rehabil Med **15**, 117-123
Elderly, MUSCLE STRENGTH

110/112   **Macleod, D., Maughan, R., Nimmo, M., Reilly, T. & Williams, C. (Eds.)**   (1987)
Exercise. Benefits, limits and adaptations
E. & F.N. Spon, London
Review

110/113   **McDonough, J.R., Kusumi, F., & Bruce, R.A.**   (1970)
Variations in maximal oxygen intake
with physical activity in middle-aged men
Circulation **41**, 743-751
Adult, AEROBIC CAPACITY, BLOOD PRESSURE, CARDIAC PERFORMANCE, Comparative, Leisure activity, LIPIDS, Male

110/114   **Mercier, J., Vago, P. & Ramonatxo, M.**   (1987)
Effect of aerobic training quantity on the
VO2 max of circumpubertal swimmers
Int J Sports Med **8**, 26-30
AEROBIC CAPACITY, Children, Comparative, Swimming

110/115   **Mirwald, R.L. Bailey, D.A., Cameron, N. & Rasmussen, R.L.**   (1981)
Longitudinal comparison of aerobic
power in active and inactive boys aged 7.0
to 17.0 years
Ann Hum Biol **8**, 405-414
AEROBIC CAPACITY, Children, Comparative, Leisure activity, Longitudinal, Male

110/116   **Miyashita, M. & Sadamoto, T.**   (1987)
The current problems of physical fitness
in Japanese children in comparison with
European and North American children
J Sports Med Phys Fitness **27**, 217-222
Children, Comparative

110/117   **Moffat, R.J., Stamford, B.A., Weltman, A. & Cuddihee, R.**   (1977)
Effects of high intensity aerobic training
on maximal oxygen uptake capacity and
field test performance
J Sports Med Phys Fitness **17**, 351-359
Adult, AEROBIC CAPACITY, Comparative, Exercise programme, Intervention, Male

110/118   **Montgomery, D.L. & Ismail, A.H.**   (1977)
The effect of a four-month physical
fitness program on high- and low- fit
groups matched for age
J Sports Med Phys Fitness **17**, 327-333.
Adult, Body composition, Exercise programme, Intervention, LIPIDS, Male

110/119   **Moore, R.L., Thacker, E.M., Kelley, G.A., Musch, T.I., Sinoway, L.I., Foster, V.L. & Dickinson, A.L.**   (1987)
Effect of training/detraining on
submaximal exercise responses in
humans
J Appl Physiol **63**, 1719-1724
Adult, AEROBIC CAPACITY, Exercise programme, Inactivity, Intervention, MUSCLE METABOLISM

110/120   **Nilsson, S., Staff, P.H. & Pruett, E.D.R.**   (1975)
Physical work capacity and the effect of
training on subjects with long-standing
paraplegia
Scand J Rehabil Med **7**, 51-56
Adult, AEROBIC CAPACITY, Exercise programme, Handicap, Intervention, MUSCLE STRENGTH,

110/121   **Nordesjo, L.-O.**   (1974)
Effect of quantitated training on the
capacity for short and prolonged work
Acta Physiol Scand (Suppl 405) **91**,
Adult, AEROBIC CAPACITY, Exercise programme, Intervention, Male

110/122   Norgan, N.G. & Ferro-Luzzi, A.
Nutrition, physical activity and physical
fitness in contrasting environments
*Dept of Human Sciences, Loughborough
University of Technology*
Review

110/123   Orlander, J., Kiessling, K. &
Ekblom, B.   (1980)
Time course of adaptation to low
intensity training in sedentary men:
dissociation of central and local effects
Acta Physiol Scand **108,** 85-90
*Adult, AEROBIC CAPACITY, Exercise
programme, Intervention, Male,
MUSCLE METABOLISM*

110/124   Pate, R.R., Hughes, R.D.,
Chandler, J.V. & Ratliffe, J.L.   (1978)
Effects of arm training on retention of
training effects derived from leg training
Med Sci Sports **10,** 71-74
*Adult, AEROBIC CAPACITY, Exercise
programme, Inactivity, Intervention, Male*

110/125   Pedersen, P.K. & Jørgensen,
K.   (1978)
Maximal oxygen uptake in young women
with training, inactivity, and retraining
Med Sci Sports **10,** 233-237
*Adult, AEROBIC CAPACITY, Exercise
programme, Female, Inactivity,
Intervention*

110/126   Pollock, M.L., Dawson, G.A.,
Miller, H.S., Ward, A., Cooper, D.,
Headley, W., Linnerud, A.C. & Nomeir,
M.M.   (1976)
Physiologic responses of men 49-65 years
of age to endurance training
J Am Geriatr Soc **24,** 97-104.
*Adult, AEROBIC CAPACITY, BLOOD
PRESSURE, Body composition, Exercise
programme, Intervention, LIPIDS, Male*

110/127   Pollock, M.L., Foster, C., Knapp,
D., Rod, J.L. & Schmidt, D.H.   (1987)
Effect of age and training on aerobic
capacity and body composition of master
athletes
J Appl Physiol **62,** 725-731
*AEROBIC CAPACITY, Athlete, Body
composition, Elderly, Leisure activity,
Longitudinal, Male*

110/128   Pollock, M.L. Foster, C., Rod,
J.L., Hare, J. & Schmidt, D.H.   (1982)
Ten year follow-up on the aerobic
capacity of champion masters track
athletes
Med Sci Sports Exerc **14,** 105
*AEROBIC CAPACITY, Adult, Athlete,
Longitudinal*

110/129   Pollock, M.L., Miller, H.S. Jr.,
Janeway, R., Linnerud, A.C., Robertson,
B. & Valentino, R.   (1971)
Effects of walking on body composition
and cardivascular function of middle-
aged men
J Appl Physiol **30,** 126-130
*Adult, Aerobic capacity, BLOOD
PRESSURE, Body composition, Exercise
programme, Intervention, Male*

110/130   Quies, W., Metze, R. & Siegmund,
S.   (1976)
Behaviour of physical endurance
capacity in boys of secondary-school age.
ii.Influence of the school sport on the
cardiopulmonary capacity of 11- to 14-
year old boys (Long-term study)
Aerztl Jugendkd **67,** 89-94
*AEROBIC CAPACITY, Children,
Longitudinal, Male*

110/131   Quirion, A., Decareful, D.,
Laurescelle, L., Method, D., Vogelaere, P.
& Du Lac, S.   (1987)
The physiological response to exercise
with special reference to age
J Sports Med **27,** 143-150
Elderly

110/132   Raju, P.S., Kumar, K.A., Reddy, S.S., Madhavi, S, Gnanakumari, K., Bhaskaracharyulu, C., Reddy, M.V., Annapurna, N., Reddy, M.E., Girijakumari, D., Sahay, B.K. & Murthy, K.J.R.   (1986)
Effect of yoga on exercise tolerance in normal healthy volunteers
Indian J Physiol Pharmacol **30**, 121-132
Adult, Exercise programme, Intervention

110/133   Robinson, S., Dill, D.B., Robinson, R.D., Tzankoff, S.P. & Wagner, J.A.   (1976)
Physiological aging of champion runners
J Appl Physiol **41**, 46-51
AEROBIC CAPACITY, Athlete, BLOOD PRESSURE, Longitudinal, Male

110/134   Rowell, L.B., Sheriff, D.D., Wyss, C.R. & Scher, A.M.   (1986)
The nature of the exercise stimulus
Acta Physiol Scand (Suppl 556) **128**, 7-14
Adult, Review

110/135   Rusko, H. & Bosco, C.   (1987)
Metabolic response of endurance athletes to training with added load
Eur J Appl Physiol **56**, 412-418
Adult, Athlete, Intervention, Leisure activity, Vigorous

110/136   Rutenfranz, J.   (1986)
Longitudinal approach to assessing maximal aerobic power during growth: the European experience
Med Sci Sports Exerc **18**, 270-275
GROWTH, Review

110/137   Rutenfranz, J., Lange Andersen, K., Seliger, V. & Masironi, R.   (1982)
Health standards in terms of exercise fitness of school children in urban and rural areas in various European countries
Ann Clin Res (Suppl) **34**, 33-36
AEROBIC CAPACITY, Children, Comparative, Cohort, Female, Male

110/138   Rutenfranz, J. & Singer, R.   (1978)
The influence of sport activity on the development of physical performance capacities of 15-17 year old boys. In: Children and Exercise IX (Eds) Berg, K. & Eriksson, B.O.
University Park Press, Baltimore
Children, Cohort, Leisure activity, Male

110/142   Saltin, B.   (1986)
Physiological adaptation to physical conditioning
Acta Med Scand (Suppl 711) **220**, 11-24
Review

110/141   Saltin, B.   (1985)
Hemodynamic adaptions to exercise
Am J Cardiol **55**, 1-170D
Review

110/140   Saltin, B.   (1977)
Adaptive responses of muscle to endurance exercise: metabolic and physiologic studies
Ann NY Acad Sci **301**, 411-454
Review

110/139   Saltin, B.   (1977)
The interplay between peripheral and central factors in the adaptive response to exercise and training
Ann N Y Acad Sci **301**, 224-231
Review

110/143   Saltin, B., Blomquist, G., Mitchell, J.H., Johnson, R.L. Jr., Wildenthal, K. & Chapman, C.B.   (1968)
Response to exercise after bedrest and training
Circulation (Suppl 7) **38**, 1-78
Adult, AEROBIC CAPACITY, CARDIAC PERFORMANCE, Exercise programme, Inactivity, Intervention, Male

110/144   **Saltin, B. & Grimby, G.**   (1968)
Physiological analysis of middle-aged
and old former athletes. Comparison
with still active athletes of the same ages
Circulation **38**, 1104-1115
Adult, AEROBIC CAPACITY,
CARDIAC PERFORMANCE,
Comparative, LIPIDS, Male

110/145   **Saltin, B., Hartley, L.H, Kilbom,**
& Åstrand, I.   (1969)
Physical training in sedentary middle-
aged and older men. II. Oxygen uptake,
heart rate, and blood lactate
concentration at sub-maximal and
maximal exercise
Scand J clin Lab Invest **24**, 323-334
Adult, AEROBIC CAPACITY,
ANAEROBIC CAPACITY, Exercise
programme, Intervention, Male

110/146   **Saltin, B., Nazar, K., Costill, D.L.,**
Stein, E., Jansson, E., Essen, B. &
Gollnick, P.D.   (1976)
The nature of the training response;
peripheral and central adaptations to
one-legged exercise
Acta Physiol Scand **96**, 289-305
Adult, AEROBIC CAPACITY, Exercise
programme, Intervention, Male,
MUSCLE METABOLISM, MUSCLE
STRENGTH

110/147   **Saltin, B. & Rowell, L.B.**   (1980)
Functional adaptions to physical activity
and inactivity
Fed Proc **39**, 1506-1513
Review

110/148   **Santiago, M.C., Alexander, J.F. &**
Stull, G.A.   (1987)
Physiological responses of sedentary
women to a 20-week conditioning
program of walking or jogging
Scand J Sports Sci **9**, 33-39
Adult, Exercise programme, Female,
Intervention

110/149   **Saris, W.H.M.**   (1985)
The assessment and evaluation of daily
physical activity in children. A review
Acta Paediatr Scand (Suppl) **318**, 37-48
Children, Review

110/150   **Saris, W.H.M.**   (1986)
Habitual physical activity in children:
methodology and findings in health and
disease
Med Sci Sports Exerc **18**, 253-263
Children, Review

110/151   **Seliger, V., Trefny, Z.,**
Bartunkova, S. & Pauer, M.   (1974)
The habitual activity and physical fitness
of 12 year old boys
Acta Paed Belg (Suppl) **28**, 54-59
Children, Customary activity

110/153   **Shephard, R.J**   (1978)
Physical Activity and Ageing
Croom Helm, London.
Review

110/152   **Shephard, R.J.**   (1968)
Intensity, duration and frequency of
exercise as determinants of the response
to a training regime
Int Z Angew Physiol **26**, 272-278
Adult, AEROBIC CAPACITY, Exercise
programme, Intervention

110/154   **Shephard, R.J., Corey, P. & Cox,**
M.   (1982)
Health hazard appraisal – the influence of
an employee fitness program
Can J Public Health **73**, 183-187
Adult, AEROBIC CAPACITY, BLOOD
PRESSURE, Body composition,
Intervention, JOINTS, LIPIDS,
MUSCLE STRENGTH

110/155   **Shindo, M., Kumergai, S. & Tanaka, H.**   (1987)
Physical work capacity and effect of endurance training in visually handicapped boys and young male adults
Eur J Appl Physiol **56**, 501-507
Adult, AEROBIC CAPACITY, Exercise programme, Handicap, Intervention, Male, MENTAL HEALTH, MUSCLE STRENGTH

110/156   **Sidney, K.H. & Shephard, R.J.**   (1978)
Frequency and intensity of exercise training for elderly subjects
Med Sci Sports **10**, 125-131
AEROBIC CAPACITY, Elderly, Exercise programme, Female, Intervention, Male

110/157   **Sidney K.H. & Shephard R.J.**   (1977)
Activity patterns of elderly men and women
J Gerontol **32**, 25-32
AEROBIC CAPACITY, Customary activity, Elderly, Intervention

110/158   **Siegel, W., Blomqvist, G. & Mitchell, J.H.**   (1970)
Effects of a quantitated physical training program on middle-aged sedentary men
Circulation **41**, 19-29
Adult, AEROBIC CAPACITY, CARDIAC PERFORMANCE, Exercise programme, Inactivity, Intervention, Male

110/159   **Skrobak-Kaczynski, J. & Vavik, T.**   (1978)
Physical fitness and trainability of young male patients with Down Syndrome. In: Children and Exercise IX (Eds) Berg, K. & Eriksson, B.O.
University Park Press, Baltimore
AEROBIC CAPACITY, Body composition, Children, Exercise programme, Handicap, Intervention, JOINTS, MUSCLE STRENGTH

110/160   **Sprynarova, S.**   (1974)
Longitudinal study of the influence of different physical activity programs on functional capacity of the boys from 11-18 years
Acta Paed Belg (Suppl) **28**, 204-213
AEROBIC CAPACITY, Children, Comparative, Longitudinal, Male

110/161   **Stamford, B.A.**   (1972)
Physiological effects of training upon institutionalized geriatric men
J Gerontol **27**, 451-455
Elderly, Exercise programme, Intervention, Male

110/162   **Stephens, T.**   (1983)
Fitness and lifestyles in Canada
Report by Canada Fitness Survey, Ottawa.
Review

110/163   **Stephens, T., Craig, C.L. & Ferris, B.F.**   (1986)
Adult physical activity in Canada: Findings from The Canada Fitness Survey I
Can J Public Health **77**, 285-290
Review

110/164   **Sundberg, S.**   (1982)
Maximal oxygen uptake in relation to age in blind and normal boys and girls
Acta Paediatr Scand **71**, 603-608
AEROBIC CAPACITY, Children, Comparative, Handicap

110/165   **Sunnegårdh, J., Bratteby, L.-E. & Sjölin, S.**   (1985)
Physical activity and sports involvement in 8- and 13-year-old children in Sweden
Acta Paediatr Scand **74**, 904-912
Children, Customary activity, Leisure activity

110/166   **Svedenhag, J.**   (1985)
The sympatho-adrenal system in physical conditioning
Acta Physiol Scand (Suppl 543) **125**, 5-73
Review

110/167   **Taggart, A.C., Taggart, J. & Siedentop, D.**   (1986)
Effects of a home-based activity program. A study with low fitness elementary school children
Behav Modif **10**, 487-507
Children

110/168   **Terjung, R.L., Baldwin, K.M., Cooksey, J., Samson, B. & Sutter, R.A.**   (1973)
Cardiovascular adaptation to twelve minutes of mild daily exercise in middle-age sedentary men
J Am Geriatr Soc **21**, 164-168
Adult, BLOOD PRESSURE, Body composition, CARDIAC PERFORMANCE, Exercise programme, Intervention, LIPIDS, Male

110/169   **The President's Council on physical fitness and sports. Washington , D.C. 2001**   (1985)
1990 Physical fitness and exercise objectives

Review

110/170   **Thomas, S.G., Cunningham, D.A., Rechnitzer, P.A., Donner, A.P. & Howard, J.H.**   (1985)
Determinants of the training response in elderly men
Med Sci Sports Exerc **17**, 667-672
AEROBIC CAPACITY, Body composition, Elderly, Exercise programme, Intervention, Male

110/171   **Tuxworth, W., Nevill, A.M., White, C. & Jenkins, C.**   (1986)
Health, fitness, physical activity, and morbidity of middle aged factory workers
Br J Ind Med **43**, 733-753
Adult, Body composition, Cohort, EPIDEMIOLOGY-CHD, Leisure activity, Male, Occupational activity

110/172   **Vaccaro, P. & Clarke, D.H.**   (1978)
Cardiorespiratory alterations in 9- to 11-year old children following a season of competitive swimming
Med Sci Sports **10**, 204-207
AEROBIC CAPACITY, Children, Comparative, Intervention, Leisure activity, RESPIRATORY FUNCTION, Swimming

110/173   **Wardlaw, G.M., Kaplan, M.L. & Lanza-Jacoby, S.**   (1986)
Effect of treadmill training on muscle oxidative capacity and accretion in young male obese and nonobese Zucker rats
J Nutr **116**, 1841-1852
Animal, Body composition, Exercise programme, Intervention

110/174   **Watkins, J.**   (1984)
Step tests of cardiorespiratory fitness suitable for mass testing
Br J Sports Med **18**, 84-89
Review

110/175   **Watkins, J., Farrally, M.R. & Powley, A.**   (1983)
The anthropometry and physical fitness of secondary schoolgirls in Strathclyde
Jordanhill College of Education, Glasgow, Scotland
Body composition, BONES, Children, Female, JOINTS, MUSCLE STRENGTH

110/176   **Watson, A.W.A. & O'Donovan, D. J.**   (1977)
Influence of level of habitual activity on physical work capacity and body composition of post-pubertal boys
Quart J Experimental Physiol **62**, 325-332
Body composition, Children, Customary activity, Male

110/177   **Watson, A.W.S. & O'Donovan, D.J.**   (1977)
A study of the relationships between somatotype, levels of habitual activity and physical working capacity in post-pubertal males
Irish J Med Sci **146,** 381-385
Body composition, Children, Customary activity, Male

110/178   **Welsh Heart Programme Directorate**   (1987)
Exercise for health: health related fitness in Wales
Heartbeat Report No 23
Adult, AEROBIC CAPACITY, BLOOD PRESSURE, Children, Customary activity, Leisure activity, LIPIDS

110/179   **Wenger, H.A.**   (1986)
The interactions of intensity, frequency and duration of exercise training in altering cardiorespiratory fitness
Sports Med **3,** 346-356
Adult, Exercise programme, Intervention,

110/180   **Yoshida, T., Ishiko, I. & Muraoka, I.**   (1980)
Effect of endurance training on cardiorespiratory functions of 5-year-old children
Int J Sports Med **1,** 91-94
Children

120 ANAEROBIC CAPACITY AND THRESHOLD

KEYWORDS are listed in the appendix in addition the following specific keywords have been used in this section:

E. stimulation (electrical stimulation)
Fibre type
Lactate

Summary of evidence: exercise ameliorates, prevents or reverses poor physical capability arising from low levels of customary activity

THE PROBLEM

Inactivity related disability was suspected to be widespread and to prejudice the quality of life especially in the elderly. Improvements are known to occur in athletic individuals in short term power output and adaptation to prolonged exercise (stamina or endurance). The latter can be assesed by finding the intensity of exercise above which aerobic resources are inadequate and lactic acid levels rise sharply (the anaerobic threshold). Raised lactic acid affects the working muscle acutely and eventually the whole body in prolonged exercise. Are the improvements also available to the sedentary, old or disabled?

SCOPE

This section contains references dealing primarily with changes produced by exercise in the ventilatory, lactate and anaerobic thresholds. These are thresholds above which anaerobic energy consumption rises steeply, their relation to endurance in prolonged activity is described. There are a few references on the effects of exercise on short term maximal power output which is a measure of anaerobic capacity. There is a large literature, this is therefore a representative selection not a comprehensive

listing. It contains references on the intensity and amount of exercise needed to raise thresholds or reduce lactate production; it contains studies of all age groups including the sedentary and the athletic. There are also some studies of the acute effects on lactate production, but only a few in which lactic acid levels are measured, without attempting to identify a threshold.

METHODOLOGICAL DIFFICULTIES

The outcome of these studies is highly dependent on the details of the protocol. This is because the concentrations of the primary variable, lactic acid, depend upon the balance between production in the working muscles and removal by other tissues. Many factors influence its rate of removal and uptake as well as its production from the working muscle. The three thresholds are not always coincident and they cannot be satisfactorily assessed in all subjects. The measurement of short term power output requires highly motivated subjects as do all maximal performances.

EVIDENCE

It is clear that exercise can raise the threshold leading to improved exercise tolerance in almost anyone. The improvement is associated with increased maximal oxygen uptake, maximal work capacity and particularly submaximal exercise performance. Fairly vigorous levels of sub-maximal work can be sustained for much longer. Because of the non-linear relation between lactic acid levels and increasing exercise intensity, improvements of up to 300% may be seen in the duration for which a moderate exercise task can be sustained. This is a marked improvement in endurance for prolonged exercise and an increase in reserve capacity for normal activities. The mechanisms are found in sections 140 and 210.

120/1   Allen, W.K., Seals, D.R., Hurley, B.F., Ehsani, A.A. & Hagberg, J.M.   (1985)
Lactate threshold and distance-running performance in young and older endurance athletes
J Appl Physiol **58**, 1281-1284
Adult, AEROBIC CAPACITY, ANAEROBIC CAPACITY, Athlete, Comparative, Lactate

120/2   Atomi, Y., Iwaoka, K., Hatta, H., Miyashita, M. & Yamamoto, Y.   (1986)
Daily physical activity levels in pre-adolescent boys related to VO2 max and lactate threshold
Eur J Appl Physiol **55**, 156-161
AEROBIC CAPACITY, Body composition, Children,Customary activity, Male

120/3   Bhambhani, Y. & Singh, M.   (1985)
The effects of three training intensities on VO2 max and VE/VO2 ratio
Can J Appl Spt Sci **10**, 44-51
Adult, AEROBIC CAPACITY, Exercise programme, Intervention, Male,

120/4   Casaburi, R., Storer, T.W., Ben-Dov, I. & Wasserman, K.   (1987)
Effect of endurance training on possible determinants of VO2 during heavy exercise
J Appl Physiol **62**, 199-207
Adult, AEROBIC CAPACITY, Exercise programme, Intervention, Lactate

120/5   Cisar, C.J., Thorland, W.G., Johnson, G.O. & Housh, T.J.   (1986)
The effect of endurance training on metabolic responses and the prediction of distance running performance
J Sports Med **26**, 234-240
Adult, AEROBIC CAPACITY, ANAEROBIC CAPACITY, Athlete, Body composition, Exercise programme, Intervention, Male

120/6   Coyle, E.F., Martin, W.H., Ehsani, A.A., Hagberg, J.M., Bloomfield, S.A., Sinacore, D.R. & Holloszy, J.O.   (1983)
Blood lactate threshold in some well-trained ischemic heart disease patients
J Appl Physiol **54**, 18-23
Adult, AEROBIC CAPACITY, Comparative, Lactate, Running

120/7   Davis, J.A., Frank, M.H., Whipp, B.J. & Wasserman, K.   (1979)
Anaerobic threshold alterations caused by endurance training in middle-aged men
J Appl Physiol **46**, 1039-1046
Adult, AEROBIC CAPACITY, Exercise programme, Intervention, Male, RESPIRATORY FUNCTION

120/8   Favier, R.J., Constable, S.H., Chen, M. & Holloszy, J.O.   (1986)
Endurance exercise training reduces lactate production
J Appl Physiol **61**, 885-889
Animal, E. stimulation, Lactate

120/9   Ferrettu, G.   (1987)
Effects of exercise on maximal instantaneous muscular power of humans
J Appl Physiol **62**, 2288-2294
Adult, Exercise programme, Intervention

120/10   Foster, V.L.   (1986)
The reproducibility of VO2max, ventilatory, and lactate thresholds in elderly women
Med Sci Sports Exerc **18**, 425-430
AEROBIC CAPACITY, ANAEROBIC CAPACITY, Elderly, Female

120/11   Gaesser, G.A. & Pooler, D.C.   (1986)
Lactate and ventilatory thresholds: disparity in time course of adaptions to training
J Appl Physiol **61**, 999-1004
Adult, AEROBIC CAPACITY, Exercise programme, Intervention, Lactate

120/12 **Girandola, R.N., Wiswell, R. A., Frisch, F. & Wood, K.** (1981)
VO2 max and anaerobic threshold in pre- and post-pubescent girls. In: WOMEN AND SPORT; an historical, biological,and sportmedical approach (Eds.) Borms, J., Hebbelinck, M., Vererando, A.
S. Karger, Basel **14**, 155-161
CARDIAC PERFORMANCE, Children, Female, Review

120/13 **Gollnick, P.D., Bayly, W.M. & Hodgson, D.R.** (1986)
Exercise intensity, training, diet and lactate concentration in muscle and blood
Med Sci Sports Exerc **18**, 334-340
Review

120/14 **Grodjinovsky, A., Inbar, O., Dotan, R. & Bar-Or, O.** (1978)
Training effect on the anaerobic performance of children as measured by the Wingate Anaerobic Test. In: Children and Exercise IX (Eds) Berg, K. & Eriksson, B.O.
University Park Press, Baltimore
Children, Exercise programme, Intervention, Male,

120/15 **Henritze, J., Weltman, A., Schurrer, R.L. & Barlow, K.** (1985)
Effect of training at and above the lactate threshold on the lactate threshold and maximal oxygen uptake
Eur J Appl Physiol **54**, 84-88
Adult, AEROBIC CAPACITY, Body composition, Exercise programme, Female, Intervention

120/16 **Hughes, E.F., Turner, S.C. & Brooks, G.A.** (1982)
Effects of glycogen depletion and pedaling speed on anaerobic threshold
J Appl Physiol **52**, 1598-1607
Adult, AEROBIC CAPACITY, Intervention, Lactate, Male

120/17 **Reybrouck, T., Weymans, W., Styns, H. & Van der Hauwaert, L.G.** (1986)
Ventilatory anaerobic threshold for evaluating exercise performance in children with congenital left-to-right intracardiac shunt
Pediatr Cardiol **7**, 19-24
Children, Handicap

120/18 **Rotstein, A., Dotan, R. & Bar-Or, O.** (1986)
Effect of training on anaerobic theshold, maximal aerobic power and anaerobic performance of preadolescent boys
Int J Sports Med **7**, 282-286
AEROBIC CAPACITY, Children, Exercise programme, Intervention, Male

120/19 **Sahlin, K.** (1986)
Muscle fatigue and lactic acid accumulation
Acta Physiol Scand (Suppl 556) **128**, 83-91
Review

120/20 **Seals, D.R., Hurley, B.F., Schultz, J. & Hagberg, J.M.** (1984)
Endurance training in older men and women: II. Blood lactate response to submaximal exercise
J Appl Physiol **57**, 1030-1033
AEROBIC CAPACITY, Body composition, Elderly, Exercise programme, Intervention, Lactate

120/21 **Simon, J., Young, J.L., Gutin, B., Blood, D.K. & Case, R.B.** (1983)
Lactate accumulation relative to the anaerobic and respiratory compensation thresholds
J Appl Physiol **54**, 13-17
Adult, Lactate, Male

120/22   **Sjodin, B., Jacobs, I. & Svendenhaag, J.**   (1982)
Changes in onset of blood lactate accumulations (OBLA) and muscle enzymes after training at OBLA
Eur J Appl Physiol **49**, 45-57
Adult, AEROBIC CAPACITY, Athlete, Exercise programme, Fibre type, Intervention, Male, MUSCLE METABOLISM

120/23   **Stainsby, W.N.**   (1986)
Biochemical and physiological bases for lactate production
Med Sci Sports Exerc **18**, 341-343
Review

120/24   **Stanly, W.C., Gertz, E.W., Wisneski, J.A., Neese, R.A., Morris, L. & Brooks, G.A.**   (1986)
Lactate extraction during net lactate release in legs of humans during exercise
J Appl Physiol **60**, 1116-1120
Adult, Lactate, Male

120/25   **Tanaka, K., Watanabe, H., Komishi, Y., Mitsuzono, R., Sumida, S., Tanaka, S., Fukuda, T. & Nakadomo, F.**   (1986)
Longitudinal associations between anaerobic threshold and distance running performance
Eur J Appl Physiol **55**, 248-252
Adult, AEROBIC CAPACITY, Athlete, Exercise programme, Intervention, Male, Running, Vigorous

120/26   **Vago, P.**   (1987)
Is ventilatory anaerobic threshold a good index of endurance capacity?
Int J Sports Med **8**, 190-195

120/27   **Wasserman, K.**   (1986)
The anaerobic threshold: definition, physiological significance and identification
Adv Cardiol **35**, 1-23
Review

120/28   **Whipp, B.J.**   (1986)
Respiratory markers of the anaerobic threshold
Adv Cardiol **35**, 47-64
Review

120/29   **Yoshida, T., Chida, M., Ichioka, M. & Suda, Y.**   (1987)
Blood lactate parameters related to aerobic capacity and endurance performance
Eur J Appl Physiol **56**, 7-11
Adult, AEROBIC CAPACITY, Female

130 MUSCLE STRENGTH

KEYWORDS are listed in the appendix in addition the following specific keywords have been used in this section:

Back pain
Body composition (includes muscle cross-sectional area)
EMG (electromyograph)
E. stimulation (electrical stimulation)
Fibre type
Isokinetic

Summary of evidence: exercise ameliorates, prevents or reverses muscle weakness arising from lack of use

THE PROBLEM

Poor physical capability including muscle weakness due to low levels of customary activity was suspected to be widespread and to prejudice the quality of life especially in the elderly. Are the improvements in performance and adaptation to exercise, well known in athletic individuals, also available to the sedentary, old or disabled?

SCOPE

This section contains references dealing primarily with changes produced by exercise in muscle strength assessed isometrically, isokinetically or as electrically evoked force. There is a large literature, this is therefore a representative selection not a comprehensive listing. Exercise in this section usually consists of strong briefly sustained muscle contractions repeated many times. The strength of the contraction must be at least 50% of the maximum for the specific muscle. There are references on the effects of exercise on muscle fibre type and muscle cross-sectional area; references on the intensity and amount of exercise needed to increase strength; and studies of all age groups including the sedentary and the athletic. There are also some references on the effects of exercise on back pain, on the effects of inactivity, of overuse, and some animal studies. (See also 140 for muscle enzymes and muscle capillarity.)

METHODOLOGICAL DIFFICULTIES

The measurement of maximal muscle strength requires highly motivated subjects and there is no objective criteria with which to assess this.

EVIDENCE

It is clear that increased strength can be obtained with exercise in almost anyone but that this may be due to improvements in neural control (skill) as well as intrinsic muscle changes. The latter include increases in the cross-sectional area of the fibres; there is no good evidence for hyperplasia. The improvements are especially useful in the elderly who will have suffered some inevitable wasting of muscle and whose safety margins for strength are therefore low. Increases in muscle strength are associated with improvements in the strength of the muscle's ligamentous attachment to bone. This is also a particular advantage in the elderly as it protects against damage due to an unexpected strain. The stability of a joint depends critically upon the strength of the muscles inserted near that joint and upon that strength being sustained when required. Well-maintained muscle strength is therefore likely to provide some protection against accidental falls and the distress of resulting fractures. There is some evidence that exercise which improves the strength of the postural muscles may prevent 'slipped discs' or ease low back pain as well as improving posture. Isometric exercise has been considered a health hazard due to the large rise in blood pressure which occurs during sustained isometric exercise. Provided the duration of the contraction is limited to five seconds or less there is no risk that the blood pressure will rise to dangerous levels; this is a sufficient duration for improvement in strength if the effort is repeated frequently. The improvements are specific to the muscle which is exercised.

130/1 **Andersen, L.B. & Henckel, P.** (1987)
Maximal voluntary isometric strength in Danish adolescents 16-19 years of age
Eur J Appl Physiol **56**, 83-91
Body composition, Children, Comparative

130/2 **Aniansson, A., Grimby, G. & Rundgren, Å.** (1980)
Isometric and isokinetic quadriceps muscle strength in 70-year-old men and women
Scand J Rehabil Med **12**, 161-168
Comparative, Customary activity, Elderly, Isokinetic

130/3 **Aniansson, A. & Gustafsson, E.** (1981)
Physical training in elderly men with special reference to quadriceps muscle strength and morphology
Clin Physiol **1**, 87-98
Elderly, Exercise programme, Intervention, Male

130/4 **Aniansson, A., Sperling, L., Rundgren, K. & Lehnberg, E.** (1983)
Muscle function in 75-year-old men and women. A longitudinal study
Scand J Rehabil Med (Suppl 9) 92-102
Elderly, Isokinetic, Longitudinal

130/5 **Armstrong, R.B.** (1984)
Mechanisms of exercise-induced delayed onset muscular soreness: a brief review
Med Sci Sports Exerc **16**, 529-538
Hazards, Review

130/6 **Asfour, S.S., Ayoub, M.M. & Mital, A.** (1984)
Effects of an endurance and strength training programme on lifting capability of males
Ergonomics **27**, 435-442
AEROBIC CAPACITY, Adult, Exercise programme, Intervention, JOINTS, Male

130/7 **Bassey, E.J., Bendall, M.J. & Pearson, M.B.** (1988)
Muscle strength in the triceps surae and objectively measured customary walking activity in men and women over 65 years of age
Clin Sci **74**, 85-89
Body composition, Customary activity, Elderly

130/8 **Biering-Sorensen, F.** (1984)
Physical measurements as risk indicators for low back trouble over a one-year period
Spine **9**, 106-118
Adult, Back pain

130/9 **Bishop, P., Cureton, K. & Collins, M.** (1987)
Sex difference in muscular strength in equally-trained men and women
Ergonomics **30**, 675-687
Adult, Comparative

130/10 **Boone, T. & Byrd, R.** (1982)
The influence of lower extremity muscular endurance training on cardiac output and related measures
J Sports Med **22**, 450
Adult, AEROBIC CAPACITY, Exercise programme, Intervention, Male

130/11 **Byrnes, W.C. & Clarkson, P.M.** (1986)
Delayed onset muscle soreness and training
Clin Sports Med **5**, 605-614
Hazards, Review

130/12   Caizzo, V.J., Perrine, J.J. &
Edgerton, V.R.   (1981)
Training-induced alterations of the in-
vivo force-velocity relationship of human
muscle
J Appl Physiol **51,** 750-754.
*Adult, Exercise programme, Intervention,
Isokinetic*

130/13   Cannon, R.J. & Cafarelli,
E.   (1987)
Neuromuscular adaptations to training
J Appl Physiol **63,** 2396-2402
*Adult, E. stimulation, Exercise
programme, Intervention, EMG*

130/14   Cauley, J.A., Petrini, A.M.,
LaPorte, R.E., Sandler, R.B., Bayles,
C.M., Robertson, R.J. & Slemenda,
C.W.   (1987)
The decline of grip strength in the
menopause: relationship to physical
activity, estrogen use and anthropometric
factors
J Chron Dis **40,** 115-120
*Adult, Body composition, Comparative,
Customary activity, Female*

130/15   Costill, D.L., Coyle, E.F., Fink,
W.F., Lesmes, G.R. & Witzmann,
F.A.   (1979)
Adaptations in skeletal muscle following
strength training
J Appl Physiol **46,** 96-99
*Adult, Exercise programme, Fibre type,
Intervention, Isokinetic, Male, MUSCLE
METABOLISM*

130/16   Cunningham, B.A., Morris, G. &
Cheney, C.L.   (1986)
Effects of resistive exercise on skeletal
muscle in marrow transplant recipients
receiving total parenteral nutrition
J Parenter Enteral Nutr **10,** 558-563
Acute exercise, Adult

130/17   Cunningham, D.A., Morrison, D.,
Rice, C.L. & Cooke, C.   (1987)
Ageing and isokinetic plantar flexion
Eur J Appl Physiol **56,** 24-29
*AEROBIC CAPACITY, Adult,
Customary activity, Isokinetic, Male*

130/18   Czerwinski, S.M., Kurowski, T.G.,
O'Neil, T.M. & Hickson, R.C.   (1987)
Initiating regular exercise protects
against muscle atrophy from
glucocorticoids
J Appl Physiol **63,** 1504-1510
*Animal, Comparative, Exercise
programme. Intervention*

130/19   Davies, C.T.M.   (1985)
Strength and mechanical properties of
muscle in children and young adults
Scand J Sports Sci **7,** 11-15
*Adult, Children, Comparative, E.
stimulation*

130/20   Davies, C.T.M., Dooley, P.,
McDonagh, M.J.N. & White,
M.J.   (1985)
Adaptation of mechanical properties of
muscle to high force training in man
J Physiol **365,** 277-284
*Adult, E. stimulation, Exercise
programme, Intervention, Male*

130/21   Davies, C.T.M., Mecrow, I.K. &
White, M.J.   (1982).
Contractile properties of the human
triceps surae with some observations of
the effects of temperature and exercise
Eur J Appl Physiol **49,** 255-269
Adult, E. stimulation, Male

130/22   Davies, C.T.M. & Sargeant,
A.J.   (1975)
Effects of exercise therapy on total and
component tissue leg volumes of patients
undergoing rehabilitation from lower
limb injury
Annals of Human Biology **2,** 327-337
*Adult, Body composition, Exercise
programme, Male*

130/23   **Davies, C.T.M. & Young, K.**   (1983)
Effects of training at 30 and 100% maximal isometric force (MVC) on the contractile properties of the triceps surae in man
J Physiol **336**, 22P-23P
Adult, E. stimulation, Exercise programme, Intervention, Male

130/24   **Davies, C.T.M., Rutherford, I.C. & Thomas, D.O.**   (1987)
Electrically evoked contractions of the triceps surae during and following 21 days of voluntary leg immobilization
Eur J Appl Physiol **56**, 306-312
Adult, E. stimulation, Female, Inactivity, Isokinetic

130/25   **Deshin, D.F.**   (1972)
Physical activity and ageing. In: A survey of Soviet literature. Gore I.Y.
Gerontol. Clin. **14**, 65-69
Elderly, Exercise programme, Intervention, Longitudinal

130/26   **Doriguzzi, C., Palmucci, L., Mongini, T. & Arnaudo, E.**   (1988)
Body building and myoglobinuria: report of three cases
Br Med J **296**, 826-827
Adult, Hazards, Intervention

130/27   **Duchateau, J. & Hainaut, K.**   (1987)
Electrical and mechanical changes in immobilized human muscle
J Appl Physiol **62**, 2168-2173
Adult, Inactivity

130/28   **Edgerton, V.R.**   (1970)
Morphology and histochemistry of the soleus muscle from normal and exercised rats
Am J Anat **127**, 81-88
Animal, Comparative, Fibre type, MUSCLE METABOLISM

130/29   **Ericson, M.O., Bratt, A., Nisell, R., Arborelius, V.P. & Ekholm, J.**   (1986)
Power output in different muscle groups during ergometer cycling
Eur J Appl Physiol **55**, 229-235
Adult, Male

130/30   **Friden, J.**   (1984)
Muscle soreness after exercise: implications of morphological changes
Int J Sports Med **5**, 57-66
Adult, Hazards

130/31   **Frontera, W.R., Meredith, C.N., O'Reilly, K.P., Knuttgen, H.G. & Evans, W.J.**   (1988)
Strength conditioning in older men: skeletal muscle hypertrophy and improved function
J Appl Physiol **64**, 1038-1044
Body composition, Elderly, Exercise programme, Fibre type, Intervention, Isokinetic, Male

130/32   **Gaffney, F.A., Grimby, G., Danneskiold-Samsoe, B. & Halskov, O.**   (1981)
Adaptation to peripheral muscle training
Scand J Rehabil Med **13**, 11-16
Adult, AEROBIC CAPACITY, Exercise programme, Fibre type, Intervention, MUSCLE METABOLISM

130/33   **Goldspink, G. & Howells K.F.**   (1974)
Work induced hypertrophy in exercised normal muscles of different ages and the reversibility of hypertrophy after cessation of exercise
J Physiol **239**, 179-193
Animal, Exercise programme, Inactivity, Intervention

130/34   **Gonyea, W.J. & Bonde-Peterson, F.**   (1978)
Alterations in muscle contractile properties and fibre composition after weight-lifting exercise in cats
Exp Neurol **59**, 75-84
Animal

130/35   **Gonyea, W.J.**   (1986)
Exercise induced increases in muscle fiber
number
Eur J Appl Physiol **55**, 137-141
***Animal, Exercise programme, Fibre type,
Intervention***

130/36   **Grimby, G. & Saltin, B.**   (1983)
The ageing muscle: mini-review
Clin Physiol **3**, 209-218
Elderly, Review

130/37   **Hakkinen, K. & Komi,
P.V.**   (1983)
Alterations of mechanical characteristics
of human skeletal muscle during strength
training
Eur J Appl Physiol **50**, 161-172
***Adult, Exercise programme, Inactivity,
Intervention, Isokinetic, Male***

130/38   **Hamel, P., Simoneau, J.A., Lortie,
G., Boulay, M.R. & Bouchard, C.**   (1986)
Heredity and muscle adaptation to
endurance training
Med Sci Sports Exerc **18**, 690-696
***Adult, AEROBIC CAPACITY, Body
composition, Exercise programme,
Intervention, MUSCLE METABOLISM***

130/39   **Herrin, G.D.**   (1980)
Standardised strength testing methods
for population descriptions. Proceedings
of NATO symposium on anthropometry
and biomechanics
Conf Proceedings, Cambridge
Review

130/40   **Howell, J.N., Chila, A.G., Ford, G.,
David, D. & Gates, T.**   (1985)
An electromyographic study of elbow
motion during postexercise muscle
soreness
J Appl Physiol **58**, 1713-1718
Adult, EMG, Hazards

130/41   **Hurley, B.F., Seals, D.R., Ehsani,
A.A., Cartier, L.J., Dalsky, G.P.,
Hagberg, J.M. & Holloszy, J.O.**   (1984)
Effects of high-intensity strength training
on cardiovascular function
Med Sci Sports Exerc **16**, 483-488
***Adult, AEROBIC CAPACITY, BLOOD
PRESSURE, Body composition,
CARDIAC PERFORMANCE, Exercise
programme, Intervention, Male***

130/42   **Ikai, M. & Fukunuga, T.**   (1970).
A study on the training effect of strength
per unit cross-sectional area of muscle by
means of ultrasonic measurement
Int. Z. Agnew Physiol. **28**, 173-180.
***Adult, Body composition, Exercise
programme, Intervention, Male***

130/43   **Ingemann-Hansen ,T. & Halkjaer-
Kristensen, J.**   (1980)
Computerized tomographic
determination of human thigh
components
Scand. J. Rehabil Med **12**, 27-31
***AEROBIC CAPACITY, Adult, Exercise
programme,Inactivity, Intervention,Male***

130/44   **Ingemann-Hansen, T. & Halkjaer-
Kristensen, J.**   (1983)
Progressive resistance exercise training of
the hypotrophic quadriceps muscle in
man
Scand J Rehabil Med **15**, 29-35
***Adult, Athlete, Body composition,
Exercise programme, Fibre type,
Inactivity, Intervention, Male, MUSCLE
METABOLISM***

130/45   **Jansson, E. & Kaijser, L.**   (1977)
Muscle adaptation to extreme endurance
training in man
Acta Physiol.Scand **100**, 315-324.
***Adult, Comparative, Fibre type,
MUSCLE METABOLISM***

130/46 **Kahanovitz, N., Nordin, M., Vederame, R., Yabut, S., Parnianpour, M., Viola, K. & Mulvihill, M.** (1987) Normal trunk muscle strength and endurance in women and the effect of exercises and electrical stimulation. Part 2: Comparative analysis of electrical stimulation and exercises to increase trunk muscle strength and endurance *Spine* **12**, 112-118 *Review*

130/47 **Kanehisa, H. & Miyashita, M.** (1983) Effect of isometric and isokinetic muscle training on static strength and dynamic power *Eur J Appl Physiol* **50**, 365-371 *Adult, Exercise programme, Intervention, Isokinetic, Male*

130/48 **Krotkiewski, M., Aniansson, A., Grimby, G., Bjorntorp, L. & Sjostrom, L.** (1979) The effect of unilateral isokinetic strength training on adipose and muscle tissue morphology. *J Appl Physiol* **42**, 271-281 *Adult, Exercise programme, Intervention, Isokinetic*

130/49 **Kuta, I., Parizkova, J. & Dycka, J.** (1970) Muscle strength and lean body mass in old men of different physical activity *J Appl Physiol* **29**, 168-171 *Body composition, Comparative, Customary activity, Elderly, Male*

130/50 **Larsson, L.** (1982) Physical training effects on muscle morphology in sedentary males of different ages *Med Sci Sports Exerc* **14**, 203-206 *Adult, Exercise programme, Fibre type, Intervention, Male*

130/51 **Leino, P., Aro, S. & Hasan, J.** (1987) Trunk muscle function and low back disorders: a ten-year follow-up study *J Chron Dis* **40**, 289-296 *Adult, Back pain, JOINTS, Longitudinal*

130/52 **Lewis, S., Nygaard, E., Sanchez, J., Egeblad, H. & Saltin, B.** (1984) Static contraction of the quadriceps muscle in man: Cardiovascular control and responses to one-legged strength training *Acta Physiol Scand* **122**, 341-353 *Adult, BLOOD PRESSURE, EMG, Exercise programme, Intervention, Male, MUSCLE METABOLISM*

130/53 **MacDougall, J.D., Elder, G.C.B., Sale, D.G. Moroz, J.R. & Sutton, J.R.** (1980) Effects of strength training and immobilization on human muscle fibres *Eur J Appl Physiol* **43**, 25-34 *Adult, Exercise programme, Fibre type, Inactivity, Intervention, Isokinetic, Male*

130/54 **MacLennan, W.J., Hall, M.R.P., Timothy, J.I. & Robinson, M.** (1980). Is weakness in old age due to muscle wasting? *Age and Ageing* **9**, 188-192. *Body composition, Elderly*

130/55 **Matoba, H. & Gollnick, P.D.** (1984). Response of skeletal muscle to training *Sports Med* **1**, 240-251 *Review*

130/56 **McDonagh, M.J.N & Davies, C.T.M.** (1984). Adaptive response of mammalian skeletal muscle to exercise with high loads *Eur J Appl. Physiol* **52**, 139-155 *Review*

130/57   **McDonagh, M.J.N., Hayward, C.M. & Davies, C.T.M.**   (1983)
Isometric training in human elbow flexor muscles. The effects of voluntary and electrically-evoked forces
J Bone Joint Surg **65-B**, 355-358
Adult, Exercise programme, E. stimulation, Intervention, Male

130/58   **McNeill, T., Warwick, D. Andersson, G. & Schultz, A.**   (1980)
Trunk strengths in attempted flexion, extension, and lateral bending in healthy subjects and patients with low-back disorders
Spine **5**, 529-538
Adult, Back pain, Comparative

130/59   **Mellin, G.**   (1986)
Chronic low back pain in men 54-63 years of age. Correlations of physical measurements with the degree of trouble and progress after treatment
Spine **11**, 421-426
Adult, Back pain, Comparative, Exercise programme, Intervention, JOINTS, Male,

130/60   **Milner-Brown, H.S., Mellenthin, M. & Miller, R.G.**   (1986)
Quantifying human muscle strength, endurance and fatigue
Arch Phys Med Rehabil **67**, 530-535
Adult, EMG

130/61   **Milner-Brown, H.S. & Miller, R.G.**   (1988)
Muscle strengthening through high-resistance weight training in patients with neuromuscular disorders
Arch Phys Med Rehabil **69**, 14-19
Adult, Exercise programme, Handicap, Intervention

130/62   **Milner-Brown, H.S. & Miller, R.G.**   (1988)
Muscle strengthening through electric stimulation combined weith low-resistance weights in patients with neuromuscular disorders
Arch Phys Med Rehabil **69**, 20-24
Adult, E. stimulation, Handicap

130/63   **Moritani, T. & de Vries, H.A.**   (1980)
Potential for gross muscle hypertrophy in older men
J Gerontol **35**, 672-682
Comparative, Elderly, EMG, Exercise programme, Intervention, Male

130/64   **Nachemson, A.**   (1976)
A critical look at conservative treatment for low back pain In: The lumbar spine and back pain (Ed.) Jayson, M.
Sector Pub Ltd, London.
Review

130/65   **Newham, D.J., Jones, D.A. & Clarkson, P.M.**   (1987)
Repeated high-force eccentric exercise: effects on muscle pain and damage
J Appl Physiol **63**, 1381-1386
Adult, E. stimulation, Exercise programme, Hazards, Intervention

130/66   **Newman, D.G., Pearn, J., Barnes, A., Young, C.M., Kehoe, M. & Newman, J.**   (1984)
Norms for hand grip strength
Arch Dis Childh **59**, 453-459
Children, Female, Male

130/67   **Nicolaisen, T. & Jorgensen, K.**   (1985)
Trunk strength, back muscle endurance and low-back trouble
Scand J Rehabil Med **17**, 121-127
Adult, Back pain, Comparative, JOINTS

130/68   Nordin, M., Kahanovitz, N., Vederame, R., Parnianpour, M., Yabut, S., Viola, K., Greenidge, N. & Mulvihill, M.   (1987)
Normal trunk muscle strength and endurance in women and the effect of exercises and electrical stimulation. Part 1: Normal endurance and trunk muscle strength in 101 women
Spine **12**, 105-111
Adult, Back pain, E. stimulation, Female, Isokinetic, JOINTS

130/69   Nygard, C.H., Luopajarvi, T.,, Cedercreutz, A. & Ilmarinen, J.   (1987)
Musculoskeletal capacity of employees aged 44 to 58 years in physical, mental and mixed types of work
Eur J Appl Physiol **56**, 555-561
Adult, Comparative, Female, JOINTS, Male, Occupational activity

130/70   Owen, B.D.   (1986)
Posture, exercise can help prevent low back injuries
Occup Health Saf **55**, 33-37
Adult, Back pain, Hazards

130/71   Pearson, M.B.   (1985).
Muscle strength, body composition and activity in the elderly
M Phil Thesis, University of Nottingham.
Body composition, Customary activity, Elderly

130/72   Plum, P. & Rehfeld, J.   (1985)
Muscular training for acute and chronic back pain
Lancet **i**, 453-454
Adult, Back pain, Exercise programme, Intervention

130/73   Radin, E.L.   (1986)
Role of muscles in protecting athletes from injury
Acta Med Scand (Suppl 711) 143-147
Hazards, Review

130/74   Rutherford, O.M.   (1986)
The determinants of human muscle strength and the effects of different high resistance training regimes
Ph.D. Thesis, University College, London
Review

130/75   Sale, D.G., MacDougall, J.D., Alway, S.E. & Sutton, J.R.   (1987)
Voluntary strength and muscle characteristics in untrained men and women and male bodybuilders
J Appl Physiol **62**, 1786-1793
Adult, Body composition, Comparative, Fibre type, Isokinetic,

130/76   Salminen, A.   (1985)
Lysosomal changes in skeletal muscles during the repair of exercise injuries in muscle fibers
Acta Physiol Scand (Suppl 539) **124**, 1-31
Review

130/77   Salmons, S. & Henriksson, J.   (1981)
The adaptive response of skeletal muscle to increased use
Muscle & Nerve **4**, 94-105
Review

130/78   Saltin, B. & Gollnick, P.D.   (1983)
Skeletal muscle adaptability significance for metabolism and performance. In: Handbook of Physiology, Section 10: Skeletal Muscle
Am Phys Soc, Bethesda, Maryland. 555-632.
Review

130/79   Saltin, B., Henriksson, J., Nygaard, E. & Anderson, P.   (1977)
Fibre type and metabolic potentials of skeletal muscles in sedentary men and endurance runners
Ann NY Acad Sci **301**, 3-29
Adult, Comparative, Fibre type, MUSCLE METABOLISM

130/80   Sargeant, A.J. & Davies,
C.T.M.   (1977)
The effect of disuse muscular atrophy on
the forces generated in dynamic exercise
Clin Sci Mol Med **53**, 183-188
Adult, Male, Inactivity

130/81   Sargeant, A.J., Davies, C.T.M.,
Edwards, R.H.T., Masunder, C. & Young,
A.   (1977)
Functional and structural changes after
disuse of human muscle
Clin Sci Mol Med **52**, 337-342
Adult, Fibre type, Inactivity, Male

130/82   Scelsi, R., Marchetti, C. & Poggi,
P.   (1980)
Histochemical and ultrastructural
aspects of m.vastus lateralis in sedentary
old people
Acta Neuropathol **51**, 99-105
Elderly

130/83   Schantz, P.G.   (1986)
Plasticity of human skeletal muscle
Acta Physiol Scand (Suppl 558) **128**, 7-62
Review

130/84   Simoneau, J.A., Lortie, G., Boulay,
M.R., Marcotte, M., Thibault, M.-C. &
Bouchard, C.   (1985)
Human skeletal muscle fibre type
alteration with high intensity intermittent
training
Eur J Appl Physiol **54**, 250-253
*Adult, Exercise programme, Fibre type,
Intervention*

130/85   Sjöström, M., Friden, J. & Ekblom,
B.   (1987)
Endurance, what is it? Muscle
morphology after an extremely long
distance run
Acta Physiol Scand **130**, 513-520
*Adult, Fibre type, Hazards, Male,
Running*

130/86   Stone, M.H. & Lipner, H.   (1978)
Response to intensive training and
methandrostenelone administration. I
Contractile and performance variables.
Pflugers Arch **375**, 141-146
*Animal, Comparative, Exercise
programme, Intervention*

130/87   Suzuki, N. & Endo, S.   (1983)
A quantitative study of trunk muscle
strength and fatigability in the low-back-
pain syndrome
Spine **8**, 69-74
Adult, Back pain

130/88   Tesch, P. A. & Larsson, L.   (1982)
Muscle hypertrophy in bodybuilders
Eur J Appl Physiol **49**, 301-306
Adult, Comparative, Fibre type, Male

130/89   Tiidus, P.M. & Ianuzzo,
C.D.   (1983)
Effects of intensity and duration of
muscular exercise on delayed soreness
and serum enzyme activities
Med Sci Sports Exerc **15**, 461-465
Adult, Hazards

130/90   Tornvall, G.   (1963)
Assessment of physical capabilities with
special reference to the evaluation of
maximal voluntary isometric muscle
strength and maximal working capacity
Acta Physiol Scand (Suppl 201) **58**, 201
*Adult, AEROBIC CAPACITY, Body
composition, Male*

130/91   Watson, A.W.S. & O'Donovan,
D.J.   (1977)
The effects of five weeks of controlled
interval training on youths of diverse pre-
training condition
J Sports Med **17**, 139-146
*Body composition, Children,
Comparative, Exercise programme,
Intervention*

130/92   **Weltman, A., Janney, C., Rians, C.B., Strand, K., Berg, B. & Tippitt, S.** (1986)
The effects of hydraulic resistance strength training in pre-pubertal males
Med Sci Sports Exerc **18**, 629-638
AEROBIC CAPACITY, Body composition, Children, Exercise programme, Hazards, Intervention, Isokinetic, Male

130/93   **Whipple, R.H., Wolfson, L.I. & Amerman, P.M.** (1987)
The relationship of knee and ankle weakness to falls in nursing home residents: an isokinetic study
J Am Geriatr Soc **35**, 13-20
Comparative, Elderly, Isokinetic

130/94   **Wilmore, J.H.** (1974)
Alterations in strength
Med Sci Sports Exerc **6**, 133-138
Adult, Body composition, Exercise programme, Intervention

130/95   **Wilmore, J.H., Parr, R.B., Girandola, R.N., Ward, P., Vodak, P.A., Barstow, T.J., Pipes, T.V., Romero, G.T. & Leslie, P.** (1978)
Physiological alterations consequent to circuit weight training
Med Sci Sports Exerc **10**, 79-84
Adult, AEROBIC CAPACITY, Body composition, Exercise programme, Intervention, Isokinetic, JOINTS

140 MUSCLE METABOLISM

KEYWORDS are listed in the appendix in addition the following specific keywords have been used in this section:

Body composition (includes muscle cross-sectional area)
Capillaries
EMG (electromyograph)
Fibre type
Isokinetic

Summary of evidence: exercise ameliorates, prevents or reverses poor physical capability arising from poor muscle function due to lack of use of the muscle

THE PROBLEM

Improvements with exercise in maximal aerobic capacity and endurance are due to a large extent to changes within the muscle. Do these changes also occur in the sedentary, old or disabled?

SCOPE

This section contains references dealing primarily with changes produced by exercise in muscle, as described in section 130, but with additional information derived from biopsies about enzyme concentrations, mitochondrial content and capillarity. Moreover the studies are mainly of the effects of rhythmic exercise although there are some studies of weight or strength training.

METHODOLOGICAL PROBLEMS

The assessment of changes within muscle requires that a piece of muscle be removed with a biopsy needle. This invasive technique restricts the number of live human subjects studied, and the number of samples which can be taken from one subject.

EVIDENCE

It is clear nevertheless that improvements in muscle enzymes and capillarity can be obtained by rhythmic exercise in almost anyone, including the elderly and that they contribute importantly to the increases in maximal oxygen uptake and exercise performance described in sections 110 and 120. It is also clear that these improvements are specific to the muscle which is exercised.

140/1 **Adolfsson, J.** (1986)
The time dependence of training-induced increase in skeletal muscle capillarization and the spatial capillary to fibre relationship in normal and neovascularized skeletal muscle of rats
Acta Physiol Scand **128**, 259-266
Animal, Capillaries, Exercise programme, Fibre type, Intervention, Swimming

140/2 **Ama, P.F.M., Simoneau, J.A., Boulay, M.R., Serresse, O., Theriault, G. & Bouchard, C.** (1986)
Skeletal muscle characteristics in sedentary Black and Caucasian males
J Appl Physiol **61**, 1758-1761
Adult, Comparative, Fibre type, Male,

140/3 **Andersen, P. & Henriksson, J.** (1977)
Capillary supply of the quadriceps femoris muscle of man; adaptive response to exercise
J Physiol **270**, 677-690
Adult, AEROBIC CAPACITY, Capillaries, Exercise programme, Fibre type, Intervention, Male

140/4   Bjorntorp, P., Fahlen, M., Holm, T., Schersten, T. & Stenberg, J.   (1971)
Changes in the activity of skeletal muscle succinic oxidase after training. In: Coronary heart disease and physical fitness (Eds) Larsen, O. A. & Sullivan, L. *Munksgaard, Copenhagen.* 138-142
Review

140/5   Blom, P.C., Vollestad, N.K. & Costill, D.L.   (1986)
Factors affecting changes in muscle glycogen concentration during and after prolonged exercise
Acta Physiol Scand (Suppl 556) **128,** 67-74
Review

140/6   Brodal, P., Ingjer, F. & Hermansen, L.   (1977)
Capillary supply of skeletal muscle fibers in untrained and endurance-trained men
Am J Physiol **232,** H705-712
Adult, AEROBIC CAPACITY, Capillaries, Comparative, Fibre type, Male

140/7   Brown, M. & Rose, S.J.   (1985)
The effects of aging and exercise on skeletal muscle-clinical considerations
Top Ger Rehabil **1,** 20-30
Elderly, Review

140/8   Burton, H.W. & Barclay, J.K.   (1986)
Metabolic factors from exercising muscle and the proliferation of endothelial cells
Med Sci Sports Exerc **18,** 390-395
Animal

140/9   Cartee, G.D. & Farrar, R.P.   (1987)
Muscle respiratory capacity and VO2 max in identically trained young and old rats
J Appl Physiol **63,** 257-261
AEROBIC CAPACITY, Animal, Comparative, Exercise programme, Intervention

140/10   Costill, D.L., Fink, W.J., Getchell, L.H., Ivy, J.L. & Witzmann, F.A.   (1979)
Lipid metabolism in skeletal muscle of endurance-trained males and females
J Appl Physiol **47,** 787-791
Adult, AEROBIC CAPACITY, Comparative, Female, Male

140/11   Cress, M.E., Byrnes, W.C., Dickinson, A.L. & Foster, V.L.   (1984)
Modification of Type II fiber atrophy and LDH isoenzymes component of an 8 week endurance training program in elderly women
Med Sci Sports Exerc **16,** 105
Elderly, Exercise programme, Female, Fibre type, Intervention

140/12   Davies, K.J.A., Packer, L. & Brooks, G.A.   (1981)
Biochemical adaptation of mitochondria, muscle and whole-animal respiration to endurance training
Arch Biochem Biophysics **209,** 539-554
AEROBIC CAPACITY, Animal, Exercise programme, Intervention

140/13   Eriksson, B.O.   (1980)
Muscle metabolism in children – A review
Acta Paediat Scand (Suppl) **283,** 20-28
Children, Review

140/14   Eriksson, B.O., Gollnick, P.D. & Saltin, B.   (1974)
The effect of physical training on muscle enzyme activities and fiber composition in 11-year-old boys
Acta Paediat Belg (Suppl) **28,** 245-252
Children, Exercise programme, Fibre type, Intervention, Male

140/15   Eriksson, B.O. & Saltin, B.   (1974)
Muscle metabolism during exercise in boys 11 to 16 years compared to adults
Acta Paed Belg (Suppl) **28,** 257-265
Children, Comparative, Male

140/16 **Gibson, H. & Edwards, R.H.T.** (1985)
Muscular exercise and fatigue
Sports Med **2**, 120-132
Review

140/17 **Gibson, J.N.A., Halliday, D., Morrison, W.L., Stoward, P.J., Hornsby, G.A., Watt, P.W., Murdoch, G. & Rennie, M.J.** (1987)
Decrease in human quadriceps muscle protein turnover consequent upon leg immobilization
Clin Sci **72**, 503-509
Adult, Fibre type, Inactivity, Male

140/18 **Gohil, K., Packer, L., De Luman, B., Brooks, G.A. & Terblanche, S.E.** (1986)
Vitamin E deficiency and vitamin C supplements: exercise and mitochondrial oxidation
J Appl Physiol **60**, 1986-1991
Animal, Comparative, Intervention

140/19 **Gollnick, P.D.** (1972)
Enzyme activity and the composition of skeletal muscle of untrained and trained men
J Appl Physiol **33**, 312-319
Adult, Athlete, Comparative, Fibre type, Male

140/20 **Gollnick, P.D.** (1986)
Metabolic regulation in skeletal muscle: influence of endurance training as exerted by mitochrondrial protein
Acta Physiol Scand (Suppl 556) **128**, 53-66
Review

140/21 **Gregory, P., Low, R.B. & Stirewalt, W.S.** (1986)
Changes in skeletal muscle myosin isoenzymes with hypertrophy and exercise
Biochem J **238**, 55-63
Animal, Intervention

140/22 **Grimby, G.** (1986)
Physical activity and muscle training in the elderly
Acta Med Scand (Suppl 711) **220**, 233-237
Review, Elderly

140/23 **Grimby, G., Saltin, B., Kaijser, L. & Renstrom, P.** (1983)
Aerobic power, muscle morphology and enzymatic capacity in a follow-up study of very old still active endurance athletes
Med Sci Sports Exerc **15**, 105
Adult, Athlete, AEROBIC CAPACITY, Fibre type, Longitudinal, Male, METABOLIC FUNCTION

140/24 **Hakkinen, K. & Komi, P.V.** (1986)
Training-induced changes in neuromuscular performance under voluntary and reflex conditions
Eur J Appl Physiol **55**, 147-155
Adult, EMG, Exercise programme, Intervention, Male, Vigorous

140/25 **Haralambie, G.** (1979)
Skeletal muscle enzyme activities in female subjects of various ages
Bull Europ Physiopath Resp **15**, 259-267
Adult, Comparative, Female

140/26 **Henriksson, J.** (1977)
Training induced adaptation of skeletal muscle and metabolism during submaximal exercise
J Physiol **270**, 661-675
Adult, AEROBIC CAPACITY, Exercise programme, Fibre type, Intervention, Male

140/27 **Henriksson, J. & Reitman, J.S.** (1976)
Quantitative measures of enzyme activities in Type i and Type ii muscle fibres of man after training
Acta Physiol Scand **97**, 392-397
Adult, AEROBIC CAPACITY, Exercise programme, Fibre type, Intervention

140/28   Herscovich, S. & Gershon, D.   (1987)
Effects of aging and physical training on the neuromuscular junction of the mouse
Gerontology **33**, 7-13
Animal, Exercise programme, Intervention

140/29   Holloszy, J.O.   (1982)
Muscle metabolism during exercise
Arch Phys Med Rehabil **63**, 231-234
Review

140/30   Horber, F.F., Hoopeler, H. & Scheidegger, J.R.   (1987)
Impact of physical training on the ultrastructure of midthigh muscle in normal subjects and patients treated with glucocorticoids
J Clin Invest **79**, 1181-1190
Adult, Body composition, Capillaries, Exercise programme, Intervention, Isokinetic

140/31   Houston, M.E., Froese, E.A., Valeriote, StP., Green, H.J. & Ranney, D.A   (1983)
Muscle performance, morphology and metabolic capacity during strength training and de-training: a one-legged model
Eur J Appl Physiol **51**, 25-35
Adult, Exercise programme, Fibre type, Inactivity, Intervention, Isokinetic, Male

140/32   Hudlicka, O.   (1982)
Growth of capillaries in skeletal and cardiac muscle
Circulation Res 50,
451-461

140/33   Hurley, B.F., Nemeth, P.M., Martin, W.H., Hagberg, J.M., Dalsky, G.P. & Holloszy, J.O.   (1986)
Muscle triglyceride utilization during exercise: effect of training
J Appl Physiol **60**, 562-567
Adult, AEROBIC CAPACITY, Exercise, Intervention, Male

140/34   Ingjer, F.   (1979)
Effects of endurance training on muscle fibre ATP-ase activity, capillary supply and mitochondrial content in man
J Physiol **294**, 419-432
Adult, AEROBIC CAPACITY, Capillaries, Female, Exercise programme, Intervention, MUSCLE STRENGTH, Vigorous

140/35   Jansson, E. & Kaijser, L.   (1987)
Substrate utilization and enzymes in skeletal muscle of extremely endurance-trained men
J Appl Physiol **62**, 999-1005
Adult, AEROBIC CAPACITY, Comparative, Male

140/36   Katz, A.   (1986)
Leg glucose uptake during maximal dynamic exercise in humans
Am J Physiol **251**, E65-70

140/37   Klausen, K., Andersen, L.B. & Pelle, I.   (1981)
Adaptive changes in work capacity, skeletal muscle capillarization and enzyme levels during training and detraining
Acta Physiol Scand **113**, 9-16
Adult, AEROBIC CAPACITY, Capillaries, Exercise programme, Fibre type, Inactivity, Intervention, Male

140/38   Kristensen, J.H., Hansen, T.I. & Saltin, B.   (1980)
Cross-sectional and fiber size changes in the quadriceps muscle of man with immobilization and physical training
Muscle & Nerve **3**, 275-276
Adult, Exercise programme, Inactivity, Intervention

140/39   Leinonen, H.   (1980)
Effects of sprint- and endurance-training on capillary circulation in human skeletal muscle
Acta Physiol Scand **108**, 425-427
Adult, Athlete, Capillaries, Comparative

140/40   MacDougall, J.D., Ward, G.R., Sale, D.G. & Sutton, J.R.   (1977)
Biochemical adaptation of skeletal muscle to heavy resistance training and immobilisation
J Appl Physiol **43**, 700-703
Adult, Exercise programme, Inactivity, Intervention

140/41   Newham, D.J., Jones, D.A., Tolfree, S.E. & Edwards, R.H.T.   (1986)
Skeletal muscle damage: a study of isotope uptake, enzyme efflux and pain after stepping
Eur J Appl Physiol **55**, 106-112
Hazards

140/42   Nygaard, E.   (1981)
Skeletal muscle fibre characteristics in young women
Acta Physiol Scand **112**, 299-304
Adult, AEROBIC CAPACITY, Capillaries, Comparative, Female, Fibre type

140/43   Orlander, J. & Aniansson, A.   (1980)
Effects of physical training on skeletal muscle metabolism and ultrastructure in 70 to 75-year-old men
Acta Physiol Scand **109**, 149-154
Elderly, Exercise programme, Intervention, Male, Muscle strength

140/44   Orlander, J., Kiessling, K.-H., Karlsson, J. & Ekblom, B.   (1977)
Low intensity training, inactivity and resumed training in sedentary men
Acta Physiol Scand **101**, 351-362
Adult, AEROBIC CAPACITY, Exercise programme, Fibre type, Inactivity, Intervention, Male

140/45   Rehunen, S., Karli, P. & Harkonen, M.   (1985)
High-energy phosphate compounds in slow-twitch and fast-twitch muscle fibres. Changes during exercise in some neuromuscular diseases
J Neurol Sci **67**, 299-306
Adult, Fibre type, Handicap

140/46   Salmons, S. & Henriksson, J.
The adaptive response of skeletal muscle to increased use
Muscle and Nerve **4**, 94-105
Review

140/47   Saltin, B., Kiens, B., Savard, G. & Pedersen, P.K.   (1986)
Role of haemoglobin and capillarization for oxygen delivery and extraction in muscular exercise
Acta Physiol Scand (Suppl 556) **128**, 21-32
Adult

140/48   Schantz, P.G., Sjoberg, B. & Svedenhag, J.   (1986)
Malate-aspartate and alpha-glycerophosphate shuttle enzyme levels in human skeletal muscle: methodological consideration and effect of endurance training
Acta Physiol Scand **128**, 397-407
Adult, Capillaries, Comparative, Exercise programme, Fibre type, Intervention

140/49   Simoneau, J.A., Lortie, G., Boulay, M.R., Marcotte, M., Thibault, M.-C. & Bouchard, C.   (1987)
Effects of two high-intensity intermittent training programs interspaced by detraining on human skeletal muscle and performance
Eur J Appl Physiol **56**, 516-521
Adult, Exercise programme, Inactivity, Intervention, MUSCLE STRENGTH

140/50   Sinoway, L.I., Musch, T.I., Minotti, J.R. & Zelis, R.   (1986)
Enhanced maximal metabolic vasodilation in the dominant forearms of tennis players
J Appl Physiol **61**, 673-678
Adult, AEROBIC CAPACITY, Intervention, Male, MUSCLE STRENGTH

140/51 Snell, P.G., Martin, W.H., Buckey, J.C. & Blomqvist, C.G. (1987) Maximal vascular leg conductance in trained and untrained men *J Appl Physiol* **62**, 606-610 *Adult, Comparative, Male*

140/52 Stebbins, C.L., Schultz, E., Smith, R.T. & Smith, E.L. (1985) Effects of chronic exercise during aging on muscle end-plate morphology in rats *J Appl Physiol* **58**, 45-51 *Animal, Fibre type, Intervention*

140/53 Suominen, H., Heikkinen, E., Liesen, H., Michel, D. & Hollman, W. (1977) Effects of 8 weeks endurance training on skeletal muscle metabolism in 56-70 year old sedentary men *Eur J Appl Physiol* **37**, 173-180 *Elderly, Exercise programme, Intervention*

140/54 Terrados, N., Melichna, J., Sylven, C. & Jansson, E. (1986) Decrease in skeletal muscle myoglobin with intensive training in man *Acta Physiol Scand* **128**, 651-652 *Adult, Athlete, Capillaries, Exercise programme, Fibre type, Intervention, Male*

140/55 Tesch, P.A. & Wright, J.E. (1983) Recovery from short term intense exercise: its relation to capillary supply and blood lactate concentration *Eur J Appl Physiol* **52**, 98-103 *Adult, Capillaries, Fibre type, Isokinetic, Male*

140/56 Thomason, D.B., Herrick, R.E. & Baldwin, K.M. (1987) Activity influences on soleus muscle myosin during hindlimb suspension *J Appl Physiol* **63**, 138-144 *Animal, Exercise programme, Intervention*

140/57 Thorstensson, A. (1976) Muscle strength, fibre types and enzyme activities in man *Acta Physiol Scand (Suppl 443)* **99**, *Adult, Customary activity, Exercise programme, Intervention, Isokinetic, Male, MUSCLE STRENGTH*

140/58 Thorstensson, A., Hultén, B., von Döbeln, W. & Karlsson, J. (1976) Effect of strength training on enzyme activities and fibre characteristics in human skeletal muscle *Acta Physiol Scand* **96**, 392-398 *Adult, Body composition, Exercise, Fibre type, Intervention, Male*

140/59 Vihko, V., Sarviharju, P.J., Havu, M., Hirsimaki, Y., Salminen, A., Rahkila, P. & Arstila, A.U. (1975) Selected skeletal muscle variables and aerobic power in trained and untrained men *J Sports Med* **15**, 294-304. *Adult, AEROBIC CAPACITY, Capillaries, Comparative, Fibre type, Male*

140/60 Wallenstein, R. & Karlsson, J. (1984) Histochemical and metabolic changes in lower leg muscles in exercise-induced pain *Int J Sports Med* **5**, 202-208 *Fibre type, Hazards*

140/61 Ward, G.R., MacDougall, J.D., Sutton, J.R., Toews, C.J. & Jones, N.L. (1986) Activation of human muscle pyruvate dehydrogenase with activity and immobilisation *Clin Sci* **70**, 207-210 *Exercise programme, Inactivity, Intervention,*

140/62   **Wilkinson, J.G. & Wenger, H.A.,** (1987)
Skeletal muscle RNA synthesis following endurance and sprint exercise
Biochem Med Metab Biol **36,** 293-299
Comparative

140/63   **Young, J.C., Chen, M. & Holloszy, J.O.**
Maintenance of the adaptation of skeletal muscle mitochondria to exercise in rat
Med Sci Sports Exerc **15,** 243-246
Animal, Exercise programme, Intervention, Swimming

KEYWORDS are listed in the appendix in addition the following specific keywords have been used in this section:

Angina
Arrhythmia
Autonomic nervous system
Cardiac output
Heart rate
Heart failure
Hypertrophy
Myocardial contractility
Stroke volume

Summary of evidence: exercise ameliorates overt or occult coronary heart disease due to a slower heart rate at a given exercise intensity

THE PROBLEM

To what extent is the improvement in maximal oxygen uptake and the reduced submaximal heart rate due to effects on cardiac muscle, such as an increase in cardiac size or an improvement in contractility? Does exercise produce changes in cardiac perfusion or in coronary arteries which are beneficial in heart disease? Coronary heart disease is the major cause of death in middle-aged men in the developed countries. It is also causes a great deal of disability.

SCOPE

This section contains references dealing primarily with changes produced by exercise in cardiac function including cardiac output, stroke volume, heart size and heart rate. There is a large literature, this is therefore a representative selection not a comprehensive listing. It contains references on the intensity and amount of exercise needed to improve cardiac function; it contains studies of all age groups and includes the sedentary and the athletic. There are some animal studies, a few studies of the acute effects of exercise and some studies of the effects of inactivity.

METHODOLOGICAL DIFFICULTIES

Assessment of small but functionally important increases in cardiac dimensions such as wall thickness in an actively beating heart poses severe difficulty. Moreover, these increases should not be confused with the hypertrophy of the left ventricle which occurs in hypertension and is a pathological adaptation. Small increases in the internal dimensions of the heart may be a secondary effect due to increased filling pressure or a slowed heart rate. Large increases which occur in heart failure compromise the myocardium because the wall tension required to generate an adequate pumping pressure rises steeply. Studies of autonomic control depend on complete blockade with drugs of one or both of the autonomic neural pathways. Assessment of very low plasma levels of catecholamines requires sophisticated equipment and the assessments are complicated by possible changes in receptor density, sensitivity or reuptake mechanisms.

EVIDENCE

It is clear that several kinds of improvement in cardiac function can be obtained with exercise. Vigorous rhythmic exercise can lead to increases in maximal stroke volume and cardiac output; this is associated with an increased maximal aerobic capacity (see section 110). The cardiac changes are sometimes associated with increased myocardial contractility and, in young subjects, small increases in cardiac dimensions. These are seen in athletes who run or swim but not in weightlifters. Repeated maximal isometric efforts used in the training of weightlifters may lead to hypertrophy of the left ventricle. This is an undesirable effect of exercise akin to that

seen in hypertension which eventually
compromises the blood supply to the
myocardium and may cause angina. There
are also increases in plasma volume which
could increase filling pressures. These
changes are associated with a reduced heart
rate and lower catecholamine levels at
submaximal levels of work despite an
unchanged cardiac output (except in cardiac
patients). This reduced heart rate reduces the
work of the myocardium and therefore
relieves symptoms of angina in a
compromised heart. This is a health benefit
for cardiac patients and for middle-aged
people many of whom will have some degree
of coronary atheroma.

210/1   (1982)
    Editorial: Cardiovascular consequences
    of sustained exercise
    Lancet **i**, 893
    *MUSCLE METABOLISM, MUSCLE
    STRENGTH, Review*

210/2   (1984)
    Editorial: Athlete's heart: Is big bad or
    can it be benign?
    Lancet **ii**, 613-614
    Hypertrophy, Review

210/3   **Adams, T.D., Yanowitz, F.G., Fisher,
    A.G., Ridges, J. D., Lovell, K. & Pryor,
    T.A.**   (1981)
    Non-invasive evaluation of exercise
    training in college-age men
    Circulation **64**, 958-965
    *Adult, AEROBIC CAPACITY, Body
    composition, Cardiac output, Exercise
    programme, HAZARDS-CVS,
    Hypertrophy, Intervention, Male,
    Running, Stroke volume, Vigorous,
    Weight*

210/4   **Amsterdam, E.A. & Laslett,
    L.J.**   (1985)
    Effects of exercise on the myocardium:
    echocardiographic studies. In: Exercise
    and the Heart, edition 2 (Ed.) Brest,
    A.N., F.A.Davis Company,
    Philadelphia
    Cardiovasc Clinics **15**, 87-94
    HAZARDS-CVS, Hypertrophy, Review

210/5   **Baldwin, K. M.**   (1985)
    Effects of chronic exercise on biochemical
    and functional properties of the heart
    Med Sci Sports Exerc **17**, 522-528
    Myocardial contractility, Review

210/6   **Bezucha, G.R., Lenser, M.C.,
    Hanson, P.G. & Nagle, F.J.**   (1982)
    Comparison of hemodynamic responses
    to static and dynamic exercise
    J Appl Physiol **53**, 1589-1593
    *Acute exercise, Adult, AEROBIC
    CAPACITY, BLOOD PRESSURE,
    Cardiac output, Comparative, Heart rate,
    Male, MUSCLE STRENGTH, Stroke
    volume*

210/7   **Breisch, E.A., White, F.C., Nimmo,
    L.E., Mckirnan, M.D. & Bloor,
    C.M.**   (1986)
    Exercise-induced cardiac hypertrophy: a
    correlation of blood flow and
    microvasculature
    J Appl Physiol **60**, 1259-1267
    *Acute exercise, AEROBIC CAPACITY,
    Animal, BLOOD PRESSURE, Cardiac
    output, COLLATERALS, Exercise
    programme, Heart rate, Hypertrophy,
    Intervention, Vigorous*

210/8   **Brundin, T. & Cernigliaro,
    C.**   (1975)
    Effect of physical training on the
    sympathoadrenal response to exercise
    Scand J clin Lab Invest **35**, 525-530
    *Adult, Autonomic nervous system,
    Endocrine, Exercise programme, Heart
    rate, Intervention, Male*

210/9   Bryhn, M. & Castenfors, J.   (1987)
Left ventricular diastolic and systolic
function during isometric exercise: an
echocardiographic study
Clin Cardiol **10**, 71-77
*Acute exercise, Adult, MUSCLE
STRENGTH*

**210/10   Butler, J., O'Brien, M., O'Malley,
K. & Kelly, J.G.**   (1982)
Relationship of β-adrenoceptor density to
fitness in athletes
Nature **298**, 60-62
*Adult, AEROBIC CAPACITY, Athlete,
Autonomic nervous system, Endocrine,
Exercise programme, Intervention,
Swimming*

210/11   Chinkin, A.S.   (1986)
Effect of physical effort levels on
hypertrophy of the heart and its
substructure
Bull Eksp Biol Med **102**, 602-604
*Adult, Comparative, HAZARDS-CVS,
Hypertrophy*

210/12   Clausen, J.P.   (1977)
The effects of physical training on
cardiovascular adjustments to exercise in
man
Physiol Rev **57**, 779-815
Review

**210/13   Cohen, J.L., Gupta, P.K., Lichstein,
E. & Chadda, K.D.**   (1980)
The heart of a dancer: Noninvasive
cardiac evaualtion of professional ballet
dancers
Am J Cardiol **45**, 959-965
*Adult, Arrhythmia, Comparative,
Dancing, HAZARDS-CVS,
Hypertrophy, Vigorous*

**210/14   Cokkinos, D.V., Perrakis, C.,
Diakoumakos, N., Papantonakos, A. &
Mamaki, S.**   (1984)
Cardiac function at treadmill exercise in
various age groups
Eur Heart J (Suppl.E) **5**, 41-45
*Acute exercise, Adult, BLOOD
PRESSURE, Comparative, Elderly,
Heart rate, Male*

**210/15   Coleman, R., Silbermann, M.,
Gershon, D. & Reznick, A.Z.**   (1987)
Effects of long-term running stress on the
ultrastructure of the aging mouse heart
Gerontology **33**, 19-33
*Animal, COAGULATION, Elderly,
Exercise programme, Intervention,
Vigorous*

**210/16   Coleman, R., Silbermann, M.,
Gershon, D. & Reznick, A.Z.**   (1987)
Giant mitochondria in the myocardium
of aging and endurance-trained mice
Gerontology **33**, 34-39
*Animal, Elderly, Exercise programme,
Intervention, Vigorous*

**210/17   Cox, M.L., Bennett, J.B. 3rd &
Dudley, G.A.**   (1986)
Exercise training-induced alterations of
cardiac morphology
J Appl Physiol **61**, 926-931
*Adult, AEROBIC CAPACITY, Cardiac
output, Cycling, Exercise programme,
Intervention, HAZARDS-CVS,
Hypertrophy, Running, Stroke volume,
Vigorous*

**210/18   Cutilletta, A.F., Edmiston, K. &
Dowell, R.T.**   (1979)
Effect of a mild exercise program on
myocardial function and the
development of hypertrophy
J Appl Physiol **46**, 354-360
*Animal, Exercise programme,
Intervention, SECONDARY
PREVENTION, Stroke volume,*

210/19   DeMaria, A.N., Neumann, A., Lee, G., Fowler, W. & Mason, D.T.   (1978)
Alterations in ventricular mass and performance induced by exercise training in man evaluated by echocardiography
Circulation **57**, 237-244
Adult, AEROBIC CAPACITY, BLOOD PRESSURE, Cardiac output, Exercise programme, Female, Hypertrophy, Intervention, Male, Myocardial contractility, Stroke volume, Vigorous

210/20   DeVries, H.A., & Adams, G.M.   (1972)
Comparison of exercise reponses on old and young men. I. The cardiac effort/total body effort relationship
J Gerontol **27**, 344-8
Adult, AEROBIC CAPACITY, BLOOD PRESSURE, Comparative, Elderly, Heart rate, Male

210/21   Dimsdale, J.E. & Moss, J.   (1980)
Plasma catecholamines in stress and exercise
J Am Med Ass **243**, 340-342
Adult, Autonomic nervous system, Customary activity, Endocrine

210/22   Ehsani, A.A.   (1986)
Adaptations to training in patients with exercise-induced left ventricular dysfunction
Adv Cardiol **34**, 148-155
Adult, Exercise programme, Intervention, SECONDARY PREVENTION

210/23   Ehsani, A.A.   (1987)
Cardiovascular adaptations to exercise training in the elderly
Fed Proc **46**, 1840-1843
AEROBIC CAPACITY, Autonomic nervous system, Cardiac output, Elderly, Heart rate, Hypertrophy, Myocardial contractility, Review

210/24   Ehsani, A.A., Hagberg, J.M. & Hickson, R.C.   (1978)
Rapid changes in left ventricular dimensions and mass in response to physical conditioning and deconditioning
Am J Cardiol **42**, 52-56
Adult, AEROBIC CAPACITY, Athlete, HAZARDS-CVS, Hypertrophy, Inactivity, Intervention, Leisure activity

210/25   Ehsani, A.A., Martin, W.H. 3rd, Heath G.W. & Coyle, E.F.   (1982)
Rapid changes in left ventricular dimensions and mass in response to physical conditioning and deconditioning
Am J Cardiol **50**, 246-254
Adult, Exercise programme, Intervention, HAZARDS-CVS, Hypertrophy, Myocardial contractility, Swimming, Training

210/26   Eriksson, B.O., Engström, I., Karlberg, P., Lundin, A., Saltin, B. & Thorén, C.   (1978)
Long-term effect of previous swimtraining in girls. A 10-year follow-up of the girl swimmers
Acta Paediatr Scand **67**, 285-292
AEROBIC CAPACITY, Athlete, Children, Female, GROWTH, Hypertrophy, Longitudinal, RESPIRATORY FUNCTION, Swimming,

210/27   Fardy, P.S., Maresh, C.M. & Abbott, R.D.   (1976)
A comparison of myocardial function in former athletes and non-athletes
Med Sci Sports **8**, 26-30
Adult, BLOOD PRESSURE, Comparative, Leisure activity, Male, Occupational activity,

210/28   **Flaim, S.F. & Minter, W.J.**   (1980)
Ventricular volume overload alters
cardiac output distribution in rats during
exercise
J Appl Physiol **49**, 482-490
*Acute exercise, Animal, BLOOD
PRESSURE, Cardiac output,
HAZARDS-CVS, Heart failure, Heart
rate, Hypertrophy*

210/29   **Galbo, H., Christenssen, N.J. &
Holst, J.J.**   (1977)
Catecholamines and pancreatic
hormones during autonomic blockade in
exercising man
Acta Physiol Scand **101**, 428-437
*Acute exercise, Adult, Autonomic nervous
system, CARBOHYDRATE
TOLERANCE, Endocrine, Male*

210/30   **Galbo, H., Holst, J.J. &
Christensen, N.J.**   (1975)
Glucagon and plasma catecholamine
responses to graded and prolonged
exercise in man
J Appl Physiol **38**, 70-76
*Acute exercise, Adult, AEROBIC
CAPACITY, Autonomic nervous system,
CARBOHYDRATE TOLERANCE,
Endocrine, Male*

210/31   **Geenen, D.L., Gilliam, T.B.,
Crowley, D., Moorehead-Steffens, C. &
Rosenthal, A.**   (1982)
Echocardiographic measures in 6 to 7
year old children after an 8 month
exercise program
Am J Cardiol **49**, 1990-1995
*Children, Exercise programme,
HAZARDS-CVS, Heart rate,
Hypertrophy, Intervention, Vigorous*

210/32   **Geenen, D.L., White, T.P. &
Lampman, R.M.**   (1987)
Papillary mechanics and cardiac
morphology of infarcted rat hearts after
training
J Appl Physiol **63**, 92-96
*Animal, Exercise programme,
Hypertrophy, Intervention, Myocardial
contractility, SECONDARY
PREVENTION*

210/33   **Gerstenblith, G., Renlund, D.G. &
Lakatta, E.G.**   (1987)
Cardiovascular response to exercise in
younger and older men
Fed Proc **46**, 1834-1839
*Autonomic nervous system, BLOOD
PRESSURE, Cardiac output, Elderly,
Review*

210/34   **Goldfarb, A.H., Bruno, J.F. &
Buckenmeyer, P.J.**   (1986)
Intensity and duration effects of exercise
on heart cAMP, phosphorylase, and
glycogen
J Appl Physiol **60**, 1268-1273
Acute exercise, Animal

210/35   **Granger, C.B., Karimeddini, M.K.,
Smith, V.E., Shapiro, H.R., Katz, A.M.,
& Riba, A.L.**   (1985)
Rapid ventricular filling in left
ventricular hypertrophy: I. Physiologic
hypertrophy
J Am Coll Cardiol **5**, 862-868
*Adult, AEROBIC CAPACITY, BLOOD
PRESSURE, Cardiac output,
Comparative, HAZARDS-CVS,
Hypertrophy, Male, Running,*

210/36   **Hagberg, J.H., Allen, W.K., Seals,
D.R., Hurley, B.F., Ehsani, A.A. &
Holloszy, J.D.**   (1985)
A haemodynamic comparison of young
and older endurance athletes during
exercise.
J Appl Physiol **58**, 2041-2046
*Adult, AEROBIC CAPACITY, Athlete,
BLOOD PRESSURE, Body composition,
Cardiac output, Comparative, Heart rate,*

210/37 **Häggendal, J., Hartley, L.H. & Saltin, B.** (1970)
Arterial noradrenaline concentration during exercise in relation to the relative work levels
Scand J clin Lab Invest **26**, 337-342
Acute exercise, Adult, AEROBIC CAPACITY, Autonomic nervous system, Endocrine, Male

210/38 **Hickson, R.C., Foster, D., Pollock, M.L., Galassi, T. & Rich, S.** (1985)
Reduced training intensities and loss of aerobic power endurance, and cardiac growth
J Appl Physiol **58**, 492-499
Adult, AEROBIC CAPACITY, Exercise programme, Hypertrophy, Intervention

210/39 **Hickson, R.C., Galassi, T.M. & Dougherty, K.A.** (1983)
Repeated development and regression of exercise-induced cardiac hypertrophy in rats
J Appl Physiol **54**, 794-797
Animal, Exercise programme, Hypertrophy, Inactivity, Intervention, Swimming

210/40 **Hollmann, W., Rost, R., De Meirleir, K., Liesen, H., Heck, H. & Mader, A.** (1986)
Cardiovascular effects of extreme physical training
Acta Med Scand (Suppl 711) **220**, 193-203
Athlete, Autonomic nervous system, Hypertrophy, Review,

210/41 **Huston, T.P., Puffer, J.C. & Rodney, W.M.** (1985)
The athletic heart syndrome
N Engl J Med **313**, 24-32
Adult, Arrhythmia, Athlete, Cardiac output, HAZARDS-CVS, Hypertrophy, Review

210/42 **Ikäheimo, M.J., Palatsi, I.J. & Takkunen, J.T.** (1979)
Noninvasive evaluation of the athletic heart: Sprinters versus endurance runners
Am J Cardiol **44**, 24-30
Adult, Athlete, Comparative, HAZARDS-CVS, Hypertrophy, Male, Leisure activity, Running

210/43 **Kenny, W.L.** (1985)
Parasympathetic control of resting heart rate: relationship to aerobic power
Med Sci Sports Exerc **17**, 451-455
Acute exercise, Adult, Arrhythmia, Autonomic nervous system, BLOOD PRESSURE, Cardiac output, Heart rate,

210/44 **Keul, J., Dickhuth, H.-H., Simon, G. & Lehmann, M.** (1981)
Effect of static and dynamic exercise on heart volume, contractility, and left ventricular dimensions
Circulation Res (Suppl) **48**, I-162-I-170
Adult, Athlete, Autonomic nervous system, BLOOD PRESSURE, Cardiac output, Comparative, Cycling, Endocrine, HAZARDS-CVS, Hypertrophy, Leisure activity, Male, MUSCLE STRENGTH, Myocardial contractility,

210/45 **Keul, J., Lehmann, M. & Staiger, J.** (1982)
The Athlete's heart – haemodynamics and structure
Int J Sports Med **3**, 33-43
HAZARDS-CVS, Hypertrophy, Review

210/46 **Kilbom, Å & Persson, J.** (1981)
Cardiovascular response to combine dynamic and static exercise
Circulation Res (Suppl) **48**, I-93-I-97
Acute exercise, Adult, AEROBIC CAPACITY, Autonomic nervous system, BLOOD PRESSURE, Comparative, Heart rate

210/47   Kosunen, K., Pakarinen, A., Kuoppasalmi, K., Näveri, H., Rehunen, S., Standerskjöld-Nordenstam, C.G., Harkönen, M. & Adlercreutz, H.   (1980) Cardiovascular function and the renin-angiotensin-aldosterone system in long-distance runners during various training periods
Scand J clin Lab Invest **40**, 429-435
Adult, Athlete, Autonomic nervous system, BLOOD PRESSURE, Endocrine, Heart rate, Intervention, Leisure activity, Running

210/48   Laird, W.P., Fixler, D.E. & Huffines, F.D.   (1979) Cardiovascular response to isometric exercise in normal adolescents
Circulation **59**, 651-654
Acute exercise, BLOOD PRESSURE, Children, Heart rate, MUSCLE STRENGTH, Stroke volume

210/49   Lakatta, E.G. & Spurgeon, H.A.   (1987) Effect of exercise on cardiac muscle performance in aged rats
Fed Proc **46**, 1844-1849
Animal, Elderly, Review

210/50   Landry, F.C., Bouchard, C. & Dumesnil, J.   (1985) Cardiac dimension changes with endurance training. Indications of a genotype dependency
J Am Med Ass **254**, 77-80
Adult, AEROBIC CAPACITY, Exercise programme, Hypertrophy, Intervention

210/51   Lengyel, M. & Gyarfas, I.   (1979) The importance of echocardiography in the assessment of left ventricular hypertrophy in trained and untrained school children
Acta Cardiol **34**, 63-69
Children, Comparative, HAZARDS-CVS, Hypertrophy

210/52   Li, Y.X., Mendelowitz, T.L.D., Grossman, W. & Wei, J.Y.   (1986) Age-related differences in effect of exercise training on cardiac muscle function in rats
Am J Physiol **251**, H12-H18
Animal, Elderly, Exercise programme, Intervention, Myocardial contractility

210/53   Liang, C-S., Tuttle, R.R., Hood, W.B., & Gavras, H.   (1979) Conditioning Effects of Chronic Infusions of Dobutamine
J Clin Invest **64**, 613-619
Animal, Autonomic nervous system, Blood pressure, Cardiac output, Endocrine, Exercise programme, Heart rate, Intervention

210/54   Lock, J.E., Einzig, S. & Moller, J.H.   (1978) Hemodynamic responses to exercise in normal children
Am J Cardiol **41**, 1278-1284
Acute exercise, Cardiac Output, Children, Stroke Volume

210/55   Longhurst, J.C., Kelly, A.R., Gonyea, W.J. & Mitchell, J.H.   (1981) Chronic training with static and dynamic exercise: cardiovascular adaptation, and response to exercise
Circulation Res (Suppl) **48**, I-171-I-178
Adult, AEROBIC CAPACITY, Athlete, BLOOD PRESSURE, Cardiac output, Comparative, Hypertrophy, Male, MUSCLE STRENGTH, Running, Vigorous

210/56   Lusiani, L., Ronsisvalle, G., Bonanome, A., Visona, A., Castellani, V., Macchia, C. & Pagnan, A.   (1986) Echocardiographic evaluation of the dimensions and systolic properties of the left ventricles in freshman athletes during physical training
Eur Heart J **7**, 196-203
Adult, Athlete, BLOOD PRESSURE, Comparative, Cycling, Hypertrophy, Intervention, Male, MUSCLE STRENGTH, Stroke volume

210/57   Maciel, B.C., Gallo, Jr, L., Neto, J.A.M., Filho, E.C.L. & Martins, L.E.B.   (1986)
Autonomic nervous control of the heart rate during dynamic exercise in normal man
Clin Sci **71**, 457-460
Acute exercise, Adult, Autonomic nervous system, Heart rate, Male

210/58   Maciel, B.C., Gallo, Jr, L., Neto, J.A.M., Filho, E.C.L. & Martins, L.E.B.   (1987)
Autonomic nervous control of the heart rate during isometric exercise in normal man
Pflugers Arch **408**, 173-177
Acute exercise, Adult, Autonomic nervous system, Heart rate, Male, MUSCLE STRENGTH

210/59   Magder, S.A., Daughters, G.T., Hung, J., Adlerman, E.L. & Ingels, N.B.   (1987)
Adaptation of human left ventricular volumes to the onset of supine exercise
Eur J Appl Physiol **56**, 467-473
Acute exercise, Adult, Cardiac output, Male, Stroke volume

210/60   Martin, W.H. 3d, Montgomery, J., Snell, P.G., Corbett, J.R., Sokolov, J.J., Buckey, J.C., Maloney, D.A. & Blomqvist, C.G.   (1987)
Cardiovascular adaptations to intense swim training in sedentary middle-aged men and women
Circulation **75**, 323-330
Adult, AEROBIC CAPACITY, BLOOD PRESSURE, Cardiac output, Exercise programme, Intervention, MUSCLE METABOLISM, Stroke volume, Swimming, Vigorous

210/61   Moore, R.L., Riedy, M. & Gollnick, P.D.   (1982)
Effect of training on β-adrenergic receptor number in rat heart
J Appl Physiol **52**, 1133-1137
Animal, Autonomic nervous system, Endocrine, Exercise programme, Heart rate, Intervention, MUSCLE METABOLISM

210/62   Morganroth, J., Maron, B.J., Henry, W.L. & Epstein, S.E.   (1975)
Comparative left ventricular dimensions in trained athletes
Ann Intern Med **82**, 521-524
Adult, Athlete, Comparative, Hypertrophy, Leisure activity, Male, MUSCLE STRENGTH, Running, Swimming, Vigorous

210/63   Murayama, M. & Kuroda, Y.   (1980)
Cardiovascular future of athletes. In: Sports Cardiology International conference (Eds.) Lubich, T. & Venerando, A.
Aulo Gaggi, Bologna
Athlete, GENERAL HEALTH, MUSCLE STRENGTH, Review

210/64   Nandi, P.S. & Spodick, D.H.   (1977)
Recovery from exercise at varying work loads. Time course of responses of heart rate and systolic intervals
Br Heart J **39**, 958-966.
Acute exercise, Adult, Heart rate, Male, Stroke volume

210/65   Niemelä, K.O., Palatsi, I.J., Ikäheimo, M.J., Takkunen, J.T. & Vuori, J.J.   (1984)
Evidence of impaired left ventricular performance after an uninterupted competetive 24 hour run
Circulation **70**, 350-356
Acute exercise, Adult, BLOOD PRESSURE, HAZARDS-CVS, Hypertrophy, Male, Marathon, Myocardial contractility, Running, Vigorous

210/66 Nishimura, T., Yamada, Y. &
Kawai, C. (1980)
Echocardiographic evaluation of long-
term effects of exercise on left ventricular
hypertrophy and function in professional
bicyclists
Circulation **61**, 832-840
Adult, Athlete, Comparative, Cycling,
HAZARDS-CVS, Hypertrophy, Male,
Myocardial contractility, Vigorous

210/67 Oakley, D. (1984)
Cardiac hypertrophy in athletes
Br Heart J **52**, 121-123
HAZARDS-CVS, Hypertrophy, Review

210/68 Ohman, M. & Kelly, J.G. (1986)
Beta-adrenoceptor changes in exercise
and physical training. In: Sports
Cardiology. Exercise in health and
cardiovascular disease (Eds.) Fagard,
R.H. & Bekaert, I.E.
136-141
Autonomic nervous system, Endocrine,
Review

210/69 Painter, P.C., Howley, E.T. & Liles,
J.N. (1982)
Change in plasma cAMP and
catecholamines in men subjected to the
same relative amount of physical work
stress
Aviat Space Environ Med **53**, 683-686
Acute exercise, Adult, AEROBIC
CAPACITY, Autonomic nervous system,
Endocrine, Male, Vigorous

210/70 Paulsen, W., Boughner, D.R., Ko,
P., Cunningham, D.A. & Persaud,
J.A. (1981)
Left ventricular function in marathon
runners: echocardiographic assessment
J Appl Physiol **51**, 881- 886
Acute exercise, Adult, AEROBIC
CAPACITY, Athlete, BLOOD
PRESSURE, Cardiac output,
Comparative, Heart rate, Leisure activity,
Male, Running, Marathon, Myocardial
contractility, Vigorous

210/71 Pearson, A.C., Schiff, M., Mrosek,
D., Labovitz, A.J. & Williams,
G.A. (1986)
Left ventricular diastolic function in
weight lifters
Am J Cardiol **58**, 1254-1259
Adult, Comparative, HAZARDS-CVS,
Hypertrophy, Male, MUSCLE
STRENGTH

210/72 Péronnet, F., Cléroux, J., Perrault,
H., Cousineau, D., De Champlain, J. &
Nadeau, R. (1981)
Plasma norepinephrine response to
exercise before and after training in
humans
J Appl Physiol **51**, 812-815
Acute exercise, Adult, AEROBIC
CAPACITY, Autonomic nervous system,
Blood pressure, Cycling, Endocrine,
Exercise programme, Intervention, Male,
Vigorous

210/73 Peronnet, F., Ferguson, R.J.,
Perrault, H., Ricci, G. & Lajoie,
D. (1981)
Echocardiography and the athletes heart
Phys Sports Med **9**, 102-112
Review

210/74 Peronnet, F., Nadeau, R., De
Champlain, J., Magrassi, P. & Chatrand,
C. (1981)
Exercise plasma catecholamines in dogs:
role of adrenals and cardiac nerve
endings
Am J Physiol **241**, H243-H247
Acute exercise, Animal, Autonomic
nervous system, Endocrine

210/75 Péronnet, F., Perrault, H., Cléroux,
J., Cousineau, D., Nadeau, R., Pham-
Huy, G., Tremblay, G. & Le Beau,
R. (1980)
Electro- and echocardiographic study of
the left ventricle in man after training
Eur J Appl Physiol **45**, 125-130
Adult, AEROBIC CAPACITY, Exercise
programme, Hypertrophy, Intervention,
Male, Vigorous

210/76   **Perrault, H., Lajoie, D., Peronnet, F., Nadeau, R, Tremblay, G. & Lebeau, R.** (1982)
Left ventricular dimensions following training in young and middle-aged men
Int J Sports Med **3**, 141-144
Adult, Exercise programme, HAZARDS-CVS, Hypertrophy, Intervention, Male

210/77   **Perski, A., Tzankoff, S.P. & Engel, B.T.** (1985)
Central control of cardiovascular adjustments to exercise
J Appl Physiol **58**, 431-435
Acute exercise, Adult, Autonomic Nervous System, Endocrine, Heart rate, Intervention, Male

210/78   **Plotnick, G.D., Becker, L.C., Fisher, M.L., Gerstenblith, G., Renlund, D.G., Fleg, J.L., Weisfeldt, M.L. & Lakatta, E.G.** (1986)
Use of the Frank-Starling mechanism during submaximal versus maximal upright exercise
Am J Physiol **251**, H1101-H1105
Acute exercise, Adult, Autonomic Nervous System, Cardiac output, Comparative, Male, Stroke Volume

210/79   **Rämö, P., Kettunene, R. & Hirvonen, L.** (1987)
Hemodynamic effects of endurance training on canine left ventricle
Am J Physiol **252**, H7-13
Animal, Exercise programme, Heart rate, Intervention, Myocardial contractility

210/80   **Raskoff, W.J., Goldman, S. & Cohn, K.** (1976)
The 'Athletic Heart'
prevalance and physiological significance of left ventricular enlargement in distance runners
J Am Med Ass **236**, 158-162
Adult, Comparative, HAZARDS-CVS, Hypertrophy, Leisure activity, Male, Marathon, Vigorous

210/81   **Renlund, D.G., Lakatta, E.G., Fleg, J.L., Becker, L.C., Clulow, J.F., Weisfeldt, M.L. & Gerstenblith, G.** (1987)
Prolonged decrease in cardiac volumes after maximal upright bicycle exercise
J Appl Physiol **63**, 1947-1955
Acute exercise, Adult, BLOOD PRESSURE, Cardiac output, Vigorous

210/82   **Rerych, S.L., Scholz, P.M., Sabiston, D.C. & Jones, R.H.** (1980)
Effects of exercise training on left ventricular function in normal subjects: A longitudinal study by radionuclide angiography
Am J Cardiol **45**, 244-252
Adult, Cardiac output, Hypertrophy, Intervention, Swimming, Vigorous

210/83   **Rockstein, M., Chesky, J.A. & Lopez, T.** (1981)
Effects of exercise on the biochemical aging of mammalian myocardium. I. Actomyosin ATPase 1
J Gerontol **36**, 294-297
Animal, Elderly, Exercise programme, Hypertrophy,Intervention, Myocardial contractility

210/84   **Rodeheffer, R.J., Gerstenblith, G., Becker, L.C., Fleg, J.L., Weisfeldt, M.L. & Lakatta, E.G.** (1984)
Exercise cardiac output is maintained with advancing age in healthy human subjects: cardiac dilatation and increased stroke volume compensate for a diminished heart rate
Circulation **69**, 203-213
Acute exercise, Adult, BLOOD PRESSURE, Cardiac output, Comparative, Elderly, Female, Heart rate, Male, Stroke volume

210/85   **Rubal, B.J., Al-Muhailani, A.-R. & Rosentswieg, J.**   (1987)
Effects of physical conditioning on the heart size and wall thickness of college women
Med Sci Sports Exerc **19**, 423-429
Adult, AEROBIC CAPACITY, Athlete, Comparative, Exercise programme, Female, Hypertrophy, Intervention, Leisure activity, Male, Stroke volume, Vigorous

210/86   **Sable, D.L., Brammell, H.L., Sheehan, M.W., Nies, A.S., Gerber, J. & Horwitz, L.D.**   (1982)
Attenuation of exercise conditioning by beta-adrenergic blockade
Circulation **65**, 679-684
Adult, AEROBIC CAPACITY, ANAEROBIC CAPACITY, Autonomic nervous system, BLOOD PRESSURE, Exercise programme, Intervention, Male

210/87   **Savic, S. Adamovic, K. & Dimitrijevic, B.**   (1973)
Relationship between heart volume and pulse rate in sportsmen and nonsportsmen
Br J Sports Med **7**, 205-208
Adult, Athlete, Comparative, Hypertrophy, Male

210/88   **Schaible, T.F., Malhotra, A., Ciambrone, G.J., & Scheuer, J.**   (1986)
Chronic swimming reverses cardiac dysfunction and myosin abnormalities in hypertensive rats
J Appl Physiol **60**, 1435-1441
Animal, BLOOD PRESSURE, Cardiac output, Exercise programme, Hypertrophy, Intervention, Swimming

210/89   **Schaible, T.F. & Scheuer, J.**   (1985)
Cardiac adaptations to chronic exercise
Prog Cardiovasc Dis **27**, 297-324
Animal, Athlete, Hypertrophy, MUSCLE STRENGTH, Review, Vigorous

210/90   **Scheuer, J. & Tipton, C.M.**   (1977)
Cardiovascular adaptations to physical training
Ann Rev Physiol **39**, 221-51
Review

210/91   **Schmid, P. & Keul, J.**   (1984)
Age- and exercise-related sympathetic activity in untrained volunteers, trained athletes and patients with impaired left-ventricular contractility
Eur Heart J (Suppl E) **5**, 1-7
Adult, Athlete, Autonomic nervous system, Comparative, Elderly, Endocrine, MUSCLE STRENGTH, Myocardial contractility, Leisure activity, SECONDARY PREVENTION,

210/92   **Schocken, D.D., Blumenthal, J.A., Port, S., Hindle, P. & Coleman, R.**   (1983)
Physical conditioning and left ventricular performance in the elderly: Assessment by radionuclinde angiocardiography
Am J Cardiol **52**, 359-364
Acute exercise, BLOOD PRESSURE, Cardiac output, Elderly, Exercise programme, Heart rate, Intervention, Myocardial contractility

210/93   **Seals, D.R., Hurley, B.F., Hagberg, J.M., Schultz, J., Linder, B.J., Natter, L. & Ehsani, A.A.**   (1985)
Effects of training on systolic time intervals at rest and during isometric exercise in men and women 61 to 64 years
Am J Cardiol **55**, 797-800
Adult, AEROBIC CAPACITY, BLOOD PRESSURE, Exercise programme, Intervention, MUSCLE STRENGTH, Myocardial contractility

210/94   Seals, D.R., Hagberg, J.M., Hurley, B.F., Ehsani, A.A. & Holloszy, J.O.   (1984)
Endurance training in older men and women I. Cardiovascular responses to exercise
J Appl Physiol **57**, 1024-1029
AEROBIC CAPACITY, BLOOD PRESSURE, Cardiac output, Customary activity, Elderly, Exercise programme, Intervention, Stroke volume, Vigorous

210/95   Shapiro, L.M.   (1984)
Physiological left ventricular hypertrophy
Br Heart J **52**, 130-135
Adult, Athlete, Comparative, Hypertrophy, Leisure activity, MUSCLE STRENGTH, Vigorous

210/96   Shepherd, J.T.   (1987)
Circulatory response to exercise in health
Circulation (Suppl 6 Pt.2) **76**, VI 3-VI 10
Review

210/97   Sheps, D.S., Gottlieb, S., Ernst, J.C., Kallos, N., Briese, F.W., Garcia, E., Myerburg, R.J. & Castellanos, A.   (1979)
Effect of a physical conditioning program on left ventricular ejection fractions determined serially by a non-invasive technique
Cardiology **64**, 256-264
Adult, BLOOD PRESSURE, Exercise programme, Hypertrophy, Intervention

210/98   Sigvardsson, K., Svanfeldt, E. & Kilbom, Å.   (1977)
Role of the adrenergic nervous system in development of training-induced bradycardia
Acta Physiol Scand **101**, 481-488
Animal, Autonomic nervous system, Exercise programme, Heart rate, Intervention

210/99   Spurgeon, H.A., Steinbach, M.F., & Lakatta, E.G.   (1983)
Chronic exercise prevents characteristic age-related changes in rat cardiac contraction
Am J Physiol **244**, H513-518
Animal, Comparative, Elderly, Exercise programme, Intervention, Myocardial contractility

210/100   Steinhagen-Thiessen, E. & Reznick, A.Z.   (1987)
Effect of short- and long-term endurance training on creatinine phosphokinase activity in skeletal and cardiac muscles of CW-1 and C57BL mice
Gerontology **33**, 14-18
Animal, Elderly, Exercise programme, Intervention, MUSCLE METABOLISM

210/101   Steinhagen-Thiessen, E., Reznick, A.Z. & Ringe, J.-D.   (1984)
Age dependent variations in cardiac and skeletal muscle during short and long term treadmill-running of mice
Eur Heart J (Suppl E) **5**, 27-30
Animal, Elderly, Exercise programme, Intervention, MUSCLE METABOLISM, MUSCLE STRENGTH

210/102   Stromme, S.B. & Ingjer, F.   (1982)
The effect of regular physical training on the cardiovascular system
Scand J Soc Med (Suppl) **29**, 37-46
Review

210/103   Sugishita, Y., Koseki, S., Matsuda, M., Yamaguchi, T. & Ito, I.   (1983)
Myocardial mechanics of athletic hearts in comparision with diseased hearts
Am Heart J **105**, 273-80
Adult, Athlete, Comparative HAZARDS-CVS, Hypertrophy, Male, Running

210/104   Taylor A.W., Schoeman J.H., Esfandiary A.R. & Russell, J.C.   (1971)
Effect of exercise on urinary catecholamine excretion in active and sedentary subjects
Rev Can Biol **30,** 97-105
Adult, AEROBIC CAPACITY, Autonomic nervous system, Endocrine, exercise programme, Intervention, Male

210/105   Underwood, R.H. & Schwade, J.L.   (1977)
Non-invasive analysis of cardiac function of elite distance runners; Echo-cardiography, vectorcardiography and cardiac intervals
Ann NY Acad Sci **301,** 297-309
Athlete, Review

210/106   Washburn, R.A., Savage, D.D., Dearwater, S.R., LaPorte, R.E., Anderson, S.J., Brenes, G., Adams, L.L., Lee, H.K.M., Holland, J., Cowan, M. & Parks, E.   (1986)
Echocardiographic left ventricular mass and physical activity: Quantification of the relation in spinal cord injured and apparently healthy active young men
Am J Cardiol **58,** 1248-1253
Adult, Comparative, Customary activity, Handicap, Hypertrophy, Inactivity, Leisure activity, Male

210/107   White, F.C., Mckirnan, M.D., Breisch, E.A., Guth, B.D., Liu, Y-M. & Bloor, C.M.   (1987)
Adaptation of the left ventricle to exercise-induced hypertrophy
J Appl Physiol **62,** 1097-1110
AEROBIC CAPACITY, Animal, Exercise programme, Hypertrophy, Intervention, Stroke volume

210/108   Wierling, W., Borghols, E.A.M., Hollander, A.P., Danner, S.A. & Dunning, A.J.   (1981)
Echocardiographic dimensions and maximum oxygen uptake in oarsmen during training
Br Heart J **46,** 190-5
Adult, AEROBIC CAPACITY, Athlete, BLOOD PRESSURE, HAZARDS-CVS, Hypertrophy, Intervention, Leisure activity,

210/109   Wieshammer, S., Delagardelle, C., Sigel, H.A., Henze, E., Kress, P., Bitter, F., Adam, W.E. & Stauch, M.   (1986)
Haemodynamic response to exercise in patients with chest pain and normal coronary angiograms
Eur Heart J **7,** 654-661
Acute exercise, Adult, Angina, BLOOD PRESSURE, HEART FUNCTION TEST, Heart rate, Myocardial contractility

210/110   Wolfe, L.A. & Cunningham, D.A.   (1982)
Effects of chronic exercise on cardiac output and its determinants
Can J Physiol Pharmacol **60,** 1089-1097
Adult, AEROBIC CAPACITY, BLOOD PRESSURE, Body composition, Cardiac output, Exercise programme, Intervention, Male, Running, Stroke volume, Weight

210/111   Wolfe, L.A., Cunningham, D.A. & Boughner, D.R.   (1986)
Physical conditioning effects on cardiac dimensions: A review of echocardiographic studies
Can J Appl Spt Sci **11,** 66-79
Adult, Athlete, Children, Hypertrophy, Review

210/112   **Wolfe, L.A., Cunningham, D.A., Davis, G.M. & Rosenfeld, H.**   (1978)
Relationship between maximal oxygen uptake and left ventricular function in exercise
J Appl Physiol **44**, 44-49.
Acute exercise, Adult, AEROBIC CAPACITY, Cardiac output, Comparative, Male, Myocardial contractility

210/113   **Wolfe, L.A., Cunningham, D.A., Rechnitzer, P.A. & Nichol P.M.**   (1979)
Effects of endurance training on left ventricular dimensions in healthy men
J Appl Physiol **47**, 207-212
Adult, AEROBIC CAPACITY, Body composition, Exercise programme, Hypertrophy, Intervention, Male, Myocardial contractility, Running, Stroke volume, Vigorous

210/114   **Wolfel, E.E., Hiatt, W.R., Brammell, H.L., Carry, M.R., Ringel, S.P., Travis, V. & Horwitz, L.D.**   (1986)
Effects of selective and nonselective β-adrenergic blockade on mechanisms of exercise conditioning
Circulation **74**, 664-674
Adult, AEROBIC CAPACITY, Autonomic nervous system, BLOOD PRESSURE, Comparative, Endocrine, Exercise programme, Heart rate, Intervention, Male, MUSCLE METABOLISM, Vigorous

210/115   **Wollen, W., Bachl, N. & Prokop, L.**   (1984)
Endurance capacity of trained older aged athletes
Eur Heart J (Suppl E) **5**, 21-25
AEROBIC CAPACITY, ANAEROBIC CAPACITY, Comparative, Elderly, Heart rate, Hypertrophy

KEYWORDS are listed in the appendix in addition the following specific keywords have been used in this section:

- Autonomic nervous system
- Hypertension
- Normotension
- Peripheral resistance
- Plasma volume

Summary of evidence: exercise ameliorates, cures and prevents mild hypertension

THE PROBLEM

Does exercise reduce blood pressure? The question is important since mild to moderate hypertension is prevalent. It is associated with complications such as heart attack and stroke, and usually needs lifelong drug therapy.

SCOPE

This section contains references dealing primarily with changes produced by exercise in arterial blood pressure in both normal subjects and those with hypertension. References range from acute studies dealing with possible mechanisms (some animal studies are included) to intervention and epidemiological studies. There are references on the intensity and amount of exercise needed to reduce blood pressure, studies of all age groups and of both the sedentary and the athletic. There are more studies on men than women.

METHODOLOGICAL DIFFICULTIES

Blood pressure is an unstable variable and therefore notoriously difficult to assess; many studies were rejected because of an inadequate run-in period for baseline data, lack of a properly matched control group or confounding factors such as weight changes or drug treatment.

EVIDENCE

It is clear from the well-controlled studies that modest reductions of about 13/7 mm Hg in resting arterial blood pressure can be obtained with exercise by patients with mild or labile primary hypertension. This is sufficient for a reduction in drug therapy. Severely hypertensive women and adolescents have shown improvements. It is probable that exercise can inhibit the age-dependent rise in resting blood pressure common in Western society. These improvements are associated with a lower systolic blood pressure at a given level of work due probably to reduced adrenalin release (cf changes in heart rate, section 210). Maximal systolic blood pressure at maximal exercise remains unchanged. Improvements in blood pressure control are associated with reduced mortality and morbidity in coronary heart disease and stroke (see section 231.1).

220/1 **Adrangna, N.C., Chang, J.L., Morey, M.C., & Williams, R.S.** (1985)
Effect of exercise on cation transport in human red cells
Hypertension **7**, 132-139
Adult, Cycling, Intervention, Leisure activity, LIPIDS, Male, Plasma Volume, Running, Vigorous

220/2 **Amery, A., Julius, S., Whitlock, L.S., & Conway, J.** (1967)
Influence of hypertension on the hemodynamic response to exercise
Circulation **36**, 231-237
Acute exercise, Adult, CARDIAC PERFORMANCE, Comparative, Hypertension, Normotension, Peripheral resistance

220/3 **Andersson, G. & Malmgren, S.** (1986)
Risk factors and reported sick leave among employees of Saab-Scania, Linkoping, Sweden, between the ages of 50 and 59
Scand J Soc Med **14**, 25-30
Adult, Cohort, EPIDEMIOLOGY-CHD, Leisure activity, Occupational activity, Weight

220/4 **Attina, D.A., Giuliano, G., Arcangeli, G., Musante, R. & Cupelli, V.** (1986)
Effects of one year of physical training on borderline hypertension: An evaluation by bicycle ergometer exercise testing
J Cardiovasc Pharm (Suppl 5) **8**, S145-S147
Acute exercise, Adult, CARDIAC PERFORMANCE, Comparative, Hypertension, Intervention, Leisure activity, Male

220/5 **Barnard, R.J. & Anthony, D.F.** (1980)
Effect of health maintenance programs on Los Angeles city firefighters
J Occupational Med **22**, 667-669
Adult, Cohort, Exercise programme, LIPIDS, Male, Weight

220/6 **Bedford, T.G. & Tipton, C.M.** (1987)
Exercise training and the arterial baroreflex
J Appl Physiol **63**, 1926-1932
AEROBIC CAPACITY, Animal, Autonomic nervous system, Intervention

220/7 **Bennett, T., Wilcox, R.G. & Macdonald, I.A.** (1984)
Post exercise reduction of blood pressure in hypertensive men is not due to acute impairment of baroreflex function
Clin Sci **67**, 97-103
Acute exercise, Adult, Comparative, Hypertension, Male, Normotension

220/8 **Berglund, G. & Wilhelmsen, L.** (1975)
Factors related to blood pressure in a general population sample of Swedish men
Acta Med Scand **198**, 291-298
Adult, Leisure activity, Male, Occupational activity, Weight

220/9 **Björntorp, P.** (1982)
Hypertension and exercise
Hypertension (Suppl 3) **4**, III-56-59
Review

220/10 **Blair, S.N., Goodyear, N.N., Gibbons, L.W. & Cooper, K.H.** (1984)
Physical fitness and incidence of hypertension in healthy normotensive men and women
J Am Med Ass **252**, 487-490
Adult, Cohort, EPIDEMIOLOGY-CHD, Hypertension, Weight

220/11 **Boyer, J.L. & Kasch, F.W.** (1970)
Exercise therapy in hypertensive men
J Am Med Ass **211**, 1668-1671
Adult, Exercise programme, Hypertension, Intervention, Male, Normotension, Running, Weight

220/12 **Cade, R., Mars, D., Wagemaker, H., Zauner, C., Packer, D., Privette, M., Cade, M., Peterson, J. & Hood-Lewis, D.** (1984)
Effect of aerobic exercise training on patients with systemic arterial hypertension
Am J Med **77**, 785-790
Adult, Hypertension, Intervention, Leisure activity, Male, Running, Weight

220/13 **Cleland, J.G.F., Dargie, H.J., Robertson, J.I.S., Ball, S.G. & Hodsman, G.F.** (1984)
Renin and angiotensin responses to posture and exercise in elderly patients with heart failure.
Eur Heart J (Suppl E) **5**, 9-11
Acute exercise, Adult, Autonomic nervous system, Elderly, SECONDARY PREVENTION

220/14   Cléroux, J., Peronnet, F. & De Champlain, J.   (1987)
The effects of exercise training on plasma catecholamines and blood pressure in labile hypertensive subjects
Eur J Appl Physiol **56**, 550-554
Adult, AEROBIC CAPACITY, Autonomic nervous system, Exercise programme, Hypertension, Intervention, Weight

220/15   Convertino, V.A., Brock, P.J., Keil, L.C., Bernauer, E.M. & Greenleaf, J.E.   (1980)
Exercise training-induced hypervolemia: role of plasma albumin, renin, and vasopressin
J Appl Physiol **48**, 665-669
Adult, AEROBIC CAPACITY, Body composition, Endocrine, Exercise Programme, Intervention, Male

220/16   Convertino, V.A., Keil, L.C., Bernauer, E.M. & Greenleaf, J.E.   (1981)
Plasma volume, osmolality, vasopressin, and renin activity during graded exercise in man
J Appl Physiol **50**, 123-128
Adult, Acute exercise, AEROBIC CAPACITY, Endocrine, Male

220/17   de Plaen, J.F. & Detry, J.M.   (1980)
Hemodynamic effects of physical training in established arterial hypertension
Acta Cardiol **3**, 179-188
Adult, AEROBIC CAPACITY, CARDIAC PERFORMANCE, Cycling, Exercise programme, Hypertension, Intervention, Peripheral resistance

220/18   Duncan, J.J., Farr, J.E., Upton, S.J., Hagan, R.D., Oglesby, M.E., & Blair, S.N.   (1985)
The effects of aerobic exercise on plasma catecholamines and blood pressure in patients with mild essential hypertension
J Am Med Ass **254**, 2609-2613
Adult, AEROBIC CAPACITY, Autonomic nervous system, Hypertension, Intervention, Leisure activity, Male, Running, Vigorous, Weight

220/19   Eckberg, D.L. & Wallin, B.G.   (1987)
Isometric exercise modifies autonomic baroreflex responses in humans
J Appl Physiol **63**, 2325-2330
Adult, Autonomic Nervous System, MUSCLE STRENGTH

220/20   Ewing, D.J., Irving, J.B., Kerr, F. & Kirby, B.J.   (1973)
Static exercise in untreated systemic hypertension
Br Heart J **35**, 413-421
Acute exercise, Adult, CARDIAC PERFORMANCE, Hypertension, MUSCLE STRENGTH

220/21   Fagard, R., Staessen, J., Vanhees, L. & Amery, A.   (1986)
Sports and hypertension. In: Sports Cardiology: Exercise in health and cardiovascular disease (Eds) Fagard, R.H. & Bekaert, I.E.
Martinus Nijhoff 195-204
Review

220/22   **Findlay, I.N., Taylor, R.S., Dargie, H.J., Grant, S., Pettigrew, A.R., Wilson, J.T., Aitchison, T., Cleland, J.G., Elliot, A.T., Fisher, B.M., Gillen, G., Manzie, A., Rumley, A.G. & Durnin, J.V.G.A.**   (1987)
Cardiovascular effect of training for a marathon run in unfit middle aged men
Br Med J **295**, 521-524
Adult, AEROBIC CAPACITY, BLOOD PRESSURE, Body composition, CARDIAC PERFORMANCE, Intervention, Leisure activity, LIPIDS, Male, Marathon, Running

220/23   **Fiocchi, R., Fagard, R., Staessen, J., Vanhees, L. & Amery, A.**   (1985)
Relationship between carotid baroreflex sensitivity, physical fitness and activity in cyclists
J Hypertension (Suppl 3) **3**, S131-S133
Acute exercise, Adult, Cycling, Leisure activity, Male

220/24   **Fitzgerald, W.**   (1981)
Labile hypertension and jogging: new diagnostic tool or spurious discovery?
Br Med J **282**, 542-544
Adult, Hypertension, Intervention, Leisure activity, Male, Running

220/25   **Fixler, D.E., Laird, P., Browne, R., Fitzgerald, V., Wilson, S. & Vance, R.**   (1979)
Response of hypertensive adolescents to dynamic and isometric exercise stress
Pediatrics **64**, 579-583
Acute exercise, CARDIAC PERFORMANCE, Children, Comparative, Hypertension

220/26   **Ghaemmaghami, F., Gauquelin, G., Favier, R., Vincent, M., Sassard, J., Legros, J.J., Allevard, A.-M. & Gharib, G.**   (1986)
Effect of swim training on systolic blood pressure, vasopressin and total neurophysins in the Lyon hypertensive rat
J Hypertens (Suppl) **4**, S475-S478
Animal, Hypertension, Intervention, Swimming

220/27   **Goldberg, A.P., Hagberg, J.M., Delmez, J.A., Florman, R.W. & Harter, H.R.**   (1979)
Effects of exercise training on coronary risk factors in hemodialysis patients
Proc Dialysis Transplant Forum **9**, 39-43
Adult, AEROBIC CAPACITY, CARBOHYDRATE TOLERANCE, Exercise programme, Intervention, Kidney disease, LIPIDS, SECONDARY PREVENTION

220/28   **Gyntelberg, F. & Meyer, J.**   (1974)
Relationship between blood pressure and physical fitness, smoking and alcohol consumption in Copenhagen males aged 40-59
Acta Med Scand **195**, 375-380
Adult, AEROBIC CAPACITY, Male, Weight

220/29   **Hagberg, J.M., Goldring, D., Ehsani, A.A., Heath, G.W., Hernandez, A., Schechtman, K. & Holloszy, J.O.**   (1983)
Effect of exercise training on the blood pressure and hemodynamic features of hypertensive adolescents
Am J Cardiol **52**, 763-768
AEROBIC CAPACITY, CARDIAC PERFORMANCE, Children, Female, Hypertension, Inactivity, Intervention, Leisure activity, Male, Peripheral resistance, Running, Vigorous, Weight,

220/30   Hagberg, J.M., Montain, S.J. &
Martin, W.H. 3rd   (1987)
Blood pressure and hemodynamic
responses after exercise in older
hypertensives
J Appl Physiol **63**, 270-276
***Acute exercise, Adult, AEROBIC
CAPACITY, CARDIAC
PERFORMANCE, Hypertension,
Plasma Volume, Peripheral Resistance***

220/31   Hagberg, J.M. & Seals,
D.R.   (1986)
Exercise training and hypertension
Acta Med Scand (Suppl) **711**, 131-136
Review

220/32   Hales, J.R.S. & Ludbrook,
J,   (1988)
Baroreflex participation in redistribution
of cardiac output at onset of exercise
J Appl Physiol **64**, 627-634
***Acute exercise, Animal, CARDIAC
PERFORMANCE***

220/33   Harrison, M.H., Edwards, R.J. &
Leitch, D.R.   (1975)
Effect of exercise and thermal stress on
plasma volume
J Appl Physiol **39**, 925-931
***Acute exercise, Adult, AEROBIC
CAPACITY, Male***

220/34   Hickey, N., Mulchay, R., Bourke,
G.J., Graham, I. & Wilson-Davies,
K.   (1975)
Study of coronary risk factors related to
physical activity in 15,171 men
Br Med J **3**, 507-509
***Adult, BLOOD PRESSURE,
Comparative, Leisure activity, LIPIDS,
Male, Occupational activity, Vigorous,
Weight***

220/35   Hofman, A., Walter, H.J.,
Connelly, P.A. & Vaughan, R.D.   (1987)
Blood pressure and physical fitness in
children
Hypertension **9**, 188-191
***Children, Female, Hypertension,
Intervention, Leisure activity, Male,
Weight***

220/36   Jennings, G.L.   (1987)
The place of exercise in the long-term
treatment of hypertension
Nephron (Suppl 1) **47**, 30-33
Hypertension, Review

220/37   Jennings, G.L. Nelson, L., Esler,
M.D., Leonard, P. & Korner, P.I.   (1984)
Effects of changes in physical activity on
blood pressure and sympathetic tone
J Hypertension (Suppl 3) **2**, 139-141
***Adult, AEROBIC CAPACITY,
CARDIAC PERFORMANCE, Exercise
programme,Intervention***

220/38   Jennings, G.L., Nelson, L., Nestel,
P., Esler, M., Korner, P.I., Burton, D. &
Bazelmans, J.   (1986)
The effects of changes in physical activity
on major cardiovascular risk factors,
hemodynamics, sympathetic function
and glucose utilization in men: a
controlled study of four levels of activity
Circulation **73**, 30-40
***Adult, AEROBIC CAPACITY,
Autonomic nervous system,
CARBOHYDRATE TOLERANCE,
CARDIAC PERFORMANCE, Exercise
programme, Inactivity, Intervention,
LIPIDS, Peripheral resistance,
PRIMARY PREVENTION***

220/39   Kaplan, N.M.   (1981)
Non-drug treatment of hypertension
Aust N Z J Med (Suppl 1) **11**, 73-75
Review

220/40   Kaufman, F.L., Hughson, R.L. &
Schaman, J.P.   (1987)
Effect of exercise on recovery blood
pressure in normotensive and
hypertensive subjects
Med Sci Sports Exerc **19**, 17-20
***Acute exercise, Adult, Hypertension,
Male, Normotension,***

220/41   Kenney, W.L. & Zambraski,
E.J.   (1984)
Physical activity in human hypertension
Sports Med **1**, 459-473
Review

220/42 **Kiyonaga, A., Arakawa, K., Tanaka, H., & Shindo, M.** (1984)
Blood pressure and hormonal responses to aerobic exercise
Hypertension **7**, 125-131
Acute exercise, Adult, Autonomic nervous system, Exercise programme, Hypertension, Intervention, Weight

220/43 **Korner, P.I.** (1952)
The normal human blood pressure during and after exercise, with some related observations on changes in heart rate and the blood flow in limbs
Aust J Exp Biol Med Sci **30**, 375-384
Acute exercise, Adult

220/44 **Kukkonen, K., Rauramaa, R., Voutilainen, E. & Lansimies, E.** (1982)
Physical training of middle-aged men with borderline hypertension
Ann Clin Res (Suppl 34) **14** , 139-145
Adult, AEROBIC CAPACITY, Body composition, Cycling, Exercise programme, Hypertension, Intervention, Male, Normotension,

220/45 **Kuroda, Y.** (1982)
Sports medical problems on physical activity in middle and old age
J Sports Med Phys Fitness **22**, 1-16
ENERGY BALANCE, HAZARDS-CVS, LIPIDS, Review

220/46 **Leibel, V., Kobrin, I. & Ben-Ishay, D.** (1982)
Exercise testing in assessment of hypertension
Br Med J **285**, 1535-1536
Acute exercise, Adult, Comparative, Hypertension, Normotension

220/47 **Ludbrook, J.** (1983)
Reflex control of blood pressure during exercise
Ann Rev Physiol **45**, 155-168
Review

220/48 **Lund-Johansen, P.** (1982)
Physical activity and hypertension
Scand J Soc Med (Suppl) **29**, 185-194
Review

220/49 **Lund-Johansen, P.** (1987)
Exercise and antihypertensive therapy
Am J Cardiol **59**, 98A-107A
CARDIAC PERFORMANCE, Review

220/50 **Mack, G.W., Shi, X., Nose, H., Tripathi, A. & Nadel, E.R.** (1987)
Diminished baroreflex control of forearm vascular resistance in physically fit humans
J Appl Physiol **63**, 105-110
Adult, AEROBIC CAPACITY, Comparative, Peripheral resistance

220/51 **Martin, J.E., Dubbert, P.M. & Cushman, W.C.** (1985)
Controlled trial of aerobic exercise in hypertension
Circulation (Suppl) **72**, III-13
Adult, Exercise programme, Hypertension, Intervention, Male

220/52 **Nelson, L., Jennings, G.L., Esler, M.D. & Korner, P.I.** (1986)
Effect of changing levels of physical activity on blood pressure and haemodynamics in essential hypertension
Lancet **ii**, 473-476
Adult, AEROBIC CAPACITY, CARDIAC PERFORMANCE, Exercise Programme, Hypertension, Intervention

220/53 **Paffenbarger, R.S. Jr, Wing, A.L., Hyde, R.T. & Jung, D.L.** (1983)
Physical activity and the incidence of hypertension on college alumni
Am J Epidemiol **117**, 245-257
Adult, Cohort, Customary activity, ENERGY BALANCE, EPIDEMIOLOGY-CHD, Hypertension, Leisure activity, Male, Vigorous, Weight

220/54 **Panico, S., Celentano, E., Krogh, V., Jossa, F., Farinaro, E., Trevisan, M. & Mancini, M.** (1987)
Physical activity and its relationship to blood pressure in school children
J Chron Dis **40**, 925-930
Acute exercise, Children, Female, Male, Weight

220/55   **Paulev, P.E., Jordal, R., Kristensen, O. & Ladefoged, J.** (1984)
Therapeutic effect of exercise on hypertension
Eur J Appl Physiol **53**, 180-185
Acute exercise, Adult, Autonomic nervous system, Female, Hypertension, Peripheral resistance

220/56   **Pedersen, E.B., Danielsen, H., Nielsen, A.H., Knudsen, F., Jensen, T., Kornerup, H.J. & Madsen, M.** (1986)
Effect of exercise on plasma concentrations of arginine vasopressin, angiotensin II and aldosterone in hypertensive and normotensive renal transplant recipients
Scand J clin Lab Invest. **46**, 151-157
Adult, Comparative, Hypertension, Kidney disease, Normotension

220/57   **Pelech, A.N., Kartodihardjo, W., Balfe, J.A., Olley, P.M. & Leenen, F.H.H.** (1986)
Exercise in children before and after coartectomy: hemodynamic, echocardiographic and biochemical assessment
Am Heart J **112**, 1263-1270
Acute exercise, Autonomic Nervous System, Children, Endocrine, Hypertension

220/58   **Penny, G., Rust, J.O. & Carlton, J.** (1981)
Effects of a 14-week jogging program on operational blood pressure
J Sports Med Phys Fitness **21**, 395-400
Adult, Exercise programme, Intervention, Male, Normotension, Running,

220/59   **Remington, R.D., Taylor, H.L. & Buskirk, E.R.** (1978)
A method for assessing volunteer bias and its application to a cardiovascular disease prevention program involving physical activity
J Epidemiol Community Health **32**, 250-255
Adult, BLOOD PRESSURE, Exercise programme, Intervention, LIPIDS, Male, Weight

220/60   **Roman, O., Camuzzi, A.L., Villalon, E. & Klenner, C.** (1981)
Physical training program in arterial hypertension; a long-term prospective follow-up
Cardiology **67**, 230-243
Acute exercise, Adult, AEROBIC CAPACITY, Cycling, Exercise programme, Female, Hypertension, Inactivity, Intervention, Running, Vigorous

220/61   **Rowlands, D.B., Stallard, T.J., Littler, W.A. & Isaacs, B.** (1984)
Ambulatory blood pressure and its response to exercise in the elderly
Eur Heart J (Suppl E) **5**, 13-16
Acute exercise, Comparative, Elderly, Hypertension, Normotension

220/62   **Rowlands, D.B., Stallard, T.J., Watson, R.D.S. & Littler, W.A.** (1980)
The influence of physical activity on arterial pressure during ambulatory recordings in man
Clin Sci **58**, 115-117
Adult, Customary activity, Hypertension

220/63   **Saar, E., Chayoth, R. & Meyerstein, N.** (1986)
Physical activity and blood pressure in normotensive young women
Eur J Appl Physiol **55**, 64-67
Adult, AEROBIC CAPACITY, Body composition, Comparative, Female, Normotension, Occupational activity, Weight

220/64   Sankaran, K., Krishnamurti,
B.S.C., Muralidhar, K. & Gupta,
G.D.   (1979)
Exercise study in hypertension
J Assoc Phys Ind **27**, 45-55
***Acute exercise, Adult, CARDIAC
PERFORMANCE, Comparative,
Hypertension, Male***

220/65   Sannerstedt, R., Wasir, H., Henning
R. & Werko, L.   (1973)
Systemic haemodynamics in mild arterial
hypertension before and after physical
training
Clin Sci Mol Med **45**, 145s-149s
***Adult, CARDIAC PERFORMANCE,
Exercise programme, Hypertension,
Intervention, Male***

220/66   Seals, D.R. & Hagberg,
J.M.   (1984)
The effect of exercise training on human
hypertension.
Med Sci Sports Exerc **16**, 207-215
Review

220/67   Shore, P.S., Bartels, R.L. &
Dujardin, J.P.   (1985)
Exercise training and the hemodymanic
profile at rest and during stress in mild
hypertensives
Med Sci Sports Exerc **17**, 264
***Adult, Acute exercise, Comparative,
Hypertension, Intervention, MOOD***

220/68   Siconolfi, S.F., Lasater, T.M.,
McKinlay, S., Boggia, P. & Carleton,
R.A.   (1985)
Physical fitness and blood pressure: The
role of age
Am J Epidemiol **122**, 452-457
***Adult, AEROBIC CAPACITY, Female,
Male***

220/69   Siconolfi, S.F., Snow, R.C.K.,
Lasater, T.M., Duck, E.A. & Carleton,
R.A.   (1985)
Exercise training attenuated the blood
pressure response to mental stress
Med Sci Sports Exerc **17**, 281
***Adult, Exercise Programme,
Hypertension, Intervention, MOOD***

220/70   Smith, M.L., Graitzer, H.M.,
Hudson, D.L. & Raven, P.B.   (1988)
Baroreflex function in endurance- and
static exercise-trained men
J Appl Physiol **64**, 585-591
***Adult, Comparative, Male, MUSCLE
STRENGTH***

220/71   Smith, M.L. & Raven, P.
B.   (1986)
Cardiovascular responses to lower body
negative pressure in endurance and static
exercise-trained men
Med Sci Sports Exerc **18**, 545-550
***Adult, Comparative, Leisure activity,
Male, MUSCLE STRENGTH,
Peripheral resistance, Running***

220/72   Staessen, J., Fiocchi, R., Fagard,
R., Hespel, P. & Amery, A.   (1987)
Progressive attenuation of the carotid
baroreflex control of blood pressure and
heart rate during exercise
Am Heart J **114**, 765-772
***Acute exercise, Adult, Autonomic nervous
system, CARDIAC PERFORMANCE,
Male.***

220/73   Strazzullo, P., Cappuccio, F.P.,
Trevisan, M., De Leo, A., Krogh, V.,
Giorgione, N. & Mancini, M.   (1988)
Leisure time physical activity and blood
pressure in schoolchildren
Am J Epidemiol **127**, 726-733
***Body composition, Children, Female,
Leisure activity, Male***

220/74   Tipton, C.M.   (1984)
Exercise, training and hypertension
Exerc Sports Sci Rev **12**, 245-306
Review

220/75   **Wei, J.Y., Li, Y.X. & Ragland, J.**   (1987)
Effect of exercise training on resting blood pressure and heart rate in adult and aged rats
J Gerontol **42,** 11-16
Animal, Intervention

220/76   **Westheim, A., Simonsen, K., Schamaun, O., Muller, O., Stokke, O. & Teisberg P.**   (1985)
Effect of exercise training in patients with essential hypertension
J Hypertension (Suppl 3) **3,** S479-S481
Adult, Exercise programme, Hypertension, Intervention, LIPIDS

220/77   **Wilcox, R.G., Bennett, T., Brown, A.M. & Macdonald, I.A.**   (1982)
Is exercise good for high blood pressure?
Br Med J **285,** 767-769
Acute exercise, Adult, Comparative, Exercise test, Hypertension, Male, Normotension

220/78   **Williams, M.A., Petratic, M.M. & Baechle, T.R.**   (1987)
Frequency of physical activity, exercise capacity, and athersclerotic heart disease risk factors in male police officers
J Occup Med **29,** 596-600
Adult, Leisure activity, LIPIDS, Male, Occupational activity

231 PRIMARY PREVENTION (REVIEWS)

All the references in this section are general reviews including metanalyses where the author has collated and systematically analysed evidence from many sources. See section 231.1 for the references describing each study and the summary notes pertinent to this section.

Keywords are listed in the appendix.

231/1   (1976)
The report of a joint working party of the Royal College of Physicians of London and the British Cardiac Society: The prevention of Coronary Heart Disease
J Royal Coll Physicians **10**, 213-275
Review

231/2 **Benestad, A.M.** (1982)
Physical activity and cardiovascular disease
Scand J Soc Med (Suppl) **29**, 179-184
Review

231/3 **Boyer, J.L.** (1974)
Coronary heart disease as a pediatric problem
Am J Cardiol **33**, 784-786
Children, Review

231/4 **Goldsmith, R.** (1977)
Report of the joint E.E.C./W.H.O. workshop on physical activity in primary prevention of ischaemic heart disease
Luxembourg
Review

231/5 **Hollmann, W., Rost, R., Liesen, H., Dufaux, B., Heck, H. & Mader, A.** (1981)
Assessment of different forms of physical activity with respect to preventive and rehabilitative cardiology
Int J Sports Med **2**, 67-80
Review

231/6 **Laporte, R.E., Dearwater, S., Cauley, J.A., Slemenda, C. & Cook, T.** (1985)
Physical activity or cardiovascular fitness: which is more important for health?
Phys Sportsmed **13**, 145-50
Children, Hazards, Review

231/7 **Levy, R.I.** (1978)
Progress in prevention of cardiovascular disease
Prev Med **7**, 464-475
Review

231/8 **Lichtenstein, M.J.** (1985)
Jogging in middle age
J Royal Coll Gen Pract **35**, 341-345
Review

231/9 **Morris, J.N., Everitt, M.G. & Semmence, A.M.** (1987)
Exercise and coronary heart disease. In: Exercise Benefits, Limits and Adaptations (Eds.) Macleod, D., Maughan, R., Nimmo, M., Reilly, T. & Williams,C.
E. & F.N. Spon 4-19
Review

231/10 **Oberman, A.** (1985)
Exercise and the primary prevention of cardiovascular disease
Am J Cardiol **55**, 10D-20D
Review

231/11 **Powell, K.E., Spain, K.G., Christenson, G.M. Mollenkamp, M.P.** (1986)
The status of the 1990 objectives for physical fitness and exercise
Public Health Rep **101**, 15-21

231/12 **Simonelli, C. & Eaton,**
R.P. (1978)
Cardiovascular and metabolic effects of
exercise – the strong case for
conditioning
Postgrad Med **63,** 71-77
BLOOD PRESSURE, Endocrine,
LIPIDS, Review

231/13 **Superko, H.R., Wood, P.D. &**
Haskell, W.L. (1985)
Coronary heart disease and risk factor
modification. Is there a threshold?
Am J Med **78,** 826-838
BLOOD PRESSURE, LIPIDS, Review

231/14 **Vuori, I.** (1983)
The potential for primary prevention of
coronary heart disease by physical
activity
Finnish Sports Exerc Med **2,** 43-53
Review

231/15 **Zohman, L.R.**
The cardiologist's guide to fitness and
health through exercise
Simon & Schuster
Review

231.1   EPIDEMIOLOGY - CHD

This section contains individual references on the epidemiological effects of exercise on coronary heart disease, for general reviews see section 231 above.

KEYWORDS are listed in the appendix in addition the following specific keywords have been used in this section:

Angina
CHD-morbidity (all manifestations of coronary heart disease)
CHD-mortality (deaths due to cornary heart disease)
Myocardial infarction
PWC (physical work capacity)
Stroke
Sudden cardiac death
Total activity (daily or weekly activity by monitor or diary)

Summary of evidence: exercise helps prevent coronary heart disease

THE PROBLEM

Coronary heart disease is a major disease in middle-aged men in the developed Western countries. It causes premature death and a great deal of disability. Is exercise of benefit in preventing heart disease? This hope has been pursued for many years.

SCOPE

These two sections (231 and 231.1) contain epidemiological references in which exercise has been studied as a factor acting directly or through other known risk factors which may reduce the incidence of coronary heart disease. Prospective and retrospective studies are included, those which deal with leisure activity or occupational activity. Most studies are of men but there are a few concerning women.

METHODOLOGICAL DIFFICULTIES

Retrospective studies inevitably yield exercise information of low reliability. Prospective studies need to run for many years because of the slow development of the disease and/or to have exceedingly large numbers because of the low reliability of assessments of the exercise content of a lifestyle especially over such a time span. There is always the uncertainty in epidemiology of the true cause of death unless there has been an autopsy.

EVIDENCE

Metanalysis of reliable references provides strong evidence of a link between a physically active lifestyle and a reduced incidence of coronary heart disease. This is found in studies of morbidity and mortality and there is tentative evidence of a graded response. The more the exercise, in both amount and intensity, the greater the reduction of risk. This strengthens the conclusion that the link is causal. The evidence for putative mechanisms is contained in sections 231.2 – 231.4. The reduction in risk is small if the exercise is moderate but since it is available to anyone at minimal cost and since the population at risk (sedentary middle-aged males) is large it constitutes an important potential preventive health measure.

231.1/1   **Albanes, D.**   (1987)
Potential for confounding physical activity risk assessment by body weight and fatness
Am J Epidemiol **125**, 745-746
Adult, Body composition, Female, Leisure activity, Male, Occupational activity

231.1/2 **Aravanis, C.M., Corcondilas, A., Dontas, A.S., LeKos, D. & Keys, A.** (1970)
The Greek Islands of Crete and Corfu
Circulation (Suppl) **46**, I-88-I-100
Adult, Angina, CHD-morbidity, CHD-mortality, Comparative, Occupational Activity, Male, Myocardial infarction

231.1/3 **Aravanis, C.M., Dontas, A.S., Lekos, D. & Keys, A.** (1966)
Rural populations in Crete and Corfu, Greece
Acta Med Scand (Suppl 460) **181**, 209-230
Adult, BLOOD PRESSURE, Body composition, Comparative, HEART FUNCTION TEST, LIPIDS, Male, Occupational activity,

231.1/4 **Bauer, R.L., Heller, R.F. & Challah, S.** (1985)
United Kingdom heart disease prevention project: 12 year follow-up of risk factors
Am J Epidemiol **121**, 563-569
Adult, Cohort, Intervention, Leisure activity, Male

231.1/5 **Brand, R.J., Paffenbarger, R.S. Jr., Sholtz, R.I. & Kampert, J.B.** (1979)
Work activity and fatal heart attack studied by multiple logistic risk analysis
Am J Epidemiol **110**, 52-62
Adult, BLOOD PRESSURE, CARBOHYDRATE TOLERANCE, CHD-mortality, Cohort, Comparative, Male, Occupational activity, Vigorous, Weight

231.1/6 **Breslow, L. & Buell, P.** (1960)
Mortality from coronary heart disease and physical activity of work in California.
J Chron Dis **11**, 421-440
Adult, CHD-mortality, Comparative, Male, Occupational activity

231.1/7 **Brunner, D., Manelis, G., Modan, M. & Levin, S.** (1974)
Physical activity at work and the incidence of myocardial infarction. An epidemiological study in Israeli kibbutzim
J Chron Dis **27**, 217-233
Adult, Angina, CHD-morbidity, CHD-mortality, Comparative, Female, LIPIDS, Male, Myocardial infarction, Occupational activity

231.1/8 **Buring, J.E., Evans, D.A., Fiore, M., Rosner, B. & Hennekens, C.H.** (1987)
Occupation and risk of death from coronary heart disease
J Am Med Ass **258**, 791-792
Adult, Case-control, CHD-mortality, Leisure activity, Male, Occupational activity

231.1/9 **Buzina, R., Keys, A. & Mohacek, I.** (1966)
Rural men in Dalmatia and Slavonia, Yugoslavia
Acta Med Scand (Suppl) **460**, 147-168
Adult, BLOOD PRESSURE, Body composition, Comparative, HEART FUNCTION TEST, LIPIDS, Male, Occupational activity,

231.1/10 **Buzina, R., Keys,. A., Mohacek, I.,Hahan, H. & Blackburn, H.** (1970)
Five year follow-up in Dalmatia and Slavonia
Circulation (Suppl) **46**, I-40-I-51
Adult, BLOOD PRESSURE, CHD-morbidity, CHD-mortality, Comparative, LIPIDS, Male, Occupational activity, Vigorous

231.1/11   Cassel, J., Heyden, S., Bartel, A.G., Kaplan, B.H., Tyroler, H.A., Cornoni, J.C. & Hames, C.G.   (1971) Occupation and physical activity and coronary heart disease
Arch Intern Med **128**, 920-928
Adult, BLOOD PRESSURE, CHD-morbidity, CHD-mortality, Comparative, Elderly, Leisure activity, LIPIDS, Male, Occupational activity

231.1/12   Chapman, J.M., Goerke, L.S., Dixon, W., Loveland, D.B. & Phillips, E.   (1957)
The clinical status of a population group in Los Angeles under observation for 2 to 3 years
Am J Pub Health (Suppl) **47**, 33-42
Adult, CHD-morbidity, Cohort, Male, Occupational activity

231.1/13   Chave, S.P.W., Morris, J.N., Moss, S. & Semmence, A.M.   (1978)
Vigorous exercise in leisure time and the death rate: a study of male civil servants
J Epidemiol Community Health **32**, 239-243
Adult, Angina, CHD-morbidity, CHD-mortality, Cohort, Leisure activity, Male, Vigorous

231.1/14   Deuster, P.A.   (1987)
Health and fitness profiles of male military officers
Milt Med **152**, 290-293
Adult, CHD-morbidity, Male, Occupational activity

231.1/15   Donahue, R.P., Abbott, R.D., Reed, D.M. & Yano, K.   (1988)
Physical activity and coronary heart disease in middle-aged and elderly men: The Honolulu heart program
Am J Pub Health **78**, 683-685
Adult, CHD-morbidity, Cohort, Elderly, Male, Total activity

231.1/16   Dyer, A.R., Persky, V., Stamler, J., Paul, O., Shekelle, R.B., Berkson, D.M., Lepper, M.H., Schoenberger, J.A. & Lindberg, H. A.   (1980)
Heart rate as a prognostic factor for coronary heart disease and mortality: Findings in three Chicago epidemiologic studies
Am J Epidemiol **112**, 736-749
Adult, BLOOD PRESSURE, CARDIAC PERFORMANCE, CHD-mortality, Cohort, Female, LIPIDS, Male, Weight

231.1/17   Eichner, E.R.   (1983)
Exercise and heart disease
Am J Med **75**, 1008-1023
HAZARDS-CVS, Review

231.1/18   Elmfeldt, D., Wilhelmsson, C., Vedin, A., Tibblin, G. & Wilhelmsen, L.   (1976)
Characteristics of representative male survivors of myocardial infarction compared with representative population samples
Acta Med Scand **199**, 387-398
Adult, BLOOD PRESSURE, Case-control, Leisure activity, LIPIDS, Male, Myocardial infarction, Occupational activity

231.1/19   Epstein, L., Miller, G.J., Stitt, F.W. & Morris, J.N.   (1976)
Vigorous exercise in leisure time, coronary risk factors and resting ECG in middle-aged male civil servants
Br Heart J **38**, 403-409
Adult, BLOOD PRESSURE, Body composition, Heart Function test, Leisure activity, LIPIDS, Male, Vigorous

231.1/20   Erikssen, J.   (1986)
Physical fitness and coronary heart disease morbidity and mortality
Acta Med Scand (Suppl) **711**, 189-192
Review

231.1/21 Fidanza, F., Puddu, V., Imbimbo, B., Menotti, A. & Keys, A. (1970)
Five-year experience in rural Italy
Circulation (Suppl 1) **46**, 63-75
Adult, CHD-morbidity, CHD-mortality, Leisure activity, LIPIDS, Male, Myocardial infarction, Occupational activity, Sudden cardiac death

231.1/22 Franck, C.W., Weinblatt, E., Shapiro, S. & Sager, R.V. (1966)
Physical inactivity as a lethal factor in myocardial infarction in man
Circulation **34**, 1022-1033
Adult, BLOOD PRESSURE, CHD-mortality, Comparative, Leisure activity, Male, Myocardial infarction,

231.1/23 Fraser, G.E., Dysinger, W., Best, C. & Chan, R. (1987)
Ischemic heart disease risk factors in middle-aged Seventh-Day Adventist men and their neighbors
Am J Epidemiol **126**, 638-646
Adult, BLOOD PRESSURE, CHD-mortality, Cohort, Comparative, LIPIDS Leisure activity, Male

231.1/24 Friedewald, W.T. (1985)
Physical activity research and coronary heart disease
Public Health Reports **100**, 115-117
Review

231.1/25 Garcia-Palmieri, M.R., Costas, R. Jr. & Cruz-Vidal, M., Sorlie, P.D. & Havlik, R.J. (1982)
Increased physical activity: a protective factor against heart attacks in Puerto Rico
Am J Cardiol **50**, 749-755
Adult, Angina, BLOOD PRESSURE, Cohort, Comparative, LIPIDS, Male, Myocardial infarction, Sudden cardiac death, Total activity, Weight

231.1/26 Heady, J.A., Morris, J.N., Kagan, A. & Raffle, P.A.B. (1961)
Coronary heart disease in London busmen: a progress report with special reference to physique
Br J Prev Soc Med **15**, 143-153
Adult, Angina, Body composition, CHD-morbidity, Male, Occupational activity, Sudden cardiac death

231.1/27 Hennekens, C.H., Rosner, B., Jesse, M.J., Drolette, M.E. & Speizer, F.E., (1977)
A retrospective study of physical activity and coronary deaths
Internat J Epidemiol **6**, 243-246
Adult, Case-control, CHD-mortality, Leisure activity, Male, Occupational activity, Weight

231.1/28 Hinkle, L.E. Jr., Thaler, H.T., Merke, D.P., Renier-Berg, D. & Morton, N.E. (1988)
The risk factors for arrhythmic death in a sample of men followed for 20 years
Am J Epidemiol **127**, 500-515
Adult, BLOOD PRESSURE, CHD-mortality, Cohort, Leisure activity, Male

231.1/29 Holme, E., Hegeland, A., Hjermann, I., Leren, P. & Lund-Larsen, P.G. (1981)
Physical activity at work and at leisure in relation to coronary risk factors and social class. A 4-year mortality follow-up. The Oslo Study
Acta Med Scand. **209**, 277-283
Adult, BLOOD PRESSURE, CHD-mortality, Cohort, Leisure activity, LIPIDS, Male, Occupational activity, Vigorous

231.1/30   **Ibsen, K.K., Lous, P. & Andersen, G.E.** (1982)
Coronary heart risk factors in 177 children and young adults whose fathers died from ischemic heart disease before age 45
Acta Paediatr Scand **71**, 609-613
BLOOD PRESSURE, Children, Comparative, Female, Leisure activity, LIPIDS, Male

231.1/31   **Ilmarinen, J. & Fardy, P.S.** (1977)
Physical activity intervention for males with high risk of coronary heart disease: A three-year follow up
Prev Med **6**, 416-425
Adult, Angina, BLOOD PRESSURE, CHD-morbidity, Exercise programme, Intervention, Leisure activity, LIPIDS, Male

231.1/32   **Kahn, H.A.** (1963)
The relationship of reported coronary disease mortality to physical activity of work
Am J Pub Health **53**, 1058-1067
Adult, CHD-mortality, Comparative, Male, Occupational activity

231.1/33   **Kannel, W.B.** (1963)
Recent findings of the Framingham Study
Resident & Staff Physician **24**, 56-71
Adult, CHD-mortality, Cohort, Male, Total activity

231.1/34   **Kannel, W.B., Belanger, A., D'Agostino, R. & Israel, I.** (1986)
Physical activity and physical demand on the job and risk of cardiovascular disease and death: The Framingham Study
Am Heart J **112**, 820-825
Adult, CHD-morbidity, CHD-mortality, Cohort, Male, Occupational activity, Total activity

231.1/35   **Kannel, W.B., Doyle, J.T., McNamara, P.M., Quickerton, P. & Gordon, T.** (1975)
Precursors of sudden coronary death. Factors related to the incidence of sudden death
Circulation **51**, 606-613
Adult, BLOOD PRESSURE, CHD-mortality, Cohort, LIPIDS, Male, Sudden cardiac death, Total activity

231.1/36   **Kannel, W.B. & Sorlie, P.** (1979)
Some health benefits of physical activity. The Framingham Study
Arch Intern Med **139**, 857-861
Adult, BLOOD PRESSURE, CARBOHYDRATE TOLERANCE, CHD-morbidity, CHD-mortality, Cohort, Female, LIPIDS, Male, Stroke, Total activity, Weight

231.1/37   **Kannel, W.B., Wilson, P. & Blair, S.N.** (1985)
Epidemiologic assessment of the role of physical activity and fitness in the development of cardiovascular disease
Am Heart J **109**, 876-885
Review

231.1/38   **Karvonen, M.J.** (1984)
Physical activity and cardiovascular morbidity
Scand J Work Environ Health **10**, 389
Review

231.1/39   **Karvonen, M.J., Rautaharju, P.M., Orma, E., Punsar, S. & Takkunen, J.** (1961)
Heart disease and employment, cardiovascular studies on lumberjacks
J Occup Med **3**, 49-53
Adult, CHD-morbidity, Cohort, Male, Occupational activity

231.1/40   **Karvonen, M.J.** (1982)
Physical activity in work and leisure time in relation to cardiovascular diseases
Ann Clin Res (Suppl 34) **14**, 118-123
Review

231.1/41   **Keys, A.**   (1970)
Coronary Heart Disease in seven
countries
Circulation (Suppl 1) **46**, I-1-I-211
***Adult, CHD-morbidity, Occupational
activity***

231.1/42   **Keys, A., Aravanis, C.M.,
Blackburn, H.W., Van Buchem, F.S.P.,
Buzina, R., Djordjevic, B.S., Dontas, A.S.,
Fidanza, F., Karvonen, M.J., Kimura, N.,
Lekos, D., Monti, M., Puddu, V. &
Taylor, H.L.**   (1966)
Epidemiological studies related to
coronary heart disease. Characteristics of
men aged 40-59 in seven countries
Acta Med Scand (Suppl 460) **181**, 1-392
***Adult, BLOOD PRESSURE, Body
composition, Comparative, HEART
FUNCTION TEST, LIPIDS, Male,
Occupational activity***

231.1/43   **Lapidus, L. & Bengtssen,
C.**   (1986)
Socioeconomic factors and physical
activity in relation to cardiovascular
disease and death
Br Heart J **55**, 295-301
***Adult, Angina, BLOOD PRESSURE,
CHD-morbidity, CHD-mortality, Cohort,
Female, Leisure activity, LIPIDS,
Occupational activity, Weight***

231.1/44   **LaPorte R.E., Adams, L.L.,
Savage, D.D., Brenes, G., Dearwater, S. &
Cook, T.**   (1984)
The spectrum of physical activity,
cardiovascular disease and health: an
epidemiologic perspective
Am J Epidemiol **120**, 507-517
Review

231.1/45   **Leon, A.S., Connett, J., Jacobs,
D.R.Jr. & Rauramaa, R.**   (1987)
Leisure-time physical activity levels and
risk of coronary heart disease and death.
The multiple risk factor intervention trial
J Am Med Ass **258**, 2388-2395
***Adult, BLOOD PRESSURE, CHD-
morbidity, CHD-mortality, Cohort,
Leisure activity, LIPIDS, Male***

231.1/46   **Leon, A.S., Connett, J., Jacobs,
D.R. Jr. & Taylor, H.L.**   (1984)
Relation of leisure time physical activity
to mortality in the Multiple Risk Factor
Intervention Trial
Circulation (Suppl 2) **70**, II-644
***Adult, BLOOD PRESSURE, CHD-
morbidity, CHD-mortality, Cohort,
Leisure activity, LIPIDS, Male***

231.1/47   **Lie, H., Mundal, R. & Erikssen,
J.**   (1985)
Coronary risk factors and incidence of
coronary death in relation to physical
fitness. 7-year follow-up study of middle-
aged and elderly men
Eur Heart J **6**, 147-157
***Adult, BLOOD PRESSURE, CHD-
mortality, Cohort, Elderly, Male, PWC***

231.1/48   **Lynch, P. & Oelman,
B.J.**   (1981)
Mortality from coronary heart disease in
the British army compared with the civil
population
Br Med J **283**, 405
***Adult, CHD-mortality, Cohort, Male,
Occupational activity***

231.1/49   **Magnus, K., Matroos, A. &
Strackee, J.**   (1979)
Walking cycling, or gardening, with or
without seasonal interruption, in relation
to acute coronary events
Am J Epidemiol **110**, 724-733
***Adult, Angina, Case-control, CHD-
morbidity, CHD-mortality, Leisure
activity***

231.1/50   **McDonough, J., Hames, C.G.,
Stulb, S. & Garrison, G.**   (1965)
Coronary heart disease among negroes
and whites in Evans County, Georgia
J Chron Dis **18**, 443-468
***Adult, Angina, BLOOD PRESSURE,
CHD-morbidity, CHD-mortality,
Comparative, LIPIDS, Male, Myocardial
infarction, Occupational activity***

231.1/51 **Menotti, A. & Puddu, V.** (1979)
Ten-year mortality from coronary heart
disease among 172,000 men classified by
occupational physical activity
Scand J Work Environ Health **5**, 100-108
*Adult, CHD-mortality, Comparative,
Male, Occupational activity*

231.1/52 **Morris, J.N.** (1960 & 1961)
Epidemiology and cardiovascular disease
of middle-age: Parts I and II
Mod Concepts Cardiovasc Dis Part I – 29,
625. Part II – 30
Review

231.1/53 **Morris, J.N.** (1974)
Physical inactivity and coronary heart
disease
Acta Cardiol (Brux.) **20**, 95-103
Review

231.1/54 **Morris, J.N., Chave, S.P.W.,
Adam, C., Sirey, C. & Epstein, L.** (1973)
Vigorous exercise in leisure time and the
incidence of coronary heart-disease
Lancet **i**, 333-339
*Adult, Angina, Case-control, CHD-
morbidity, Cohort, Leisure activity, Male,
Vigorous, Weight*

231.1/55 **Morris, J.N. & Crawford,
M.D.** (1958)
Coronary heart disease and physical
activity of work
Br Med J **2**, 1485-1496
*Adult, Autopsy, CHD-morbidity, Male,
Occupational activity*

231.1/56 **Morris, J.N., Everitt, M.G.
Pollard, R. & Chave, S.P.W.** (1980)
Vigorous exercise in leisure-time:
protection against coronary heart disease
Lancet **ii**, 1207-1210
*Adult, Angina, CHD-morbidity, CHD-
mortality, Cohort, Leisure activity, Male,
Vigorous*

231.1/57 **Morris, J.N., Heady, J.A., Raffle,
P.A.B., Roberts, C.G. & Parks,
J.W.** (1953)
Coronary heart disease and physical
activity of work
Lancet **265**, 1053-1057,1111-1120
*Adult, Angina, CHD-morbidity, CHD-
mortality, Comparative, Male,
Myocardial infarction, Occupational
activity, Sudden cardiac death*

231.1/58 **Morris, J.N., Kagan, A., Pattison,
D.C., Gardner, M.J. & Raffle,
P.A.B.** (1966)
Incidence and prediction of ischaemic
heart disease in London busmen
Lancet **2**, 553-559
*Adult, CHD-morbidity, CHD-mortality,
Comparative, Male, Occupational activity*

231.1/59 **Mortensen, J.M., Stevenson, T.T.
& Whitney, L.H.** (1959)
Mortality due to coronary disease
analyzed by broad occupational groups
Arch Indust Health **19**, 1-4
*Adult, CHD-mortality, Male,
Occupational activity*

231.1/60 **Paffenbarger, R.S. Jr. & Hale,
W.E.** (1975)
Work activity and coronary heart
mortality
N Eng J Med **292**, 545-550
*Adult, CHD-mortality, Cohort, Male,
Occupational activity*

231.1/61 **Paffenbarger, R.S. Jr., Hale,
W.E., Brand, R.J. & Hyde, R.T.** (1977)
Work-energy level, personal
characteristics and fatal heart attack : a
birth cohort effect
Am J Epidemiol **105**, 200-213
*Adult, BLOOD PRESSURE, CHD-
mortality, Cohort, LIPIDS, Male,
Occupational activity, Vigorous*

231.1/62   Paffenbarger, R.S. Jr., Hyde,
R.T., Hsieh, C.-C. & Wing, A.L.   (1986)
Physical activity, other life-style patterns,
cardiovascular disease and longevity
Acta Med Scand (Suppl) **711**, 85-91
Review

231.1/63   Paffenbarger, R.S. Jr. & Hyde,
R.T.   (1980)
Exercise as protection against heart
attack
N Eng J Med **302**, 1026-1027
Review

231.1/64   Paffenbarger, R.S., Jr., Hyde,
R.T., Wing, A.L. & Hsieh, C.   (1986)
Physical activity, all-cause mortality, and
longevity of college alumni
N Eng J Med **314**, 605-613
*Adult, BLOOD PRESSURE, Cohort,
Customary activity, GENERAL
HEALTH, Leisure activity, Male,
RESPIRATORY FUNCTION, Weight*

231.1/65   Paffenbarger, R.S., Jr., Hyde,
R.T., Wing, A.L. & Steinmetz,
C.H.   (1984)
A natural history of athleticism and
cardiovascular health
J Am Med Ass **252**, 491-495
*Adult, BLOOD PRESSURE, CHD-
mortality, Cohort, Leisure activity, Male,
Weight*

231.1/66   Paffenbarger, R.S., Jr., Wing,
A.L., & Hyde, R.T.   (1978)
Physical activity as an index of heart
attack risk in college alumni
Am J Epidemiol **108**, 161-175
*Adult, Angina, BLOOD PRESSURE,
CHD-morbidity, CHD-mortality, Cohort,
Customary activity, Leisure activity,
Male, Weight, Vigorous*

231.1/67   Paffenbarger, R.S. Jr., Laughlin,
M.E., Gima, A.S. & Black, R.A.   (1970)
Work activity of longshoremen as related
to death from coronary heart disease and
stroke
N Eng J Med **282**, 1109-1114
*Adult, BLOOD PRESSURE, CHD-
mortality, Comparative, Male,
Occupational activity, Stroke, Weight*

231.1/68   Paffenbarger, R.S. Jr., Notkin, J.,
Krueger, D.E., Wolf, P.A., Thorne, M.C.,
Lebauer, E.J. & Williams, J.L.   (1966)
Chronic disease in former college
students. II. Methods of study and
observations on mortality from coronary
heart disease
Am J Pub Health **56**, 962-971
*Adult, BLOOD PRESSURE, Case-
control, CHD-mortality, Leisure activity,
Male, Weight*

231.1/69   Paffenbarger, R.S. Jr., Wolf,
P.A., Notkin, J. & Thorne, M.C.   (1966)
Chronic disease in former college
students; 1, Early precursors of fatal
coronary heart disease
Am J Epidemiol **83**, 314-328
*Adult, BLOOD PRESSURE, Case-
control, CHD-mortality, Leisure activity,
Male, RESPIRATORY FUNCTION,
Weight*

231.1/70   Paul, O., Lepper, M.H., Phelan,
W.H., Dupertuis, G.W., MacMillan, A.,
McKean, H. & Park, H.   (1963)
A longitudinal study of coronary heart
disease
Circulation **28**, 20-31
*Adult, Angina, BLOOD PRESSURE,
Cohort, CHD-mortality, Leisure activity,
LIPIDS, Male, Myocardial infarction*

231.1/71   Persson, C., Bengtsson, C.,
Lapidus, L., Rybo, E., Thiringer, G. &
Wedel, H.   (1986)
Peak expiratory flow and risk of
cardiovascular disease and death. A 12-
year follow-up of participants in the
population study of women in
Gothenburg, Sweden
Am J Epidemiol **124**, 942-948
Adult, Angina, BLOOD PRESSURE,
CARBOHYDRATE TOLERANCE,
CHD-mortality, Cohort, Female, Leisure
activity, LIPIDS, Myocardial infarction,
RESPIRATORY FUNCTION, Stroke

231.1/72   Peters, R.K., Cady, L.D., Jr.,
Blachoff, D.P., Bernstein, L. & Pike,
M.C.   (1983)
Physical fitness and subsequent
myocardial infarction in healthy workers
J Am Med Ass **249**, 3052-3056
Adult, BLOOD PRESSURE, Cohort,
LIPIDS, Male, Myocardial infarction,
PWC, Sudden cardiac death, Weight

231.1/73   Polednak, A.P.   (1972)
Longevity and cause of death among
Harvard College athletes and their
classmates
Geriatrics **27**, 53-64
Review

231.1/74   Pomrehn, P.R., Wallace, R.B. &
Burmeister, L.   (1982)
Ischemic heart disease mortality in Iowa
farmers. The influence of lifestyle
J Am Med Ass **248**, 1073-1076
Adult, BLOOD PRESSURE, CHD-
mortality, Comparative, LIPIDS, Male,
Occupational activity, PWC

231.1/75   Powell, K.E., Thompson, P.D.,
Casperson, C.J. & Kendrick, J.S.   (1987)
Physical activity and the incidence of
coronary heart disease
Ann Rev Public Health **8**, 253-287
Review

231.1/76   Prat, G., Guzman, R., Silva, L. &
Chamorro, G.   (1980)
Physical activity and risk of coronary
heart disease in a sedentary working
population: Preliminary report. In: Sports
Cardiology International conference
(Eds.) Lubich, T. & Venerando, A.
Aulo Gaggi, Bologna 631-638
Adult, CHD-morbidity, Cohort, Male

231.1/77   Punsar, S. & Karvonen,
M.J.   (1976)
Physical activty and coronary heart
disease in populations from east and west
Finland
Adv Cardiol **18**, 196-207
Adult, CHD-mortality, Cohort, Male,
Occupational activity

231.1/78   Reed, D.M., MacLean, C.J. &
Hayashi, T.   (1987)
Predictors of atherosclerosis in the
Honolulu heart program.I. Biologic,
dietary and lifestyle characteristics
Am J Epidemiol **126**, 214-225
Adult, Autopsy, BLOOD PRESSURE,
Body composition, CHD-morbidity,
Cohort, LIPIDS, Male, Total activity

231.1/79   Rose, G., Reid, D.D., Hamilton,
P.J.S., McCartney, P., Keen, H. &
Jarrett, R.J.   (1977)
Myocardial ischaemia, risk factors and
death from coronary heart disease
Lancet **1**, 105-110
Adult, Angina, BLOOD PRESSURE,
CHD-mortality, Cohort, Leisure activity,
Male

231.1/80   Rosenman, R.H., Bawol, R.D., &
Oscherwitz, M.   (1977)
A 4-year prospective study of the
relationship of different habitual
vocational physical activity to risk and
incidence of coronary heart disease in
volunteer male federal employees
Ann NY Acad Sci **301**, 627-641
Adult, Angina, BLOOD PRESSURE,
CHD-morbidity, CHD-mortality, Cohort,
LIPIDS, Male, Occupational activity

231.1/81 **Rosenman, R.H., Brand, R.J., Jenkins, C.D., Friedman, M., Straus, R. & Wurm, M.** (1975)
Coronary heart disease in the Western Collaborative Group Study. Final follow-up experience of 8 1/2 years
J Am Med Ass **233.** 872-877
Adult, BLOOD PRESSURE, CHD-morbidity, CHD-mortality, Cohort, Leisure activity, LIPIDS, Male, Occupational activity,

231.1/82 **Salonen, J.T., Puska, P. & Tuomilehto, J.** (1982)
Physical activity and risk of myocardial infarction, cerebral stroke and death: A longitudinal study in Eastern Finland
Am J Epidemiol **115,** 526-537
Adult, BLOOD PRESSURE, CHD-morbidity, CHD-mortality, Cohort, Female, Leisure activity, LIPIDS, Male, Myocardial infarction, Occupational activity, Stroke, Weight

231.1/83 **Salonen, J.T., Slater, J.S., Toumilehto, J. & Rauramaa, R.** (1988)
Leisure time and occupational physical activity: risk of death from ischemic heart disease
Am J Epidemiol **127,** 87-94
Adult, BLOOD PRESSURE, CHD-mortality, Cohort, Female, Leisure activity, LIPIDS, Male, Occupational activity, Weight

231.1/84 **Schettler, G.** (1976)
Risk factors of coronary heart disease: West German Data
Prev Med **5,** 216-225
Adult, Cohort, Female, Male, Myocardial infarction, Occupational activity, Sudden cardiac death

231.1/85 **Scragg, R., Stewart, A., Jackson, R. & Beaglehole, R.** (1987)
Alcohol and exercise in myocardial infarction and sudden coronary death in men and women
Am J Epidemiol **126,** 77-85
Adult, Case-control, Female, Leisure activity, Male, Myocardial infarction, Sudden cardiac death

231.1/86 **Shapiro, S., Weinblatt, E., Frank, C.W. & Sager, R.V.** (1965)
The H.I.P. study of incidence and prognosis of coronary heart disease: Preliminary findings on incidence of myocardial infarction and angina
J Chron Dis **18,** 527-558
Adult, Angina, Cohort, Female, Leisure activity, Male, Myocardial infarction, Occupational activity

231.1/87 **Siscovick, D.S., Weiss, N.S., Fletcher, R.H., Schoenbach, V.J. & Wagner, E.H.** (1984)
Habitual vigorous exercise and primary cardiac arrest: Effect of other risk factors on the relationship
J Chron Dis **37,** 625-631
Adult, BLOOD PRESSURE, Case-control, CHD-mortality, Leisure activity, Male, Vigorous, Weight

231.1/88 **Siscovick, D.S., Weiss, N.S., Hallstrom, A.P., Inui, T.S. & Peterson, D.R.** (1982)
Physical activity and primary cardiac arrest
J Am Med Ass **248,** 3113-3117
Adult, BLOOD PRESSURE, Case-control, CHD-morbidity, Leisure activity, Male, Vigorous

231.1/89 **Slattery, M.L. & Jacobs, D.R. Jr.** (1988)
Physical fitness and cardiovascular disease mortality: The U.S. Railroad study
Am J Epidemiol **127,** 571-580
Adult, BLOOD PRESSURE, CHD-mortality, Cohort, LIPIDS, Male, PWC

231.1/90   **Sobolski, J.C., DeBacker, G. &
Degré, S.G.**   (1981)
Physical activity, physical fitness and
cardiovascular diseases
Cardiology **67**, 38-51
*Adult, CHD-morbidity, CHD-mortality,
Cohort, Leisure activity, Occupational
activity, PWC, Weight*

231.1/91   **Sobolski, J.C., Kornitizer, M.,
DeBacker, G. Dramaix, M., Abramowicz,
M., Degré, S. & Denolin, H.**   (1987)
Protection against ischemic heart disease
in the Belgian Physical Fitness Study:
Physical fitness rather than physical
activity?
Am J Epidemiol **125**, 601-610
*Adult, BLOOD PRESSURE, CHD-
morbidity, CHD-mortality, Cohort,
Leisure activity, LIPIDS, Occupational
activity, PWC, Weight*

231.1/92   **Spain, D.M. & Bradess,
V.A.**   (1960)
Occupational physical activity and the
degree of coronary atherosclerosis in
normal men
Circulation **22**, 239-242
*Adult, Autopsy, CHD-morbidity, Male,
Occupational activity*

231.1/93   **Stamler, J. & Kjelsberg,
M.**   (1960)
Epidemiologic studies on cardiovascular
renal diseases: I. Analysis of mortality by
age-race-sex-occupation
J Chron Dis **12**, 440-453
*Adult, CHD-mortality, Cohort, Female,
Kidney disease, Male, Occupational
activity*

231.1/94   **Stamler, J., Lindberg, H.A.,
Berkson, D.M., Shaffer, A., Miller, W. &
Poindexter, A.**   (1960)
Prevalence and incidence of coronary
heart disease in strata of the labor force of
a Chicago industrial corporation
J Chron Dis **11**, 405-420
*Adult, BLOOD PRESSURE, CHD-
morbidity, CHD-mortality, Comparative,
Male, Occupational activity, Sudden
cardiac death*

231.1/95   **Taylor, H.L., Klepetar, E., Keys,
A., Parlin, W., Blackburn, H. & Puchner,
T.**   (1962)
Death rates among physically active and
sedentary employees of the railroad
industry
Am J Pub Health **52**, 1697-1707
*Adult, CHD-mortality, Comparative,
Male, Occupational activity*

231.1/96   **Wilhelmsen, L., Bjure, J.,
Ekstrom-Jodal, B., Aurell, M. & Cromby,
C.**   (1981)
Nine years' follow-up of a maximal
exercise test in a random population
sample of middle-aged men
Cardiology (Suppl 2) **68**, 1-8
*Adult, Male, Myocardial infarction,
PWC, Sudden cardiac death*

231.1/97   **Wilhelmsen, L.,Tibblin, G.,
Aurell, M.,Bjure, J., Ekstrom-Jodal, B. &
Grimby, G.**   (1976)
Physical activity, physical fitness and the
risk of myocardial infarction
Adv Cardiol **18**, 217-230
*Adult, BLOOD PRESSURE, Cohort,
Leisure activity, LIPIDS, Male,
Myocardial infarction, Sudden cardiac
death*

231.1/98   **Wilson, P.W.F., Paffenbarger,
R.S., Morris, J.N. & Havlik,
R.J.**   (1986)
Assessment methods for the physical
activity and physical fitness in population
studies: Report of a NHLBI workshop
Am Heart J **111**, 1177-1192
Review

231.1/99   **Wingard, D.L., Berkman, L.F. & Brand, R.J.**   (1982)
A multivariate analysis of health-related practices. A nine-year mortality follow-up of the Alameda county study
Am J Epidemiol **116,** 765-775
Adult, CHD-mortality, Cohort, Female, Leisure activity, Male

231.1/100   **Yamamoto, L., Yano, K., & Rhoads, G.G.**   (1983)
Characteristics of joggers among Japanese men in Hawaii
Am J Publ Health **73,** 147-152
Adult, BLOOD PRESSURE, CHD-morbidity, Comparative, Leisure activity, LIPIDS, Male, RESPIRATORY FUNCTION

231.1/101   **Yano, K., Reed, D.M. & McGee, D.L.**   (1984)
Ten-year incidence of coronary heart disease in the Honolulu Heart Program
Am J Epidemiol **119,** 653-666
Adult, Angina, BLOOD PRESSURE, CHD-morbidity, CHD-mortality, Cohort, LIPIDS, Male, Myocardial infarction, Total activity, Weight

231.1/102   **York, E., Mitchell, R.E. & Graybiel, A.**   (1986)
Cardiovascular epidemiology, exercise, and health: 40-year followup of the U.S.Navy's
Aviat Space Environ Med **57,** 597-599
Adult, BLOOD PRESSURE, Case-control, CHD-mortality, Leisure activity, LIPIDS, Male

231.1/103   **Zukel, W.J., Lewis, R.H., Enterline, P.E., Painter, R.C., Ralston, L.S., Fawcett, R.M., Meredith, A.P. & Peterson, B.**   (1959)
A short-term community study of the epidemiology of coronary heart disease
Am J Pub Health **49,** 1630-1639
Adult, Angina, CHD-mortality, Comparative, Male, Myocardial infarction, Occupational activity, Sudden cardiac death

231.2   COLLATERALS AND MYOCARDIAL PERFUSION

KEYWORDS are listed in the appendix
Summary of evidence: exercise does not promote the development of collaterals in humans

THE PROBLEM

Is the observed reduction in the incidence of coronary heart disease attributed to exercise (see 231 and 231.1) due to an improved perfusion of the myocardium?

SCOPE

This section contains references dealing with the effects of exercise on myocardial perfusion and the development of collateral coronary blood vessels especially after occlusion of major vessels. Most are animal studies because of the neccessarily invasive nature of the investigations.

METHODOLOGICAL DIFFICULTIES

Animal evidence is not always transferable, and human studies which allow biopsies of heart tissue are rare. Recent angiographic studies using labelled isotopes have failed to demonstrate improvements attributable to exercise. These techniques have now reached a level of reliability which would allow relevant improvements to be seen.

EVIDENCE

Although some studies found significant positive effects in animals, there is overall no clear evidence for improvement in either myocardial perfusion, which is already abundant, or the development of collateral vessels in humans.

231.2/1   **Anversa, P. Ricci, R. & Olivetti, G.**   (1987)
Effects of exercise on the capillary vasculature of the rat heart
Circulation (Suppl) **75**, I12-118
Animal, Exercise programme, Intervention

231.2/2   **Barmeyer, J.**   (1976)
Physical activity and coronary collateral development
Adv Cardiol **18**, 104-112.
Review

231.2/3   **Cohen, M.V.**   (1983)
Coronary and collateral blood flows during exercise and myocardial vascular adaptations to training
Exerc Sport Sci Rev **11**, 55-98
Review

231.2/4   **Cohen, M.V. & Steingart, R.M.**   (1987)
Lack of effect of prior training on subsequent ischaemia and infarcting myocardium and collateral development in dogs with normal hearts
Cardiovascular Res **2**, 269-278
Animal, Exercise programme, Intervention

231.2/5   **Cohen, M.V. & Yipintsoi, T.**   (1981)
Restoration of cardiac function and myocardial flow by collateral development in dogs
Am J Physiol **240**, H811-819
Animal, Exercise programme, Intervention

231.2/6   Cohen, M.V., Yipintsoi, T., Malhotra, A., Penpargkul, S. & Scheuer, J.   (1978)
Effect of exercise on collateral development in dogs with normal arteries
J Appl Physiol **45**, 797-805
Animal, CARDIAC PERFORMANCE, Exercise programme, Intervention,

231.2/7   Cohen, M.V., Yipintsoi, T. & Scheuer, J.   (1982)
Coronary collateral stimulation by exercise in dogs with stenotic coronary arteries
J Appl Physiol **52**, 664-671
Animal, Exercise programme, Intervention

231.2/8   Conner, J.F., LaCamera, F., Swanick, E.J., Oldham, M.J., Holzaepfel, D.W. & Lyczkowskyj, O.   (1976)
Effects of exercise on coronary collateralization – angiographic studies of six patients in a supervised exercise program
Med Sci Sports **8**, 145-151
Adult, CARDIAC PERFORMANCE, Exercise programme, Intervention, Male, SECONDARY PREVENTION

231.2/9   Ferguson, R.J., Peticlerc, R., Choquette, G., Chaniotis, L., Gauthier, P., Hout, R., Allard, C., Jankowski, L.& Campeau, L.   (1974)
Effect of physical training on treadmill exercise capacity, collateral circulation and progression of coronary disease
Am J Cardiol **34**, 764-769
Adult, Exercise programme, Intervention, Male, SECONDARY PREVENTION

231.2/10   Froelicher, V.F.   (1987)
The effect of exercise on myocardial perfusion and function in patients with coronary heart disease
Eur Heart J (Suppl G) **8**, 1-8
Review

231.2/11   Froelicher, V.F., Jensen, D., Atwood, J.E., McKirnan, M.D., Gerber, K., Slutsky, R., Battler, A., Ashburn, W. & Ross J.   (1980)
Cardiac rehabilitation: Evidence for improvement in myocardial perfusion and function
Arch Phys Med Rehabil **61**, 517-522
Adult, AEROBIC CAPACITY, CARDIAC PERFORMANCE, Exercise programme, Intervention, SECONDARY PREVENTION

231.2/12   Fujita, M., Sasayama, S., Asanoi, H., Nakajima, H., Sakai, O. & Ohno, A.   (1988)
Improvement of treadmill capacity and collateral circulation as a result of exercise with heparin pretreatment in patients with effort angina
Circulation **77**, 1022-1029
Adult, CARDIAC PERFORMANCE, Exercise programme, Intervention, SECONDARY PREVENTION

231.2/13   Hellerstein, H.K.   (1977)
Acceleration of collaterals due to physical activity – Dogma or fact. A misguided goal or unrealized objective? In: Critical Evaluation of cardiac rehabilitation (Eds) Kellermann, J.J. & Denolin, H. S. *Karger (Basel), Switzerland* **125**, *Review*

231.2/14   Hung, J., Gordon, E.P., Houston, N., Haskell, W.L., Goris, M.L. & DeBusk, R.F.   (1984)
Changes in rest and exercise myocardial perfusion and left ventricular function 3 to 26 weeks after clinically uncomplicated acute myocardial infarction: effects of exercise training
Am J Cardiol **54**, 943-950
Adult, CARDIAC PERFORMANCE, Exercise programme, Intervention, Male, SECONDARY PREVENTION

231.2/15 **Kennedy, C.C., Spiekerman, R.E., Lindsay, M.I. Jr, Mankin, H.T., Frye, R.L. & McCallister, B.D.** (1976)
One-year graduated exercise program for men with angina pectoris: evaluation by physiologic studies and coronary arteriography
Mayo Clin Proc **51**, 231.2-236
Adult, CARDIAC PERFORMANCE, Exercise programme, Intervention, LIPIDS, Male, SECONDARY PREVENTION

231.2/16 **Koerner, J.E. & Terjung, R.L.** (1982)
Effects of physical training on coronary collateral circulation of the rat
J Appl Physiol **52**, 376-387
Animal, CARDIAC PERFORMANCE, Exercise programme, Intervention

231.2/17 **Laughlin, M.H.** (1985)
Effects of exercise training on coronary transport capacity
J Appl Physiol **58**, 468-476
Animal, Exercise programme, Intervention

231.2/18 **Laughlin, M.H. & Tomanek, R.J.** (1987)
Myocardial capillarity and maximal capillary diffusion capacity in exercise-trained dogs
J Appl Physiol **63**, 1481-1486
Animal, Exercise programme, Intervention

231.2/19 **Neill, W.A. & Oxendine, J.M.** (1979)
Exercise can promote coronary collateral development without improving perfusion of ischemic myocardium
Circulation **60**, 1513-1519
Animal, Exercise programme, Intervention

231.2/20 **Nolewajka, A.J., Kostuk, W.J., Rechnitzer, P.A. & Cunnningham, D.A.** (1979)
Exercise and human collateralization: An angiographic and scintigraphic assessment
Circulation **60**, 114-121
Adult, CARDIAC PERFORMANCE, Exercise programme, Intervention, Male, SECONDARY PREVENTION

231.2/21 **Sanders, M., White, F.C., Peterson, T.M. & Bloor, C.M.** (1978)
Effects of endurance exercise on coronary collateral blood flow in miniature swine
Am J Physiol **234**, H614-619
Animal, Exercise programme, Intervention

231.2/22 **Scheel, K.W., Ingram, L.A. & Wilson, J.L.** (1981)
Effects of exercise on the coronary and collateral vasculature of beagles with and without coronary occlusion
Circulation Res **48**, 523-530
Animal, Exercise programme, Intervention

231.2/23 **Scheuer, J.** (1982)
Effects of physical training on myocardial vascularity and perfusion
Circulation **66**, 491-495
Review

231.2/24 **Sebrechts, C.P., Klein, J.L. & Ahnve, S.** (1986)
Myocardial perfusion changes following 1 year of exercise training assessed by thallium-201 circumferential count profiles
Am Heart J **112**, 1217-1226
Adult, AEROBIC CAPACITY, BLOOD PRESSURE, CARDIAC PERFORMANCE, Exercise programme, Intervention, Male, SECONDARY PREVENTION

231.2/25   **Stone, H.L.**   (1980)
Coronary flow, myocardial oxygen
consumption, and exercise training in
dogs
J Appl Physiol **49**, 759-768
***Animal, Exercise programme,
Intervention***

231.2/26   **Tharp, G.D. & Wagner,
C.T.**   (1982)
Chronic exercise and cardiac
vascularization
Eur J Appl Physiol **48**, 97-104
***Animal, Exercise programme,
Intervention***

231.2/27   **Tubau, J., Witztum, K.,
Froelicher, V., Jensen, D., Atwood, E.,
McKirnan, M.D., Reynolds, J. &
Ashburn, W.**   (1982)
Noninvasive assessment of changes in
myocardial perfusion and ventricular
performance following exercise training
Am Heart J **104**, 238-248
***Adult, CARDIAC PERFORMANCE,
Exercise programme, Intervention, Male,
SECONDARY PREVENTION***

231.2/28   **Verani, M.S., Hartung, G.H.,
Hoepfel-Harris, J., Welton, D.E., Pratt,
C.M. & Miller, R.R.**   (1981)
Effects of exercise training on left
ventricular performance and myocardial
perfusion in patients with coronary artery
disease
Am J Cardiol **47**, 797-803
***Adult, AEROBIC CAPACITY,
CARDIAC PERFORMANCE, Exercise
programme, Intervention, Male,
SECONDARY PREVENTION***

231.2/29   **Wolf, R. & Lichtlen, P.**   (1986)
Coronary collaterals: protective effects
during physical training? In: Sports
Cardiology Exercise in health and
cardiovascular disease (Eds) Fagard,
R.H. & Bekaert, I.E.
Martinus Nijhoff 181-187
***Adult, Exercise programme, HEART
FUNCTION TEST, Intervention, Male,
SECONDARY PREVENTION***

231.2/30   **Wyatt, H.L. & Mitchell,
J.**   (1978)
Influences of physical conditioning and
deconditioning on coronary vasculature
of dogs
J Appl Physiol **45**, 619-625
***Animal, CARDIAC PERFORMANCE,
Exercise programme, Intervention***

231.3   COAGULATION

KEYWORDS are listed in the appendix in addition the following specific keywords have been used in this section:

> Fibrin
> Fibrinolysis
> Immune response
> Platelets
> Prostaglandins

Summary of evidence: exercise helps prevent coronary heart disease, stroke, deep vein thrombosis.

THE PROBLEM

Under certain circumstances, blood forms internal clots or thrombi and thus, depending on the site, causes stroke, myocardial infarction or deep vein thromboses (DVT). These are common causes of morbidity and mortality in both men and women. The recognition that DVT is one of the health hazards of the inactivity of bedrest has already led to early mobilisation of patients. Does exercise reduce the tendency for blood to clot?

SCOPE

This section deals with the effects of exercise on the large number of factors involved in blood clotting. Some of these factors affect the formation of clots and some their dissolution.

METHODOLOGICAL DIFFICULTIES

The multiplicity of interacting factors makes it difficult to achieve controlled studies which lead to clear conclusions.

EVIDENCE

The effects of exercise are not simple; some factors promote clotting while others decrease it; fibrinolytic factors also change. The effects during exercise may differ from those found after exercise. However the overall effect appears to be a reduction in the tendency of the blood to clot during exercise and for some time afterwards thus exercise taken regularly may be of long term benefit. This may be one of the mechanisms whereby exercise reduces the incidence of coronary heart disease (see 231 and 231.1)

231.3/1   (1981)
   Blood and sports (Editorial)
   Lancet **ii,** 847-848
   Review

231.3/2   **Andrew, M., Carter, C., O'Brodovich, H. & Heigenhauser, G.**   (1986)
   Increases in factor VIII complex and fibrinolytic activity are dependent on exercise intensity
   J Appl Physiol **60,** 1917-1922
   Acute exercise, Adult, Fibrinolysis, Male, Vigorous

231.3/3   **Baele, G., Bogaerts, H., Clement, D.L., Pannier, R. & Barbier, F.**   (1981)
   Platelet activation during treadmill exercise in patients with chronic peripheral arterial disease
   Thromb Res **23,** 215-223
   Acute exercise, Adult, ARTERIES, HAZARDS-CVS, Platelets

231.3/4   **Cash, J.D.**   (1966)
   Effect of moderate exercise on the fibrinolytic system in normal young men and women
   Br Med J **2,** 502-506.
   Acute exercise, Adult, Female, Fibrinolysis, Male, MENSTRUAL FUNCTION

231.3/5   **Collen, D., Semeraro, N., Tricot, J.P. & Vermylen, J.** (1977)
Turnover of fibrinogen, plasminogen, and prothrombin during exercise in man
J Appl Physiol **42**, 865-873
Acute exercise, Adult, Female, Fibrinolysis, Male

231.3/6   **Davidson, R.J.L., Robertson, J.D., Galea, G. & Maughan, R.J.** (1987)
Hematological changes associated with marathon running
Int J Sports Med **8**, 19-25
Acute exercise, Adult, ARTERIES, Female, Hazards, Leisure activity, Male, Marathon, Platelets, Running

231.3/7   **Davis, G.L., Abildgaard, C.F., Bernauer, E.M. & Britton, M.** (1976)
Fibrinolytic and hemostatic changes during and after maximal exercise in males
J Appl Physiol **40**, 287-292
Acute exercise, Adult, AEROBIC CAPACITY, Fibrinolysis, Male, Platelets, Vigorous

231.3/8   **Dimitriadou, C., Dessypris, A., Louizou, C. & Mandalaki, T.** (1977)
Marathon run II: Effects on platelet aggregation
Thromb Haemostasis **37**, 451
Acute exercise, Adult, Male, Marathon, Platelets, Running, Vigorous

231.3/9   **Dischinger, P., Tyroler, H.A., McDonagh, R. Jr. & Hames, C.G.** (1980)
Blood fibrinolytic activity, social class and habitual physical activity – I. A study of black and white men in Evans County Georgia
J Chron Dis **33**, 283-290
Adult, BLOOD PRESSURE, Body composition, Comparative, Fibrinolysis, LIPIDS, Male, Occupational activity,

231.3/10   **Drygas, W.K.**
Changes in blood platelet function and fibrolytic activity in response to moderate exhaustive and prolonged exercise in normal men
Proceedings of IVth Eur Congr Sports Med, Praha
Acute exercise, Adult, Fibrinolysis, Male, Platelets, Vigorous

231.3/11   **Dufaux, B., Order, U. & Hollman, W.** (1984)
Can physical exercise induce an effective fibrinolysis
Thromb Res **36**, 37-43
Adult, Athlete, Comparative, Elderly, Female, Fibrinolysis, Intervention, Leisure activity, Male, Running

231.3/12   **Egeberg, O.** (1963)
The effect of exercise on the blood clotting system
Scand J clin Lab Invest **15**, 8-13
Acute exercise, Adult, Fibrinolysis, Male

231.3/13   **Eichner, E.** (1984)
Platelets, carotids, and coronaries. Critique on antithrombotic role of antiplatelet agents, exercise and certain diets
Am J Med **77**, 513-523
Platelets, Review

231.3/14   **Ferguson, E.W., Barr, C.F. & Bernier, L.L.** (1979)
Fibrinogenolysis and fibrinolysis with strenuous exercise
J Appl Physiol **47**, 1157-1161
Acute exercise, Adult, Fibrinolysis, Male, Vigorous

231.3/15   **Ferguson, E.W., Bernier, L.L., Banta, G.R., Yu-Yahiro, J. & Schoomaker, E.B.** (1987)
Effects of exercise and conditioning on clotting and fibrinolytic activity in men
J Appl Physiol **62**, 1416-1421
Acute exercise, Adult, Comparative, Fibrinolysis, Leisure activity, Male, Vigorous

231.3/16   Gimenez, M., Mohan-Kumar, T., Humbert, J.C., De Talance, N., Teboul, M. & Arino Belenguer, F.J.   (1987)
Training and leucocyte, lymphocyte and platelet response to dynamic exercise
J Sports Med Phys Fitness **27**, 172-177
Acute exercise, Adult, AEROBIC CAPACITY, Comparative, Endocrine, GENERAL HEALTH, Immune response, Male, Platelets

231.3/17   Gimenez, M., Mohan-Kumar, T., Humbert, J. C., De Talance, N. & Buisine, J.   (1986)
Leukocyte, lymphocyte and platelet response to dynamic exercise. Duration or intensity effect?
Eur J Appl Physiol **55**, 465-470
Acute exercise, Adult, Endocrine, Immune system, Male, Platelets, Vigorous

231.3/18   Green, L.H., Seroppian, E. & Handin, R.I.   (1980)
Platelet activation during exercise-induced myocardial ischemia
N Engl J Med **302**, 193-197
Acute exercise, Adult, HAZARDS-CVS, Male, Platelets, SECONDARY PREVENTION

231.3/19   Gurewich, V., Lipinska, I. & Lipinski, B.   (1974)
Exercise-induced fibrinolytic activity and its effect on the degradation of fibrinogen, fibrin and fibrin-like precipitates
Thromb Res **5**, 647-656.
Acute exercise, Adult, Fibrinolysis, Male, Vigorous

231.3/20   Hawkey, C.M., Britton, B.J., Wood, W.G., Peele, M. & Irving, M.H.   (1975)
Changes in blood catecholamine levels and blood coagulation and fibrinolytic activity in response to graded exercise in man
Br J Haematol **29**, 377-384.
Acute exercise, Adult, Endocrine, Fibrinolysis, Male, Platelets

231.3/21   Hedlin, A.M., Loh, A.Y. & Osmond, D.H.   (1979)
Fibrinolysis, renin activity, and prorenin in normal women: Effects of exercise and oral contraceptive medication
J Clin Endocrinol Metab **49**, 663
Acute exercise, Adult, Female, Fibrinolysis

231.3/22   Huisveld, I.A., Kluft, C., Hospers, A.J.H., Bernink, M.J.E., Erich, W.B.M. & Bouma, B.N.   (1984)
Effect of exercise and oral contraceptive agents on fibrolytic potential in trained females
J Appl Physiol **56**, 906-913
Acute exercise, Adult, AEROBIC CAPACITY, Body composition, Comparative, Female, Fibrinolysis, REPRODUCTIVE HORMONES, Vigorous

231.3/23   Hyers, T.M., Martin, B.J., Pratt, D.S., Dreisin, R.B. & Franks, J.J.   (1980)
Enhanced thrombin and plasmin activity with exercise in man
J Appl Physiol **48**, 821-825
Acute exercise, Adult, AEROBIC CAPACITY, Fibrinolysis, Male, Platelets

231.3/24   Iatridis, S.G. & Ferguson, J.H.   (1963)
Effect of physical exercise on blood clotting and fibrinolysis
J Appl Physiol **18**, 337-344.
Acute exercise, Adult, Fibrinolysis, Male

231.3/25   Joye, J., DeMaria, A.N., Giddens, J., Kaku, R., Amsterdam, E.A., Mason, D.T. & Lee, G.   (1978)
Exercise induced decreases in platelet aggregation: comparison of normals and coronary patients showing similar physical activity related effects
Am J Cardiol **41**, 432
Acute exercise, Adult, Comparative, Male, Platelets, SECONDARY PREVENTION

231.3/26   **Karp, J.E. & Bell, W.R.**   (1974)
Fibrinogen-fibrin degradation products
and fibrinolysis following exercise in
humans
Am J Physiol **227**, 1212-1215.
Acute exercise, Adult, Athlete,
Fibrinolysis, Male, Vigorous

231.3/27   **Keber, D., Stegnar, M., Keber, I.**
& Accetto, B.   (1979)
Influence of moderate and strenuous
daily physical activity on fibrinolytic
activity of blood: Possibility of
plaminogen activator stores depletion
Thrombo Haemostasis **41**, 745-755
Acute exercise, Adult, Fibrinolysis,
Intervention, Leisure activity, Male,
Vigorous

231.3/28   **Khanna, P.K., Seth ,H.N.,**
Balasubramanian, V. & Hoon,
R.S.   (1975)
Effect of submaximal exercise on
fibrinolytic activity in ischemic heart
disease
Br Heart J **37**, 1273-1276.
Acute exercise, Adult, Comparative,
Fibrinolysis, Male, Platelets,
SECONDARY PREVENTION

231.3/29   **Knudsen, J.B., Brodthagen, U.,**
Gormsen, J., Jordal, R. Norregaard-
Hansen, K. & Paulev, P-E.   (1982)
Platelet function and fibrolytic activity
following distance running
Scand J Haematol **29**, 425-430
Acute exercise, Adult, Comparative,
Fibrinolysis, Male, Marathon, Platelets,
Running

231.3/30   **Kopitsky, R.G., Switzer, M.E.P.**
Williams, R.S. & McKee, P.A.   (1983)
The basis for the increase in factor VIII
procoagulant activity during exercise
Thromb Haemostasis **49**, 53-57
Acute exercise, Adult, Male

231.3/31   **Kovalcikova, J.**   (1975)
Effect of physical exercise on the
fibrinolytic activity of serum of healthy
pregnant women
Cesk Gynekol **40**, 125-127
Acute exercise, Adult, Female,
Fibrinolysis, PREGNANCY

231.3/32   **Lockette, W., McCurdy, R.,**
Smith, S. & Carretero, O.   (1987)
Endurance training and human alpha 2-
adrenergic receptors on platelets
Med Sci Sports Exerc **19**, 7-10
Adult, Athlete, Comparative, Endocrine,
Leisure activity, Platelets, Running

231.3/33   **Mant, M.J., Kappagoda, C. T. &**
Quinlan, J.   (1984)
Lack of effect of exercise on platelet
activation and platelet reactivity
J Appl Physiol **57**, 1333-1337
Acute exercise, Adult, Male, Platelets,
Vigorous

231.3/34   **Marsh, N.A. & Gaffney,**
P.J.   (1980)
Some observations on the release of
intrinsic and extrinsic plasminogen
activators during exercise in man
Haemostasis **9**, 238-247
Acute exercise, Adult

231.3/35   **Marsh, N.A. & Gaffney,**
P.J.   (1982)
Exercise-induced fibrinolysis – fact or
fiction?
Thromb Haemostasis **48**, 201-203
Acute exercise, Adult, Fibrinolysis, Male

231.3/36   **Masuhara, M., Kami, K.,**
Umebayashi, K. & Tatsumi, N.   (1987)
Effect of strenuous exercise on platelets
J Sports Med Phys Fitness **27**, 178-183
Acute exercise, Adult, AEROBIC
CAPACITY, Endocrine, Male, Platelets

231.3/37   Meade,T.W., Brozovic,M.,
Chakrabarti, R.R., Haines, A.P., Imeson,
J.D., Mellows, S., Miller, G.J., North,
W.R.S., Stirling, Y. & Thompson,
S.G.   (1986)
Haemostatic function and ischaemic
heart disease: Principal results of the
Northwick Park Heart Study
Lancet ii, 533-537
Adult, BLOOD PRESSURE, Cohort,
EPIDEMIOLOGY-CHD, Fibrin,
LIPIDS, Male

231.3/38   Meade,T.W., Chakrabarti, R.R.,
Haines, A.P., Miller, G.J., North, W.R.S.
& Stirling, Y.   (1979)
Characteristics affecting fibrinolytic
activity and plasma fibrinogen
concentrations
Br Med J 1, 153-156
Acute exercise, Adult, Cohort,
EPIDEMIOLOGY-CHD, Female,
Fibrinolysis, Male

231.3/39   Menon, I.S., Burke, F. & Dewar,
H.A.   (1967)
Effect of strenuous and graded exercise
on fibrinolytic activity
Lancet i, 700-702.
Acute exercise, Adult, Athlete,
Comparative, Fibrinolysis, Vigorous

231.3/40   Moxley, R.T., Brakman, P. &
Astrup, T.   (1970)
Resting levels of fibrinolysis in blood in
inactive and exercising men
J Appl Physiol 28, 549-552.
Adult, Comparative, Fibrinolysis, Leisure
activity, Male

231.3/41   Myreng, Y., Lande, K., Kjeldsen,
S.E., Eide, I., Grendahl, H. & Gjesdal,
K.   (1987)
Increase in beta-thromboglobulin during
exercise
Thromb Res 48, 111-115
Acute exercise, Adult, Endocrine,
SECONDARY PREVENTION

231.3/42   Ogston, D. & Fullerton,
H.W.   (1961)
Changes in fibrinolytic activity produced
by physical activity
Lancet ii, 730-733.
Acute exercise, Adult, Comparative,
Female, Fibrinolysis, Male

231.3/43   Ohri, V.C., Chatterji, J.C., Das,
B.K., Akhtar, M., Tewari, S.C.,
Bhattacharji, P. & Behl, A.   (1983)
Effect of submaximal exercise on
haemocrit, platelet count, platelet
aggregation and blood fibrinogen levels
J Sports Med Phys Fitness 23, 127-130
Acute exercise, Adult, Fibrinolysis, Male,
Platelets,

231.3/44   Rauramaa, R., Salonen, J.T.,
Seppanen, K., Salonen, R., Venalainen,
J.M., Ihanainen, M. & Rissanen,
V.   (1986)
Inhibition of platelet aggregability by
moderate-intensity physical exercise: a
randomized clinical trial in overweight
men
Circulation 74, 939-944
Adult, Exercise programme, Intervention,
Male, Platelets, Weight

231.3/45   Ritter, J.M., Barrow, S.E., Blair,
I.A., & Dollery, C.T.   (1983)
Release of prostacyclin in vivo and its
role in man
Lancet i, 317-319
Acute exercise, Adult, Male, Platelets,
Prostaglandins, Running, Vigorous

231.3/46   Rocker, L., Drygas, W.K. &
Heyduck, B.   (1986)
Blood platelet activation and increase in
thrombin activity following a marathon
race
Eur J Appl Physiol 55, 374-80
Acute exercise, Adult, Fibrin,
HAZARDS-CVS, Leisure activity, Male,
Marathon, Platelets, Running, Vigorous

231.3/47 **Rosing, D.R., Brakman, P., Redwood, D.R., Goldstein, R.E., Beiser, G.D., Astrup, T. & Epstein, S.E.** (1970)
Blood fibrinolytic activity in man. Diurnal variation and the response to varying intensities of exercise
Circulation Res **27**, 171-184
Acute exercise, Adult, Female, Fibrinolysis, Male, Vigorous

231.3/48 **Sarajas, H.S.S.** (1976)
Reaction patterns of blood platelets in exercise
Adv Cardiol **18**, 176-195.
Review

231.3/49 **Scheele, K. & Muller, K.** (1980)
Acute cardiac death caused by an increase of platelet aggregation during and after maximal physical test. In: Sports Cardiology (Eds.) Lubrich, T. & Venerando, A.
Aulo Gaggi Publisher, Bologna 449-454
Acute exercise, Adult, HAZARDS-CVS, Male, Platelets

231.3/50 **Siess, W., Lorenz, R., Roth, P. & Weber, P.C.** (1982)
Plasma catecholamines, platelet aggregation and associated thromboxane formation after physical exercise, smoking or norepinephrine infusion
Circulation **66**, 44-48
Acute exercise, Adult, Endocrine, Male, Platelets

231.3/51 **Szczeklik, A., Dischinger, P., Kueppers, F., Tyroler, H.A., Hames, C.G., Cassel, J.C. & Creagan, S.** (1980)
Blood fibrinolytic activity, social class and habitual physical activity – II. A study of black and white men southern Georgia
J Chron Dis **33**, 291-299
Adult, BLOOD PRESSURE, Body composition, Comparative, Fibrinolysis, LIPIDS, Male, Leisure activity,

231.3/52 **Vogt, A., Hofmann, V. & Straub, P.W** (1979)
Lack of fibrin formation in exercise induced coagulation
Am J Physiol **236**, H577-H579
Acute exercise, Adult, Fibrinolysis, Male, Vigorous

231.3/53 **Williams, R.S., Logue, E.E., Lewis, J.L., Barton, T., Stead, N.W., Wallace, A.G. & Pizzo, S.V.** (1980)
Physical conditioning augments the fibrinolytic response to venous occlusion in healthy adults
N Engl J Med **302**, 987-991
Adult, Exercise programme, Female, Fibrinolysis, Intervention, LIPIDS, Male

231.4 LIPIDS

KEYWORDS are listed in the appendix in addition the following specific keywords have been used in this section:

Apoproteins
HDL (High density lipoproteins)
Hyperlipidaemia
LDL (Low density lipoproteins)
Lipolytic enzymes
Myocardial infarction
T-cholesterol (total cholesterol measurements)
Triglycerides
Uric acid

Summary of evidence: exercise improves lipid profiles which may reduce risk of coronary heart disease

THE PROBLEM

High levels of cholesterol in blood have long been recognised as the most important risk factor in the development of coronary heart disease (see 231 and 231.1). The blood concentration of cholesterol represents the resultant of input from metabolic processes and diet on the one hand and catabolism in the liver on the other. The resulting levels are controlled in part by genetic factors and it has been found difficult to change them either by dietary manipulation or exercise. Recently it has become clear that it is the way in which cholesterol and other fats are transported by carrier-proteins in the blood which is crucial. Attention has turned to the effects of exercise on the ratio in plasma between two classes of these carrier-proteins, high and low density lipoproteins (HDL/LDL). Higher ratios are known to be associated with a lower incidence of coronary heart disease (see 231.1)

SCOPE

This section contains references to the effects of exercise on the level of lipid carrying blood proteins of varying density and the ratios between them. They are mainly studies in middle-aged men, but both sedentary and active groups are represented. There are a number of studies on the acute effects of exercise on lipid profiles.

METHODOLOGICAL DIFFICULTIES

Studies report the measurements of several different sub-fractions of lipoproteins. It has proved difficult to establish which of the different sub-fractions is critically linked to the natural history of arterial wall damage by cholesterol. Studies are needed with a control group which can account for effects of dietary change or seasonal variation, baseline data which has been accurately assessed, a starting level for HDL/LDL which is undesirably high (otherwise no changes will be seen) and an activity level which is undesirably low (so that it can be increased by the exercise programme).

EVIDENCE

The least amount of vigorous exercise which has been observed to improve lipid profiles and produce a significant increase in the HDL/LDL ratio is a programme which involved running 8 miles a week. The improvement appears to be related to the amount and intensity of the exercise a beneficial effect from more modest amounts has not been excluded. The improvement occurs due to an increase in the plasma levels of HDL, and a decrease in LDL. Cholesterol levels sometimes decrease but not consistently. These changes are associated with a reduced risk of coronary heart disease which may be due to a lower rate of deposition of fatty material in the walls of arteries.

231.4/1   **Adner, M.M. & Castelli, W.P.**   (1980)
Elevated high-density lipoprotein levels in marathon runners
J Am Med Ass **243**, 534-536
Adult, BLOOD PRESSURE, Comparative, HDL, LDL, Leisure activity, Marathon, Running, T-Cholesterol, Triglycerides, Vigorous, Weight

231.4/2   **Allen, D., Willcox, K.K., Teague-Baker, T.S., & Lei, K.Y.**   (1985)
Alterations in HDL lipoprotein and apolipoprotein profiles consequent to 20 weeks of aerobic training in older men
Med Sci Sports Exerc **17**, 275
Adult, AEROBIC CAPACITY, Apoproteins, Body composition, Exercise programme,. HDL, Intervention, LDL, Male, Running, T-cholesterol, Vigorous

231.4/3   **Arnold, J.D., Shephard, R.J. & Kakis, G.**   (1985)
Lipid profile, physical fitness, and job activity of Canadian postal workers
J Cardiopulmonary Rehabil **5**, 373-377
Adult, Occupational activity

231.4/4   **Baker, T.T., Allen, D., Lei, K.Y. & Willcox, K.K.**   (1986)
Alterations in lipid and protein profiles of plasma lipoproteins in middle-aged men consequent to an aerobic exercise program.
Metabolism **35**, 1037-1043
Adult, AEROBIC CAPACITY, Apoproteins, Body composition, Exercise programme, HDL, Intervention, LDL, Male, Running, Vigorous

231.4/5   **Ball, M. & Mann, J.I.**   (1986)
Apoproteins: predictors of coronary heart disease?
Br Med J **293**, 769-770
Review

231.4/6   **Ballantyne, D., Clark, R.S., & Ballantyne, F.C.**   (1981)
The effect of physical training on plasma lipids and lipoproteins
Clin Cardiol **4**, 1-4
Review

231.4/7   **Berg, A., Frey, I. & Keul, J.**   (1986)
Apoliprotein profile in healthy males and its relation to maximum aerobic capacity (MAC)
Clin Chim Acta **161**, 165-171
Adult, AEROBIC CAPACITY, Apoproteins, Male

231.4/8   **Blair, S.N., Cooper, K.H., Gibbons, L.W., Gettman, L.R., Lewis, S. & Goodyear, N.**   (1983)
Changes in coronary heart disease risk factors associated with increased treadmill time in 753 men
Am J Epidemiol **118**, 352-359
Adult, BLOOD PRESSURE, Cohort, HDL, Leisure activity, Male, T-Cholesterol, Triglycerides, Uric acid, Weight,

231.4/9   **Blair, S.N., Piserchia, P.V., Wilbur, C.S. & Crowder, J.H.**   (1986)
A public health intervention model for worksite health promotion
J Am Med Ass **255**, 921-926
Adult, AEROBIC CAPACITY, BLOOD PRESSURE, Body composition, Cohort, Female, HDL, Leisure activity, Male, T-cholesterol, Weight

231.4/10   **Brenes, G., Dearwater, S., Shapera R., LaPorte, R.E. & Collins, E.**   (1986)
High density lipoprotein cholesterol concentrations in physically active and sedentary spinal cord injured patients
Arch Phys Med Rehabil **67**, 445-450
Adult, Comparative, Female, Handicap, HDL, Inactivity, Leisure activity, Male, T-Cholesterol, Triglycerides, Vigorous

231.4/11   **Brownell, K.D., Bachorik, P.S., & Ayerle, R.S.**   (1982)
Changes in plasma lipid and lipoprotein levels in men and women after a program of moderate exercise
Circulation **65**, 477-484
Adult, Exercise programme, Female, HDL, Intervention, LDL, Male, T-Cholesterol, Triglycerides, Weight

231.4/12   **Brunner, D. & Lobl, K.**   (1958)
Serum cholesterol, electrophoretic lipid pattern, diet and coronary heart disease. A study in coronary patients and in healthy men of different origin and occupations in Israel
Ann Intern Med **49**, 732-750
Adult, Comparative, HDL, LDL, Male, Occupational activity, T-cholesterol

231.4/13   **Campbell, D.E.**   (1965)
Influence of several physical activities on serum cholesterol concentrations in young men
J Lipid Res **6**, 478-480.
Adult, Comparative, Intervention, Leisure activity, Male, Muscle strength, Running, T-Cholesterol

231.4/14   **Campbell, D.E. & Lumsden,T.B.**   (1967)
Serum cholesterol concentrations during physical training and during subsequent detraining
Am J Med Sci **253**, 155-162
Adult, Body composition, Exercise programme, Inactivity, Intervention, Male, T-cholesterol

231.4/15   **Cardus, D., McTaggart, W.G. & Ribas-Cardus, F.**   (1980)
Exercise training in ischemic heart disease: Effect on physical performance and plasma lipids, ACTH and cortisol
Arch Phys Med Rehabil **61**, 303-310
Adult, AEROBIC CAPACITY, BLOOD PRESSURE, Endocrine, Exercise programme, HDL, Intervention, LDL, Leisure activity, Male, SECONDARY PREVENTION, T-cholesterol, Triglycerides

231.4/16   **Casal, D.C., Leon, A.S., Moy, J.S., Shaw, G., McNally, C. & Hughes, J.**   (1983)
Effects of treadmill walking and stairclimbing on coronary risk factors
Med Sci Sports Exerc **15**, 149
Adult, AEROBIC CAPACITY, Body composition, BLOOD PRESSURE, Exercise programme, HDL, Intervention, Male, T-cholesterol, Triglycerides, Weight

231.4/17   **Castelli, W.P.**   (1979)
Exercise and high-density lipoproteins
J Am Med Ass **242**, 2217
Review

231.4/18   **Castelli, W.P., Garrison, R.J.,Wilson, P.W.F., Abbott R.D., Kalousdian, S. & Kannel, W.B.**   (1986)
Incidence of coronary heart disease and lipoprotein cholesterol levels. The Framingham Study
J Am Med Ass **256**, 2835-2838
Adult, BLOOD PRESSURE, Cohort, EPIDEMIOLOGY, Female, HDL, Male, T-Cholesterol, Weight

231.4/19   **Cauley, J.A., Kriska, A.M., LaPorte, R.E., Sandler, R.B. & Pambianco, G.**   (1987)
A two year randomized exercise trial in older women: effects on HDL-cholesterol
Atherosclerosis **66**, 247-258
Adult, BLOOD PRESSURE, Body composition, Customary activity, Female, HDL, Longitudinal, T-cholesterol, Triglycerides

231.4/20   **Cauley, J.A., La Porte, R.E., Sandler, R.B., Orchard, T.J., Slemenda, C.W., & Petrini, A.M.**   (1986)
The relationship of physical activity to high density lipoprotein cholesterol in postmenopausal women
J Chron Dis **39**, 687-697
Adult, Body composition, CARBOHYDRATE TOLERANCE, Customary activity, Female, HDL, Leisure activity, T-Cholesterol, Triglycerides

231.4/21   **Clarkson, P., Hintemister, R., Fillyaw, M. & Stylos, L.**   (1981)
High density lipoprotein cholesterol in young adult weight lifters, runners and untrained subjects
Hum Biol **53**, 251-257
Adult, Athlete, Comparative, HDL, Leisure activity, MUSCLE STRENGTH, Running, T-cholesterol

231.4/22   **Cook, T.C., Laporte, R.E., Washburn, R.A., Traven, N.D., Slemenda, C.W. & Metz, K.F.**   (1986)
Chronic low level physical activity as a determinant of high density lipoprotein cholesterol and subfractions
Med Sci Sports Exerc **18**, 653-657
Adult, HDL, Longitudinal, Male, Occupational activity, Weight

231.4/23   **Cooper, K.H., Pollock, M.L., Martin, R.P., White, S.R., Linnerud, A.C. & Jackson, A.**   (1976)
Physical fitness levels versus selected coronary risk factors. A cross-sectional study
J Am Med Ass **236**, 166-169
Adult, AEROBIC CAPACITY, BLOOD PRESSURE, Body composition, Comparative, HEART FUNCTION TEST, Male, RESPIRATORY FUNCTION, T-cholesterol, Triglycerides, Uric Acid

231.4/24   **Cowan, G.O.**   (1983)
Influence of exercise on high-density lipoprotein
Am J Cardiol **52**, 13B-16B
Adult, Exercise programme, HDL, Intervention, Male, Myocardial infarction, SECONDARY PREVENTION, T-Cholesterol, Vigorous

231.4/25   **Cullinane, E.M., Lazarus, B. & Thompson, P.D.**   (1981)
Acute effects of a single exercise session on serum lipids in untrained men
Clin Chim Acta **109**, 341-344
Acute exercise, Adult, Male, T-cholesterol

231.4/26   **Cullinane, E.M., Siconolfi, S., Saritelli, A. & Thompson, P.D.**   (1982)
Acute decrease in serum triglycerides with exercise: Is there a threshold for an exercise effect?
Metabolism **31**, 844-847
Acute exercise, Adult, AEROBIC CAPACITY, ANAEROBIC CAPACITY, Athlete, Comparative, Cycling, HDL, LDL, Male, T-cholesterol, Triglycerides, Vigorous

231.4/27   **Dressendorfer, R.H., Wade, C.E., Hornick, C. & Timmis, G.C.**   (1982)
High-density lipoprotein-cholesterol in marathon runners during a 20-day road race
J Am Med Ass **247**, 1715-1717
Acute exercise, Adult, Body composition, HDL, LDL, Male, Marathon, Running, T-cholesterol, Triglycerides, Vigorous

231.4/28   **Dufaux, B., Assmann, G. & Hollmann, W.**   (1982)
Plasma lipoproteins and physical activity
Int J Sports Med **3**, 58-60
Review

231.4/29   **Dufaux, B., Assmann, G., Schachten, H. & Hollmann, W.**   (1982)
The delayed effects of prolonged physical exercise and physical training on cholesterol level
Eur J Appl Physiol **48**, 25-29
Acute exercise, Adult, Exercise programme, HDL, Intervention, Male, Running, T-cholesterol

231.4/30   **Dufaux, B., Order, U., Müller, R & Hollmann, W.**   (1986)
Delayed effects of prolonged exercise on serum lipoproteins
Metabolism **35**, 105-109
Acute exercise, Adult, Apoproteins, HDL T-cholesterol, Triglycerides

231.4/31   Durstine, J.L., Miller, W.,
Farrell, S., Sherman, W.M. & Ivy,
J.L.   (1983)
Increases in HDl-cholesterol and the
HDL/LDL cholesterol ratio during
prolonged endurance exercise
Metabolism **32,** 993-997
Acute exercise, Adult, AEROBIC
CAPACITY, HDL, LDL, Male, T-
cholesterol, Triglycerides

231.4/32   Enger, S.C., Stromme, S.B. &
Refsum, H.E.   (1980)
High density lipoprotein cholesterol,
total cholesterol and triglycerides in
serum after a single exposure to
prolonged heavy exercise
Scand J clin Lab Invest **40,** 341-345
Acute exercise, Adult, HDL, LDL, Male,
T-Cholesterol, Triglycerides

231.4/33   Enger, S., Herbjørnsen, K.,
Erikssen, J., & Fretland A.   (1977)
High density lipoproteins (HDL) and
physical ability: the influence of physical
exercise, age and smoking on HDL-
cholesterol and the HDL-/ total
cholesterol ratio
Scand J clin Lab Invest **37,** 251-255
Adult, Comparative, Female, HDL,
Leisure activity, Male, T-cholesterol,
Triglycerides

231.4/34   Erkelens, D.W., Albers, J.J.,
Hazzard, W.R., Frederick, R.C. &
Bierman, E.L.   (1979)
High-density lipoprotein-cholesterol in
survivors of myocardial infarction
J Am Med Ass **242,** 2185-2189
Adult, Body composition, Comparative,
Exercise programme, HDL, Intervention,
LDL, Lipolytic enzymes, Male, Running,
SECONDARY PREVENTION, T-
cholesterol, Triglycerides, Weight

231.4/35   Faber, M. Benade, A.J. & van
Eck, M.   (1986)
Dietary intake, anthropometric
measurements, and blood lipid values in
weight training athletes (body builders)
Int J Sports Med **7,** 342-346
Adult, Athlete, Body compostion,
ENERGY BALANCE, MUSCLE
STRENGTH, T-cholesterol

231.4/36   Farrell, P.A. & Barboriak,
J.   (1980)
The time course of alterations in plasma
lipid and lipoproteins concentrations
during eight weeks of endurance training
Atherosclerosis **37,** 231.4-238
Adult, AEROBIC CAPACITY, Body
composition, Exercise programme, HDL,
Intervention, Running, T-Cholesterol,
Triglycerides, Weight

231.4/37   Farrell, P.A., Maksud, M.G.,
Pollock, M.L., Foster, C., Anholm, J.,
Hare, J. & Leon, A.S.   (1982)
A comparison of plasma cholesterol,
triglycerides, and high density
lipoprotein-cholesterol in speed skaters,
weightlifters and non-athletes
Eur J Appl Physiol **48,** 77-82
Adult, AEROBIC CAPACITY,
Comparative, HDL, Leisure activity,
Male, MUSCLE STRENGTH, T-
cholesterol, Triglycerides, Weight

231.4/38   Fitzgerald, O., Heffernan, A. &
McFarlane, R.   (1965)
Serum lipids and physical activity in
normal subjects
Clin Sci **28,** 83-89.
Acute exercise, Adult, Exercise
programme, Intervention, Male, T-
cholesterol

231.4/39   Folsom, A.R., Casperson, C.J., Taylor, H.L., Jacobs, D.R., Luepker, R.V., Gomez-Marin, O., Gillum, R.F. & Blackburn, H.   (1985)
Leisure time physical activity and its relationship to coronary risk factors in a population-based sample
Am J Epidemiol **121**, 570-579
Adult, BLOOD PRESSURE, Comparative, Female, HDL, Leisure activity, Male, MOOD, T-cholesterol, Vigorous, Weight

231.4/40   Førde, O.H., Thelle, D.S., Arnesen, E. & Mjøs, O.D.   (1986)
Distribution of high density lipoprotein cholesterol according to relative body weight, cigarette smoking and leisure time physical activity
Acta Med Scand **219**, 167-171
Adult, BLOOD PRESSURE, CARBOHYDRATE TOLERANCE, Comparative, Female, HDL, Leisure activity, Male, T-cholesterol, Weight

231.4/41   Frey, M.A.B., Doerr, B.M., Laubach, L.L., Mann, B.L. & Glueck, C.J.   (1982)
Exercise does not change high-density lipoprotein cholesterol in women after ten weeks of training
Metabolism **31**, 1142-1146
Adult, AEROBIC CAPACITY, Body composition, Exercise programme, Female, HDL, Intervention, LDL, T-Cholesterol, Triglycerides, Weight

231.4/42   Frey, M.A.B., Doerr, B.M., Shrivastava, L.S. & Glueck, C.J.   (1983)
Exercise training, sex hormones and lipoprotein relationships in man
J Appl Physiol **54**, 757-762
Adult, AEROBIC CAPACITY, ANAEROBIC CAPACITY, Body composition, Exercise programme, HDL, Intervention, LDL, Male, REPRODUCTIVE HORMONES, T-cholesterol, Triglycerides, Vigorous

231.4/43   Fripp, R.R. & Hodgson, J.L.   (1987)
Effect of resistive training on plasma lipid and lipoprotein levels in male adolescents
J Pediatr **111**, 926-931
AEROBIC CAPACITY, BLOOD PRESSURE, Body composition, Children, Exercise programme, HDL, Intervention, LDL, Male, T-cholesterol

231.4/44   Gale, D.G., Butts, N.K., Kirkendall, D. & Hosler, C.F.   (1982)
Effects of training on the blood lipids and lipoproteins of intercollegiate swimmers
Med Sci Sports Exerc **14**, 103
Adult, Exercise programme, Female, HDL, Intervention, Male, Swimming, T-Cholesterol, Triglycerides,

231.4/45   Garcia-Palmieri, M.R., Costas, R., Schiffman, J., Colon, A.A., Torres, R. & Nazario, E.   (1972)
Interrelationship of serum lipids with relative body weight, blood glucose and physical activity
Circulation **45**, 829-836
Adult, Comparative, ENERGY BALANCE, Male, Occupational activity, T-cholesterol, Triglycerides, Weight

231.4/46   Gibbons, L.W., Blair, S.N., Cooper, K.H. & Smith, M.   (1983)
Association between coronary heart disease risk factors and physical fitness in healthy adult women
Circulation **67**, 977-983
Adult, AEROBIC CAPACITY, BLOOD PRESSURE, Female, HDL, T-cholesterol, Triglycerides, Weight

231.4/47   Gillespie, W.J., Klein, E. &
Eagan-Bengston, E   (1983)
Modification of physiologic and
psychologic indices of coronary risk in
male employees in an aerobic exercise
program
Med Sci Sports Exerc **15**, 149
*Adult, AEROBIC CAPACITY, Body
composition, BLOOD PRESSURE,
Exercise programme, HDL, Intervention,
Male, MOOD, PERSONALITY, T-
cholesterol, Triglycerides, Vigorous*

231.4/48   Gilliam, T.B. & Burke,
M.B.   (1978)
Effects of exercise on serum lipids and
lipoproteins
Artery **4**, 203-213
*Children, Exercise programme, Female,
HDL, Intervention, T-Cholesterol*

231.4/49   Goldberg, A.P., Hagberg, J.M.,
Delmez, J.A., Haynes, M.E. & Harter,
H.R.   (1980)
Metabolic effects of exercise training in
hemodialysis patients
Kidney Int **18**, 754-761
*Adult, AEROBIC CAPACITY, BLOOD
PRESSURE, CARBOHYDRATE
TOLERANCE, Exercise programme,
HDL, Intervention, Kidney disease, LDL,
T-cholesterol, Triglycerides*

231.4/50   Gordon, D.J., Leon, A.S.,
Ekelund, L.-G., Sopko, G., Probstfield,
J.L., Rubenstein, C. & Sheffield,
L.T.   (1987)
Smoking, physical activity, and other
predictors of endurance and heart rate
response to exercise in asymptomatic
hypercholesterolemic men. The Lipid
Research Clinics Coronary Primary
Prevention Trial
Am J Epidemiol **125**, 587-600
*Acute exercise, Adult, BLOOD
PRESSURE, HDL, Hyperlipidaemia,
Male, T-cholesterol, Triglycerides,
Weight*

231.4/51   Gordon, D.J., Wiztum, J.L.,
Hunninghake, D., Gates, S. & Glueck,
C.J..   (1983)
Habitual physical activity and high
density lipoprotein cholesterol in men
with primary hypercholesterolemia
Circulation **67**, 512-520
*Adult, Cohort, HDL, Hyperlipidaemia,
LDL, Leisure activity, Male,
Occupational activity, T-cholesterol,
Triglycerides, Vigorous*

231.4/52   Gyntelberg, F., Brennan R.,
Holloszy, J.O., Schonfeld, G., Rennie,
M.J. & Weidman, S.W.   (1977)
Plasma triglyceride lowering by exercise
despite increased food intake in patients
with type IV hyperlipoproteinemia
Am J Clin Nutr **30**, 716-720
*Acute exercise, Adult, Endocrine,
Hyperlipidaemia, Male, T-cholesterol,
Triglycerides*

231.4/53   Hämäläinen, E., Tikkanen, H.,
Härkönen, M., Närveri, H. & Adlercreutz,
H.   (1987)
Serum lipoproteins, sex hormones and
sex hormone binding globulin in middle-
aged men of different physical fitness and
risk of coronary heart disease
Atherosclerosis **67**, 155-162
*Adult, Apoproteins, Comparative, HDL,
LDL, Leisure activity, Male,
REPRODUCTIVE HORMONES,
Running, SECONDARY
PREVENTION, T-cholesterol,
Triglycerides, Weight*

231.4/54   **Hartung, G.H., Farge, E.J. & Mitchell, R.E.**   (1981)
Effects of marathon running, jogging, and diet on coronary risk factors in middle-aged men
Prev Med **10**, 316-323
Adult, AEROBIC CAPACITY, BLOOD PRESSURE, Body composition, Comparative, HDL, Leisure activity, Male, Marathon, MOOD, Running, T-cholesterol, Triglycerides, Vigorous, Weight

231.4/55   **Hartung, G.H., Foreyt, J.P., Mitchell, R.E., Mitchell, J.G., Reeves, R.S. & Gotto, A.M.**   (1983)
Effect of alcohol intake on high density lipoprotein cholesterol levels in runners and inactive men
J Am Med Ass **249**, 747-750
Adult, Comparative, HDL, Leisure activity, Male, Marathon, Running, T-Cholesterol

231.4/56   **Hartung, G.H., Foreyt, J.P., Mitchell, R.E., Vlasek, I. & Gotto, A.M.**   (1980)
Relation of diet to HDL-cholesterol in middle-aged marathon runners, joggers and inactive men
N Engl J Med **302**, 357-361
Adult, BLOOD PRESSURE, Body composition, Comparative, LDL, Leisure activity, Male, Marathon, Running, T-cholesterol, Triglycerides, Weight

231.4/57   **Hartung, G.H., Jackson, A.S., North, S., Reeves, R.S., & Foreyt, J.P.**   (1985)
HDL cholesterol in professional golfers compared with runners and inactive men
Med Sci Sports Exerc **17**, 220
Adult, Athlete, Comparative, HDL, Leisure activity, Male, Running, T-Cholesterol, Triglycerides

231.4/58   **Hartung, G.H., Reeves, R.S., Sigurdson, A.,Traweek, M.S., Foreyt, J.P. & Blocker, W.P.**   (1983)
Effects of a low-fat diet and exercise on plasma lipoproteins and cardiac dysrhythmia in middle-aged men
Circulation (Suppl) **68**, III-226
Adult, CARDIAC PERFORMANCE, Comparative, HDL, LDL, Leisure activity, Male, Running, T-Cholesterol, Triglycerides,

231.4/59   **Hartung, G.H., Squires, W.G. & Gotto, A.M.**   (1981)
Effect of exercise training on plasma high-density lipoprotein cholesterol in coronary disease patients
Am Heart J **101**, 181-184
Adult, AEROBIC CAPACITY, Exercise programme, HDL, Intervention, LDL, Male, SECONDARY PREVENTION, T-cholesterol, Vigorous, Weight

231.4/60   **Hartung, G.H., Reeves, R.S., Foreyt, J.P., Patsch, W. & Gotto, A.M.**   (1986)
Effect of alcohol intake and exercise on plasma high-density lipoprotein cholesterol subfractions and apolipoprotein A-1 in women
Am J Cardiol **58**, 148-151
Adult, Apoproteins, Comparative, Female, HDL, LDL, Leisure activity, Running, T-cholesterol, Triglycerides, Weight

231.4/61   **Haskell, W.L.**   (1984)
Exercise-induced changes in plasma lipids and lipoproteins
Prev Med **13**, 23-36
Review

231.4/62   **Haskell, W.L.**   (1986)
The influence of exercise training on plasma lipids and lipoproteins in health and disease
Acta Med Scand (Suppl) **711**, 25-37
Review

231.4/63   Haskell, W.L., Taylor, H.L., Wood, P.D., Scrott, H. & Heiss, G.   (1980)
Strenuous physical activity, treadmill exercise test performance and high density lipoprotein cholesterol. The lipid research clinics program prevalence study
Circulation (Suppl 4) **62**, 53-61
Adult, Female, HDL, Leisure activity, Male, Vigorous, Weight

231.4/64   Herbert, P.N., Bernier, D.N., Cullinane, E.M., Edelstein, L., Kantor, M.A. & Thompson, P.D.   (1984)
High-density lipoprotein metabolism in runners and sedentary men
J Am Med Ass **252**, 1034-1037
Adult, AEROBIC CAPACITY, Apoproteins, Body composition, Comparative, HDL, Leisure activity, Lipolytic enzymes, Male, Running, T-cholesterol, Triglycerides, Weight

231.4/65   Hicks, A.L., MacDougall, J.D. & Muckle, T.J.   (1987)
Acute changes in high-density lipoprotein cholesterol with exercise of different intensities
J Appl Physiol **63**, 1956-1960
Acute exercise, Adult, Apoproteins, HDL, Male, T-Cholesterol, Triglycerides

231.4/66   Hietanen, E. (Ed.)   (1982)
Regulation of serum lipids by physical exercise
CRC Press, Boca Raton, Fl
Review

231.4/67   Hietanen, E., Hamalainen, H., Maki, J., Seppanen, A., Kallio, V. & Marniemi, J.   (1986)
Beta-blockers, diuretics and physical fitness as determinants of serum lipids in myocardial infarction patients
Scand J clin Lab Invest **46**, 97-106
Adult, Comparative, Female, HDL, Leisure activity, Male, Occupational activity, SECONDARY PREVENTION, T-cholesterol, Triglycerides

231.4/68   Higuchi, M. & Hashimoto, I.   (1982)
Effects of physical exercise on lipid metabolism in men maintained at constant weight
Med Sci Sports Exerc **14**, 113
Adult, AEROBIC CAPACITY, Apoproteins, Body composition, Exercise programme, HDL, Intervention, Male, Running, T-cholesterol, Triglycerides, Weight

231.4/69   Hoffman, A.A., Nelson, W.R. & Goss, F.A.   (1967)
Effects of an exercise program on plasma lipids of senior Air Force officers
Am J Cardiol **20**, 516-524.
Adult, HDL, Intervention, LDL, Leisure activity, Male, T-cholesterol, Triglycerides, Weight

231.4/70   Holloszy, J.O., Skinner, J.S., Toro, G. & Cureton, T.K.   (1964)
Effects of a six-month program of endurance exercise on the serum lipids of middle-aged men
Am J Cardiol **14**, 753-760
Adult, Intervention, Leisure Activity, Male, Running, T-cholesterol, Triglycerides, Weight

231.4/71   Holm, G., Björntorp, P. & Jagenburg, R.   (1978)
Carbohydrate, lipid, and amino acid metabolism following physical exercise in man
J Appl Physiol **45**, 128-131
Acute exercise, Adult, Body composition, CARBOHYDRATE TOLERANCE, ENERGY BALANCE, T-Cholesterol, Triglycerides

231.4/72   **Horby-Petersen, J., Grande, P. &
Christiansen, C.**   (1982)
Effect of physical training on serum lipids
and serum HDL cholesterol in young
men
Scand J clin Lab Invest **42**, 387-390
*Adult, AEROBIC CAPACITY, Exercise
programme, HDL, Intervention, Male, T-
cholesterol, Triglycerides, Weight*

231.4/73   **Hurley, B.F., Hagberg, J.M.,
Seals, D.R., Ehsani, A.A., Goldberg, A.P.
& Holloszy, J.O.**   (1987)
Glucose tolerance and lipid-lipoprotein
levels in middle-aged powerlifters
Clin Physiol **7**, 11-19
*Adult, AEROBIC CAPACITY, Body
composition, CARBOHYDRATE
TOLERANCE, Comparative, HDL,
LDL, Leisure activity, Male, MUSCLE
STRENGTH, PRIMARY
PREVENTION, Running, T-cholesterol,
Triglycerides,*

231.4/74   **Hurley, B.F., Seals, D.R.,
Hagberg, J.M., Goldberg, A.C., Ostrove,
S.M., Holloszy, J.O., Wiest, W.G. &
Goldberg, A.P.**   (1984)
High-density-lipoprotein cholesterol in
bodybuilders v powerlifters. Negative
effects of androgen use
J Am Med Ass **252**, 507-513
*Adult, Athlete, Body composition,
Comparative, Hazards, Male, MUSCLE
STRENGTH*

231.4/75   **Huttunen, J.K., Lansimiers, E.,
Voutilainen, E., Ehnholm, C., Hietanen,
E., Penttila, I., Siitonen, O. & Rauramaa,
R.**   (1979)
Effect of moderate physical exercise on
serum lipoproteins. A controlled trial
with special reference to serum high-
lipoproteins
Circulation **60**, 1220-1229
*Adult, AEROBIC CAPACITY,
Apoproteins, Exercise programme, HDL,
Intervention, LDL, Male, T-cholesterol,
Triglycerides, Weight*

231.4/76   **Israel, R.G., Davidson, P.C. &
Albrink, M.J.**   (1981)
Exercise effects on fitness, lipids, glucose
tolerance and insulin levels in young
adults
Arch Phys Med Rehabil **62**, 336-341
*Adult, BLOOD PRESSURE, Body
composition, CARBOHYDRATE
TOLERANCE, Endocrine, Exercise
programme, Intervention, Male, Running,
T-Cholesterol, Triglycerides*

231.4/77   **Jefferson, B.**   (1985)
Effects of exercise on blood lipids
Med Sci Sports Exerc **17**, 220
*Children, Comparative, Leisure, HDL,
LDL, Swimming, T-cholesterol,
Triglycerides,*

231.4/78   **Jobin, J., Lapien, P.J., Moorjani,
S., Fleury, L.A., Dagenais, G.R., Rochon,
J. & Robitaille, N.M.**   (1985)
Total weekly leisure energy expenditure
and HDL subfractions in free living
middle-aged men. Is rate of expenditure
important?
Med Sci Sports Exerc **17**, 220-221
*Adult, Comparative, HDL, Leisure
activity, LDL, Male, T-Cholesterol,
Triglycerides*

231.4/79   **Kantor, M.A., Cullinane, E.M.,
Sady, S.P., Herbert, P.N. & Thompson,
P.D.**   (1987)
Exercise acutely increases high density
lipoprotein-cholesterol and lipoprotein
lipase activity in trained and untrained
men
Metabolism **36**, 188-192
*Acute exercise, Adult, Comparative,
HDL, Lipolytic enzymes, Male,
Triglycerides, Vigorous*

231.4/80   Keys, A., Anderson, J.T., Aresu,
M., Biork, M., Brock, J.F., Bronte-
Stewart, B., Fidanza, F., Keys, M.F.,
Malmros, H., Poppi, A., Posteli, A.,
Swahn, B. & Del Vecchio, A.   (1956)
Physical activity and the diet in
populations differing in serum
cholesterol
J Clin Invest **35**, 1173-1181
*Adult, Comparative, EPIDEMIOLOGY,
LDL, Male, Occupational activity, T-
cholesterol*

231.4/81   Kiens, B., Jorgensen, I., Lewis, S.,
Jensen, G., Lithell, H., Vessby, B., Hoe, S.
& Schoner, P.   (1980)
Increased plasma HDL-cholesterol and
apo A-1 in sedentary middle-aged men
after physical conditioning
Europ J Clin Invest **10**, 203-209
*Adult, AEROBIC CAPACITY,
Apoproteins, BLOOD PRESSURE,
CARBOHYDRATE TOLERANCE,
Exercise programme, HDL, Intervention,
Male, T-cholesterol, Triglycerides,
Vigorous, Weight*

231.4/82   Kiens, B. & Lithell, H.   (1985)
Lipoprotein metabolism related to
adaptations in human skeletal muscle
Clin Physiol (Suppl) **5**, 108
*Adult, Exercise programme, HDL,
Intervention, LDL, Lipolytic enzymes,
Male, MUSCLE METABOLISM*

231.4/83   Kiens, B., Lithell, H. & Vessby,
B.   (1984)
Further increase in high density
lipoprotein in trained males after
enhanced training
Eur J Appl Physiol **52**, 426-430
*Adult, AEROBIC CAPACITY,
Apoproteins, Exercise programme, HDL,
Intervention, LDL, Male, T-cholesterol*

231.4/84   Kramsch, D.M., Aspen, A.J.,
Abramovitz, B.M., Kreimendahl, T. &
Hood, W.B.Jr.   (1981)
Reduction of coronary atherosclerosis by
moderate conditioning exercise in
monkeys on an atherogenic diet
N Engl Med J **305**, 1483-1489
*Animal, BLOOD PRESSURE,
CARDIAC PERFORMANCE,
Coronary heart disease, Exercise
programme, HDL, Intervention, LDL,
Triglycerides*

231.4/85   Krauss, R.M.   (1982)
Regulation of high density lipoprotein
levels
Med Clin N A **66**, 403-430
Review

231.4/86   Kuusela, P.J., Voutilainen, E.,
Kukkonen, K. & Rauramaa, R.   (1980)
Lipoprotein patterns in lumberjacks
Scand J Sports Sci **2**, 13-16
*Adult, AEROBIC CAPACITY, Body
composition, Comparative, HDL, LDL,
Lipolytic enzymes, Male, Occupational
activity, T-cholesterol, Triglycerides,
Vigorous*

231.4/87   Kuusi, T., Nikkilä, E.A.,
Saarinen, P., Varjo, P. & Laitinen,
L.A.   (1982)
Plasma high density lipoproteins HDL2,
HDL3, and postheparin plasma lipases in
relation to parameters of physical fitness
Atherosclerosis **41**, 209-219
*Adult, AEROBIC CAPACITY, Body
composition, CARBOHYDRATE
TOLERANCE, Endocrine, Exercise test,
HDL, LDL, Lipolytic enzymes, Male, T-
cholesterol, Triglycerides, Weight*

231.4/88   **Lampman, R.M., Santinga, J.T., Bassett, D.R. Mercer, N., Block, W.D., Flora, J.D., Foss, M.L. & Thorland, W.G.**   (1978)
Effectiveness of unsupervised and supervised high intensity physical training in normalizing serum lipids in men with type IV hyperlipoproteinemia
Circulation **57**, 172-180
Adult, AEROBIC CAPACITY, Body composition, Endocrine, Exercise programme, Hyperlipidaemia, Intervention, Leisure activity, Male, METABOLIC FUNCTION, T-Cholesterol, Triglycerides, Vigorous, Weight

231.4/89   **Lampman, R.M., Santinga, J.T., Hodge, M.F., Block, W.D., Flora, J.D. & Bassett, D.R.**   (1977)
Comparative effects of physical training and diet in normalizing serum lipids in men with type IV hyperlipoproteinemia.
Circulation **55**, 652
Adult, Body composition, Endocrine, Exercise programme, Hyperlipidaemia, Intervention, Leisure activity, Male, Metabolic Function, Running, T-Cholesterol, Triglycerides,

231.4/90   **LaRosa, J.C., Cleary, P., Muesing, R.A., Gorman, P., Hellerstein, H.K. & Naughton, J.**   (1982)
Effect of long-term moderate physical exercise on plasma lipoproteins: The National Exercise and Heart Disease Project
Arch Intern Med **142**, 2269-2274
Adult, Body composition, HDL, Intervention, LDL, Leisure activity, Male, SECONDARY PREVENTION, T-cholesterol, Triglycerides, Weight

231.4/91   **Lehtonen, A. & Viikari, J.**   (1978)
Serum triglycerides and cholesterol and serum high-density lipoprotein cholesterol in highly physically active men
Acta Med Scand **204**, 111-114
Adult, Comparative, Female, HDL, Hyperlipidaemia, LDL, Leisure activity, Male, Running, T-Cholesterol, Triglycerides, Vigorous, Weight

231.4/92   **Lehtonen, A. & Viikari, J.**   (1978)
The effect of vigorous physical activity at work on serum lipids with a special reference to serum high-density lipoprotein cholesterol
Acta Physiol Scand **104**, 117-121.
Adult, Comparative, HDL, LDL, Male, Occupational activity, T-Cholesterol, Triglycerides, Weight

231.4/93   **Lehtonen, A., Viikari, J. & Ehnholm, C.**   (1979)
The effect of exercise on high density (HDL) lipoprotein apoproteins
Acta Physiol Scand **106**, 487-488
Adult, Apoproteins, Athlete, Comparative, HDL, Leisure activity, Running, Vigorous

231.4/94   **Lennon, D., Stratman, F.W., Shrago, E., Nagle, F.J., Hanson, P.G., Madden, M. & Spennetta, T.**   (1983)
Total cholestrol and HDL-cholesterol changes during acute, moderate-intensity exercise in men and women
Metabolism **32**, 244-249
Acute exercise, Adult, AEROBIC CAPACITY, Comparative, Female, HDL, LDL, Male, T-cholesterol, Triglycerides

231.4/95 Linder, C.W., DuRant, R.H. & Mahoney, O.M. (1983)
The effect of physical conditioning on serum lipids and lipoproteins in white male adolescents
Med Sci Sports Exerc 15, 232-236
BLOOD PRESSURE, Body composition, Children, Exercise programme, HDL, Intervention, Leisure activity, LDL, Male, Running, T-Cholesterol, Triglycerides, Vigorous, Weight

231.4/96 Lipson, L.O., Bonow, R.O., Schaefer, E.J., Brewer, H.B. & Lindgren, F.T. (1980)
Effect of exercise conditioning on plasma high density lipoproteins and other lipoproteins
Atherosclerosis 37, 529-538
Adult, AEROBIC CAPACITY, Exercise programme, HDL, Intervention, LDL, T-cholesterol, Triglycerides, Weight

231.4/97 Lithell, H., Cedermark, M., Fröberg, J, Tesch, P. & Karlsson J. (1981)
Increase of lipoprotein-lipase activity in skeletal muscle during heavy exercise. Relation to epinephrine excretion
Metabolism 30, 1130-34
Adult, AEROBIC CAPACITY, Endocrine, Lipolytic enzymes, Male, MUSCLE METABOLISM, MUSCLE STRENGTH, Occupational activity, Triglycerides, Vigorous

231.4/98 Lithell, H., Örlander, J., Schéle, R., Sjördin, B. & Karlsson, J. (1979)
Lipoprotein lipase activity of human skeletal muscle and adipose tissue after intensive physical exercise
Acta Physiol Scand 107, 257-261
Acute exercise, Adult, AEROBIC CAPACITY, Endocrine, Lipolytic enzymes, Male, MUSCLE STRENGTH, T-cholesterol, Triglycerides

231.4/99 Lobstein, D.D., Ismail, A.H., & El-Naggar, A.M. (1982)
Circulating lipoprotein-cholesterol and multivariate adaptation to regular exercise training of middle-aged men
J Sports Med Phys Fitness 22, 440-449
Adult, AEROBIC CAPACITY, Exercise programme, HDL, Intervention, LDL, Male, T-cholesterol, Triglycerides

231.4/100 Logan, R.L., Riemersma, R.A., Thomson, M., Oliver, M.F., Olsson, A.G., Walldius, G., Rossner, S., Kaijser, L., Callmer, E., Carlson, L.A., Lockerbie, L. & Lutz, W. (1978)
Risk factors for ischaemic heart-disease in normal men aged 40. Edinburgh-Stockholm study
Lancet 1, 949-954
Adult, BLOOD PRESSURE, Body composition, CARBOHYDRATE TOLERANCE, Comparative, HDL, HEART FUNCTION TEST, LDL, Male, T-cholesterol, Triglycerides, Uric Acid, Weight

231.4/101 Marley, W.P., Smith, W.E., Linnerud, A.C., Sonner,W.H., Royster, C.L.& Chasson, A.L. (1974)
A five-year study of uric acid, cholesterol and selected fitness variables in professional men
N C Med J 35, 730-735.
Adult, Body composition, Exercise programme, Leisure activity, Longitudinal, Male, T-cholesterol

231.4/102 Marniemi, J., Dahlstrom, S., Kvist, M., Seppanen, A. & Hietanen, E. (1982)
Dependence of serum lipid and lecithin: Cholesterol acyltransferase levels on physical training in young men
Eur J Applied Physiol 49, 25-35
Adult, AEROBIC CAPACITY, Body composition, Comparative, HDL, Intervention, Leisure activity, Lipolytic enzymes, Male, Occupational activity, T-Cholesterol, Triglycerides

231.4/103   **Marniemi, J., Peltonen, P., Vuori, I. & Hietanen, E.**   (1980)
Lipoprotein lipase of human post-heparin plasma and adipose tissue in relation to physical training
Acta Physiol Scand **110**, 131-135
Adult, Comparative, Leisure activity, Lipolytic enzymes, Male, Vigorous

231.4/104   **Masarei, J.R.L., Pyke, J.E. & Pyke, F.S.**   (1982)
Physical fitness and plasma HDL cholesterol concentrations in male business executives
Atherosclerosis **42**, 77-83
Adult, BLOOD PRESSURE, Body composition, HDL, Male, RESPIRATORY FUNCTION, T-cholesterol, Triglycerides, Weight

231.4/105   **Melicher, F.**   (1965)
Plasma cholesterol and phospholipids in various occupational groups
J Atheroscler Res **5**, 432-435
Adult, Comparative, Occupational activity, T-Cholesterol

231.4/106   **Miller, N.E., Forde, D.H., Thelle, D.S. & Mjos, O.D.**   (1977)
The Tromso Heart Study; high density lipoprotein and coronary heart disease; a prospective case-control study
Lancet **i**, 965-968.
Adult, BLOOD PRESSURE, Case-control, EPIDEMIOLOGY, HDL, LDL, Male, T-cholesterol, Triglycerides

231.4/107   **Moll, M.E., Williams, R.S., Lester, R.M., Quarfordt, S.H. & Wallace, A.G.**   (1979)
Cholesterol metabolism in non-obese women: Failure of physical conditioning to alter levels of high density lipoprotein cholesterol
Atherosclerosis **34**, 159-166
Adult, Exercise programme, Female, HDL, Intervention, T-cholesterol

231.4/108   **Montoye, H.J., Block, W.D. & Gayle, R.**   (1978)
Maximal oxygen uptake and blood lipids
J Chron Dis **31**, 111-118.
Adult, AEROBIC CAPACITY, Body composition, Female, Male, T-Cholesterol, Triglycerides

231.4/109   **Montoye, H.J., Block, W.D., Metzner, H.L. & Keller, J.B.**   (1976)
Habitual physical activity and serum lipids: males, age 16-64 in a total community
J Chron Dis **29**, 697-709
Adult, Body composition, Children, Cohort, Elderly, Leisure activity, Male, Occupational activity, T-cholesterol, Triglycerides, Weight

231.4/110   **Montoye, H.J., Mikkelsen, W.M., Block, W.D. & Gayle, R.**   (1978)
Relationship of oxygen uptake capacity, serum uric acid and glucose tolerance in males and females, age 10-69
Am J Epidemiol **108**, 274-282
Acute exercise, Adult, AEROBIC CAPACITY, Body composition, CARBOHYDRATE TOLERANCE, Children, Female, Male, Uric acid, Vigorous, Weight

231.4/111   **Moore, C.E., Hartung, G.H., Mitchell, R.E., Kappus, C.M. & Hinderlitter, J.**   (1983)
The relationship of exercise and diet on high density lipoprotein cholesterol levels in women
Metabolism **32**, 189-96
Adult, Body composition, Comparative, Female, HDL, Leisure activity, LDL, Running, T-Cholesterol, Triglycerides,

231.4/112   Moore, R.A., Penfold, W.A.,
Simpson, R.D., Simpsom, R.W., Mann,
J.I. & Turner, R.C.   (1979)
High-density lipoprotein, lipid and
carbohydrate metabolism during
increasing fitness
Ann Clin Biochem **16**, 76-80
Adult, CARBOHYDRATE
TOLERANCE, Exercise programme,
HDL, Intervention, Male, T-cholesterol,
Triglycerides

231.4/113   Morgan, D.W., Cruise, R.J.,
Girardin, B.W., Lutz-Schneider, V.,
Morgan, D.H. & Wang, M.Q.   (1986)
HDL-C Concentrations in weight-
trained, endurance-trained, and
sedentary females
Phys Sports Med **14**, 166
Adult, Body composition, Comparative.
Female, Leisure activity

231.4/114   Myhre, K., Mjøs, O.D.,
Bjørsvik, G. & Strømme, S.B.   (1981)
Relationship of high density lipoprotein
cholesterol concentration to the duration
and intensity of endurance training
Scand J clin Lab Invest **41**, 303-309
Adult, Comparative, HDL, Intervention,
LDL, Leisure activity, T-cholesterol,
Triglycerides

231.4/115   Naughton, J. &
Balke,B.   (1964)
Physical working capacity in medical
personnel and the response of serum
cholesterol to acute exercise and to
training
Am J Med Sci **247**, 286-292
Acute exercise, Adult, BLOOD
PRESSURE, Comparative, Intervention,
Leisure activity, Male, T-cholesterol,
Weight

231.4/116   Naughton, J. & McCoy,
J.F.   (1966)
Observations on the relationship of
physical activity to the serum cholesterol
concentration of healthy men and cardiac
patients
J Chron Dis **19**, 727-733.
Adult, Exercise programme, Intervention,
Male, SECONDARY PREVENTION,
T-cholesterol, Weight

231.4/117   Nikkilå, E.A., Kuusi, T. &
Myllynen, P.   (1980)
High-density lipoprotein and
apolipoprotein A-1 during physical
inactivity
Atherosclerosis **37**, 457-462
Adult, Apoproteins, Comparative, Female,
Handicap, HDL, Inactivity, LDL, Male,
T-Cholesterol, Triglycerides,

231.4/118   Nikkilå, E.A., Taskinen, M-R.,
Rehunen, S. & Harkonen, M.   (1978)
Lipoprotein lipase activity in adipose
tissue and skeletal muscle of runners:
Relation to serum lipids
Metabolism **27**, 1661-1671
Adult, Athlete, Body composition,
Comparative, Female, Leisure activity,
Male, MUSCLE METABOLISM,
Running, Vigorous, Weight

231.4/119   Nye, E.R., Carlson, K., Kirstein,
P. & Rossner, S.   (1981)
Changes in high density lipoprotein
subfractions and other lipoproteins
induced by exercise
Clin Chim Acta **113**, 51-57
Adult, HDL

231.4/120   **Oehlsen, G. & Gaesser, G.A.** (1982)
Time course of changes in VO2 max, percent body fat and blood lipids during a seven-week, high intensity exercise program
Med Sci Sports Exerc **14**, 110
Adult, AEROBIC CAPACITY, Body composition, ENERGY BALANCE, Exercise programme, HDL, Intervention, LDL, Male, T-cholesterol, Triglycerides, Vigorous

231.4/121   **Paulev, P.-E.** (1984)
Exercise and risk factors for arteriosclerosis in 42 married couples followed over four years
J Chron Dis **37**, 545-553
Adult, AEROBIC CAPACITY, BLOOD PRESSURE, CARBOHYDRATE TOLERANCE, Exercise programme, Female, Leisure activity, Longitudinal, Male, Running, T-cholesterol, Triglycerides, Uric acid, Weight

231.4/122   **Pelletier, D.L. & Baker, P.T.** (1987)
Physical activity and plasma total- and HDL-cholesterol levels in Western Samoan men
Am J Clin Nutr **46**, 577-585
Adult, Body composition, Comparative, HDL, Leisure activity, Male, Occupational activity, T-cholesterol, Weight

231.4/123   **Peltonen, P., Marniemi, J., Hietanen, E., Vuori, I. & Ehnholm, C.** (1981)
Changes in serum lipids, lipoproteins, and hepatic releasable lipolytic enzymes during moderate physical training in man: A longitudinal study
Metabolism **30**, 518-526
Adult, CARBOHYDRATE TOLERANCE, HDL, Intervention, LDL, Leisure activity, Lipolytic enzymes, Male, T-cholesterol, Weight

231.4/124   **Perry, A.C., Tapp, J. & Weeks, L.** (1986)
The effects of interval aerobic training on plasma lipid fractions of male and post-menopausal sedentary faculty
J Sports Med Phys Fitness **26**, 186-193
Adult, AEROBIC CAPACITY, BLOOD PRESSURE, Body composition, Exercise programme, Female, HDL, Intervention, LDL, Male, T-cholesterol, Triglycerides

231.4/125   **Pérusse, L., LeBlanc, C., Tremblay, A., Allard, C., Theriault, G., Landry, F., Talbot, J. & Bouchard, C.** (1987)
Familial aggregation in physical fitness, coronary heart disease risk factors, and pulmonary function measurements
Prev Med **16**, 607-615
Adult, BLOOD PRESSURE, Body composition, Children, HDL, LDL, MUSCLE STRENGTH, RESPIRATORY FUNCTION, T-cholesterol, Triglycerides,

231.4/126   **Rauramaa, R., Salonen, J.T., Kukkonen-Harjula, K., Seppanen, K., Seppala, E., Vapaatalo, H. & Huttunen, J.** (1984)
Effects of mild physical exercise on serum lipoproteins and metabolites of arachidonic acid: a controlled randomised trial in middle age men
Br Med J **288**, 603-606
Adult, AEROBIC CAPACITY, COAGULATION, Endocrine, Exercise programme, HDL, Intervention, LDL, Male, T-cholesterol, Running, Weight

231.4/127   **Rotkis, T.C., Cote, R., Coyle, C. & Wilmore, J.H.** (1982)
Relationship between high-density lipoprotein cholesterol and weekly running mileage
J Cardiac Rehab **2**, 109-112
Adult, Exercise programme, Female, HDL, Intervention, Running, T-cholesterol, Weight

231.4/128   Rotkis, T.C., Stanforth, P.R., Boyden, T.W. & Wilmore, J.H.   (1982)
Cholesterol, HDL-C, and body composition changes in women during a 15-month training program
Med Sci Sports Exerc **14**, 106
Adult, Body composition, ENERGY BALANCE, Female, HDL, Intervention, Leisure activity, Running, T-cholesterol, Weight

231.4/129   Sady, S.P., Berg, K., Beal, D., Smith, J.L., Savage, M.P., Thomson, W.H. & Nutter, J.   (1984)
Aerobic fitness and serum high-density lipoprotein cholesterol in young children
Hum Biol **56**, 771-781
AEROBIC CAPACITY, Body composition, Children, Female, HDL, Male

231.4/130   Sady, S.P., Thompson, P.D., Cullinane, E.M., Kantor M.A., Domagala, E. & Herbert, P.N.   (1986)
Prolonged exercise increases the clearance of intravenous fat
Clin Res **34**, 553A.
Acute exercise, Adult, Apoproteins, HDL, LDL, Lipolytic enzymes, Male, Marathon, Running, Triglycerides

231.4/131   Sallis, J.F., Haskell, W.L., Fortmann, S.P., Wood, P.D. & Vranizan, K.M.   (1986)
Moderate-intensity physical activity and cardiovascular risk factors: The Stanford five-city project
Prev Med **15**, 561-568
Adult, BLOOD PRESSURE, Comparative, Customary activity, EPIDEMIOLOGY-CHD, Female, HDL, LDL, Male, T-cholesterol, Triglycerides, Vigorous, Weight

231.4/132   Sallis, J.F., Haskell, W.L., Wood, P.D., Fortmann, S.P. & Vranizan, K.M.   (1986)
Vigorous physical activity and cardiovascular risk factors in young adults
J Chron Dis **39**, 115-120
Adult, BLOOD PRESSURE, Comparative, Female, HDL, Intervention, LDL, Leisure activity, Male, Triglycerides, Vigorous, Weight,

231.4/133   Sallis, J.F., Patterson, T.L., Buono, M.J. & Nader, P.R.   (1988)
Relation of cardiovascular fitness and physical activity to cardiovascular disease risk factors in children and adults
Am J Epidemiol **127**, 933-941
Adult, BLOOD PRESSURE, AEROBIC CAPACITY, Children, Customary activity, HDL, Female, LDL, Leisure activity, Male, Weight

231.4/134   Salonen, J.T., Happonen, P., Salonen, R., Korhonen, H., Nissinen, A., Puska, P., Tuomilehto, J. & Vartiainen, E.   (1987)
Interdependence of associations of physical activity, smoking, and alcohol and coffee consumption with serum high-density lipoprotein and non-high-density lipoprotein cholesterol – A population study in Eastern Finland
Prev Med **16**, 647-658
Adult, Comparative, Female, HDL, Leisure activity, Male, Occupational activity, T-Cholesterol

231.4/135 Saris, W.H.M., Binkhorst, R.A., Cramwinckel, A.B., van Waesberghe, F. & van der Veen-Hezemans, A.M. (1978)
The relationship between working physical performance, daily physical activity, fatness, blood lipids and nutrition in schoolchildren. In: Children and Exercise IX (Eds) Berg, K. & Eriksson, B.O.
University Park Press, Baltimore
Body composition, Children, Customary activity, HDL, T-cholesterol, Triglycerides, Weight

231.4/136 Savage, M.P., Petratis, M.M., Thomson, W.H., Berg, K., Smith, J.L. & Sady, S.P. (1986)
Exercise training effects on serum lipids of prepubescent boys and adult men
Med Sci Sports Exerc **18**, 197-204
Adult, AEROBIC CAPACITY, Body composition, Children, Exercise programme, HDL, Intervention, LDL, Male, Running, T-cholesterol, Triglycerides, Vigorous, Weight

231.4/137 Schnabel, A. & Kindermann, W. (1982)
Effect of maximal oxygen uptake and different forms of physical training on serum lipoproteins
Eur J Appl Physiol **48**, 263-277
Adult, AEROBIC CAPACITY, CARDIAC PERFORMANCE, Comparative, HDL, LDL, Leisure activity, Male, MUSCLE STRENGTH, Running, T-cholesterol

231.4/138 Schuler, G., Schlierf, G., Wirth, A., Mautner, H.-P., Scheurlen, H., Thumm, M., Roth, H., Schwarz, F., Kohlmeier, M., Mehmel, H.C. & Kübler, W. (1988)
Low-fat diet and regular, supervised physical exercise in patients with symptomatic coronary artery disease: reduction of stress-induced myocardial ischemia
Circulation **77**, 172-181
Adult, Exercise programme, HDL, Hyperlipidaemia, Intervention, LDL, Male, Triglycerides, T-cholesterol, Vigorous

231.4/139 Schwartz, R.S. (1987)
The independent effects of dietary weight loss and aerobic training on the high density lipoproteins and apolipoprotein A-I concentrations in obese men
Metabolism **36**, 165-171
Adult, AEROBIC CAPACITY, Apoproteins, Body composition, ENERGY BALANCE, Exercise programme, HDL, Intervention, Male, T-Cholesterol, Triglycerides, Vigorous

231.4/140 Sedgwick, A.W., Brotherhood, J., Harris-Davidson, A., Taplin, R.E. & Thomas, D.W. (1980)
Long-term effects of physical training programme on risk factors for coronary heart disease in otherwise sedentary men
Br Med J **281**, 7-10
Adult, BLOOD PRESSURE, Exercise programme, Leisure activity, Longitudinal, Male, T-cholesterol, Triglycerides, Weight

231.4/141 Shephard, R.J., Youldon, P.E., Cox, M. & West, C. (1980)
Effects of a six-month industrial fitness programme on serum lipid concentrations
Atherosclerosis **35**, 277-286
Adult, AEROBIC CAPACITY, Body composition, Exercise programme, Female, HDL, Intervention, LDL, Male, Running, T-cholesterol, Triglycerides

231.4/142   **Shorey, R.A.L., Sewell, B. & O'Brien, M.**   (1976)
Efficacy of diet and exercise in the reduction of serum cholesterol and triglycerides in free living adult males
Am J Clin Nutr **29**, 512-521.
Adult, Hyperlipidaemia, Intervention, Leisure activity, Male, T-cholesterol, Triglycerides

231.4/143   **Skinner, E.R., Black, D. & Maughan, R. J.**   (1985)
Variability in the response of different male subjects to the effect of marathon running on the increase in plasma high density lipoprotein
Eur J Appl Physiol **54**, 488-493
Acute exercise, Adult, HDL, Male, Marathon, Running, T-cholesterol

231.4/144   **Skinner, E.R., Watt, C. & Maughan, R.J.**   (1987)
The acute effect of marathon running on plasma lipoproteins in female subjects
Eur J Appl Physiol **56**, 451-456
Acute exercise, Adult, Apoproteins, Female, HDL, LDL, Marathon, Running

231.4/145   **Smith, B.W., Sparrow, A.W., Heusner, W.W., Van Huss, W.D. & Conn, C.**   (1985)
Serum lipid profiles of pre-teenage swimmers
Med Sci Sports Exerc **17**, 220
Children, Comparative, HDL, LDL, Leisure activity, Swimming, T-cholesterol, Triglycerides

231.4/146   **Sopko, G., Leon, A.S., Jacobs, D.R., Foster, N., Moy, J., Kuba, K., Anderson, J.T., Casal, D., McNally, C. & Frantz, I.**   (1985)
The effects of exercise and weight loss on plasma lipids in young obese men
Metabolism **34**, 227-236
Adult, Body composition, ENERGY BALANCE, Exercise programme, HDL, Intervention, LDL, Male, T-cholesterol, Triglycerides, Weight

231.4/147   **Stamford, B.A., Matter, S., Fell, R.D., Sady, S.P., Cresanta, M.K. & Papanek, P.**   (1984)
Cigarette smoking, physical activity, and alcohol consumption: relationship to blood lipids and lipoproteins in premenopausal females
Metabolism **33**, 585-590
Adult, Body composition, Female, HDL, LDL, Leisure activity, T-cholesterol, Triglycerides

231.4/148   **Stamler, J., Wentworth, D. & Neaton, J.D.**   (1986)
Is relationship between serum cholesterol and risk of premature death from coronary heart disease continuous and graded? Findings in 356,222 primary screenees of the Multiple Risk Factor Intervention Trial (MRFIT)
J Am Med Ass **256**, 2823-2828
Adult, Cohort, EPIDEMIOLOGY, Male, T-cholesterol

231.4/149   **Streja, D. & Mymin, D.**   (1979)
Moderate exercise and high-density lipoprotein-cholesterol: observations during a cardiac rehabilitation program
J Am Med Ass **242**, 2190-2192
Adult, BLOOD PRESSURE, Body composition, CARBOHYDRATE TOLERANCE, Endocrine, Exercise programme, HDL, Intervention, LDL, Male, SECONDARY PREVENTION, T-Cholesterol, Triglycerides,

231.4/150   **Stubbe, I., Hansson, P., Gustafson, A. & Nilsson-Ehle, P.**   (1983)
Plasma lipoproteins and lipolytic enzyme activities during endurance training in sedentary men: changes in high- density lipoprotein subfractions and composition
Metabolism **32**, 1120-1128
Adult, AEROBIC CAPACITY, Apoproteins, Body composition, Exercise programme, HDL, LDL, Lipolytic enzymes, Male, MUSCLE METABOLISM, T-cholesterol, Weight

231.4/151   **Superko, H.R., Haskell, W.L. & Wood, P.D.**   (1985)
Modification of plasma cholesterol through exercise
Postgraduate Med **78**, 64-75
Review

231.4/152   **Sutherland, W.H.F. & Woodhouse, S.P.**   (1980)
Physical activity and plasma lipoprotein lipid concentrations in men
Atherosclerosis **37**, 285-292
Adult, AEROBIC CAPACITY, Body composition, HDL, Intervention, LDL, Leisure activity, Lipolytic enzymes, Male, Marathon, Running, T-Cholesterol, Vigorous

231.4/153   **Sutherland, W.H.F., Woodhouse, S.P., Williamson, S. & Smith, B.**   (1981)
Decreased and continued physical activity and plasma lipoprotein lipids in previously trained men
Atherosclerosis **39**, 307-311
Adult, Exercise programme, HDL, Inactivity, Intervention, LDL, Male, Marathon, Leisure activity, Running, T-cholesterol, Triglycerides

231.4/154   **Svedenhag, J., Lithell, H., Juhlin-Dannfelt, A. & Henriksson, J.**   (1983)
Increase in skeletal muscle lipoprotein lipase following endurance training in man
Atherosclerosis **49**, 203-207
Adult, AEROBIC CAPACITY, Exercise programme, Intervention, Lipolytic enzymes, Male, MUSCLE METABOLISM

231.4/155   **Swank, A.M., Robertson, R.J. & Deitrich, R.W.**   (1987)
The effect of acute exercise on high density lipoprotein-cholesterol and the subfractions in females
Atherosclerosis **63**, 187-192
Acute exercise, Adult, AEROBIC CAPACITY, Female, HDL, Triglycerides

231.4/156   **Tater, D., Leglise, D. & Person, B.**   (1987)
Lipoprotein status in professional football players after a period of vacation and one month after a new intensive training program
Horm Metab Res **19**, 24-27
Adult, Athlete, HDL, Inactivity, Intervention, LDL, Leisure activity, Male, Vigorous

231.4/157   **Thompson, P.D., Cullinane, E.M., Henderson, L.O. & Herbert, P.N.**   (1980)
Acute effects of prolonged exercise on serum lipids
Metabolism **29**, 662-665
Acute exercise, Adult, Apoproteins, HDL, Male, Marathon, Running, T-Cholesterol, Triglycerides

231.4/158   **Thompson, P.D., Kantor, M.A., Cullinane, E.M., Sady, S.P., Saritelli, A. & Herbert, P.N.**   (1986)
Postheparin plasma lipolytic activities in physically active and sedentary men after varying and repeated doses of intravenous heparin
Metabolism **35**, 999-1004
Adult, Comparative, Lipolytic enzymes, Male

231.4/159   **Thompson, P.D., Lazarus, B., Cullinane, E.M., Henderson, L.O., Musliner, T., Eshleman, R. & Herbert, P.N.**   (1983)
Exercise, diet or physical charcteristics as determinants of HDL-levels in endurance athletes
Atherosclerosis **46**, 333-339
Adult, Apoproteins, Body composition, Comparative, HDL, LDL, Leisure activity, Male, Running, T-cholesterol, Triglycerides, Vigorous, Weight,

231.4/160   **Thorland, W.G., & Gilliam, T.B.**   (1981)
Comparison of serum lipids between habitually high and low active pre-adolescent males
Med Sci Sports Exerc **13**, 316-321
Body composition, Children, Comparative, Customary activity, HDL, Leisure activity, Male, T-cholesterol, Triglycerides

231.4/161   **Tran, Z.V. & Weltman, A.**   (1985)
Differential effects of exercise on serum lipids and lipoprotein levels with changes in body weight. A Meta-analysis
J Am Med Ass **254**, 919-924
Review

231.4/162   **Tuomilehto, J., Marti, B., Salonen, J.T., Virtala, E., Lahti, T. & Puska, P.**   (1987)
Leisure-time physical activity in inversely related to risk factors for coronary heart disease in middle-aged Finnish men
Eur Heart J **8**, 1047-1055
Adult, BLOOD PRESSURE, HDL, Leisure activity, Male, T-cholesterol, Weight

231.4/163   **Vodak, P.A., Wood, P.D., Haskell, W.L. & Williams, P.T.**   (1980)
HDL-cholesterol and other plasma lipid and lipoprotein concentrations in middle-aged male and female tennis players
Metabolism **29**, 745
Adult, Comparative, Female, HDL, LDL, Leisure activity, Male, T-cholesterol, Triglycerides, Weight

231.4/164   **Walter, H.J., Hoffman, A., Connelly, P.A., Barrett, L.T. & Kost, K.L.**   (1985)
Primary prevention of chronic disease in childhood: Changes in risk factors after one year of intervention
Am J Epidemiol **122**, 772-781
BLOOD PRESSURE, Body composition, Children, Cohort, HDL, Leisure activity, T-cholesterol

231.4/165   **Watt, E.W., Wiley, J. & Fletcher, G.F.**   (1976)
Effect of dietary control and exercise training on daily food intake and serum lipids in post-myocardial infarction patients
Am J Clin Nutr **29**, 900-904
Adult, Exercise programme, Intervention, Male, SECONDARY PREVENTION, T-cholesterol, Triglycerides, Weight

231.4/166   **Weber, F., Barnard, R.J. & Roy, D.**   (1982)
Effects of an intensive, short-term nutrition and exercise program on individuals age 70 and older
Med Sci Sports Exerc **14**, 179-180
BLOOD PRESSURE, Elderly, Exercise programme, Intervention, T-cholesterol, Triglycerides, Weight

231.4/167   **Weltman, A., Henderson, N., Brammell, H., Chaffee, C. & Hume, G.**   (1982)
Relationship between training, serum lipids and menopause
Med Sci Sports Exerc **14**, 154
Adult, AEROBIC CAPACITY, Body composition, Exercise programme, Female, HDL, Intervention, REPRODUCTIVE HORMONES, T-cholesterol, Triglycerides, Weight

231.4/168   **Weltman, A., Janney, C., Rians, C.B., Strand, K., Berg, B., Tippitt, S., Wise, J., Cahill, B.R. & Katch, F.I.**   (1986)
The effects of hydraulic resistance strength training in pre-pubertal males
Med Sci Sports **6**, 629-638
Adult, Occupational activity

231.4/169   Weltman, A., Matter, S. &
Stamford, B.A.   (1980)
Caloric restriction and/or mild exercise:
Effects on serum lipids and body
composition
Am J Clin Nutr **33**, 1002-1009
*Adult, Body composition, ENERGY
BALANCE, Exercise programme, HDL,
Intervention, LDL, Male, T-cholesterol*

231.4/170   Williams, P.T., Haskell, W.L.,
Vranizan, M.A., Blair, S.N., Krauss,
R.M., Superko, H.R., Albers, J.J., Frey-
Hewitt, B.S. & Wood, P.D.   (1985)
Associations of resting heart rate with
concentrations of lipoprotein
subfractions in sedentary men
Circulation **71**, 441-449
*Adult, AEROBIC CAPACITY,
Apoproteins, HDL, Inactivity, LDL,
Male, T-cholesterol, Triglycerides*

231.4/171   Williams, P.T., Krauss, R.M.,
Wood, P.D., Lindgren, F.T., Giotas, C. &
Vranizan, K.M.   (1986)
Lipoprotein subfractions of runners and
sedentary men
Metabolism **35**, 45-52
*Adult, Comparative, HDL, LDL, Leisure
activity, Lipolytic enzymes, Male,
Running, Vigorous*

231.4/172   Williams, P.T., Wood, P.D.,
Haskell, W.L. & Vranizan, K.   (1982)
The effects of running mileage and
duration on plasma lipoprotein levels.
J Am Med Ass **247**, 2674-2679
*Adult, AEROBIC CAPACITY, Body
composition, Exercise programme, HDL,
Intervention, LDL, Male, Running, T-
Cholesterol, Triglycerides*

231.4/173   Williams, P.T., Wood, P.D.,
Krauss, R.M., Haskell, W.L., Vranizan,
K., Blair, S.N., Terry, R. & Farquhar,
J.W.   (1983)
Does weight loss cause the exercise
induced increase in plasma high density
lipoproteins?
Atherosclerosis **47**, 173-185
*Adult, Exercise programme, HDL,
Intervention, Male, Running, Weight*

231.4/174   Wirth, A., Diehm, C., Kohlmeier,
M., Heuck, C.C. & Vogel, I.   (1983)
Effect of prolonged exercise on serum
lipids and lipoproteins
Metabolism **32**, 669-672
*Acute exercise, Adult, Apoproteins, HDL,
Intervention, LDL, Leisure activity, Male,
T-cholesterol, Triglycerides, Vigorous,
Weight*

231.4/175   Wood, P.D., Haskell, W.L.,
Klein, H., Lewis, S., Stern, M.P. &
Farquhar, J.W.   (1976)
The distribution of plasma lipoproteins
in middle-aged male runners
Metabolism **25**, 1249-1257
*Adult, Body composition, Comparative,
HDL, LDL, Leisure activity, Male,
Running, T-cholesterol, Triglycerides,
Weight*

231.4/176   Wood, P.D. & Haskell,
W.L.   (1982)
Interrelation of physical activity and
nutrition on lipid metabolism. In: (Eds.)
White, P.L. & Mohdicka, T., Diet and
Exercise: Synergism in Health
Maintenance
American Medical Ass, Chicago, Illinois
39-47.
Review

231.4/177   **Wood, P.D., Haskell, W.L.,**
Blair, S.N., Williams, P.T., Krauss, R.M.,
Lindgren, F.T., Albers, J.J., Ho, P.H. &
Farquhar, J.W. (1983)
Increased exercise level and plasma
lipoprotein concentrations: A one-year,
randomized, controlled study in
sedentary, middle-aged men
Metabolism **32,** 31-39
Adult, AEROBIC CAPACITY,
Apoproteins, Body composition,
ENERGY BALANCE, Exercise
programme, HDL, Intervention, LDL,
Male, Running, T-cholesterol,
Triglycerides, Vigorous, Weight

231.4/178   **Wood, P.D., Haskell, W.L.,**
Stern, M.P., Lewis, S. & Perry,
C. (1977)
Plasma lipoprotein distributions in male
and female runners
Ann NY Acad Sci **301,** 748-763
Adult, BLOOD PRESSURE, Body
composition, Comparative, Female, HDL,
Leisure activity, LDL, Male, Running, T-
Cholesterol, Triglycerides, Vigorous,
Weight

232 SECONDARY PREVENTION

KEYWORDS are listed in the appendix in addition the following specific keywords have been used in this section:

- Angina
- Arrhythmia
- Recurrence rate (any incident whether fatal or not)
- Stroke

Summary of evidence: exercise ameliorates symptoms and signs of coronary heart disease

THE PROBLEM

Can exercise reverse the process of coronary atheroma which causes coronary heart disease? Does it promote improvements which protect against further acute episodes of disease ? Since exercise has a preventive role in the initial development of coronary heart disease it seemed likely that it would have beneficial effects in secondary prevention. Can exercise reduce symptoms such as breathlessness, fatigue and angina thus enabling the individual to return to normal life?

SCOPE

This section contains references on the effects of exercise on established coronary heart disease and in cardiac patients. Some references are epidemiological and deal with recurrence rates of fatal or non-fatal infarction. There are many references on the effects of rehabilitation programmes in cardiac patients chosen from an extensive literature to cover aspects ranging from cardiac function to quality of life.

METHODOLOGICAL DIFFICULTIES

Properly controlled epidemiological studies are difficult to mount when the damage to the heart and the stage of the disease are variable. It is also difficult to control for the effects of exercise in rehabilitation where there are drop-in as well as drop-out problems and an ethical barrier against withholding a potential benefit.

EVIDENCE

Although exercise can reduce the coronary heart disease risk factors in these patients this does not appear to result in a consistent and significant reduction in mortality. Met-analysis of six exercise-based rehabilitation studies shows a reduction due to exercise in the risk of death from coronary heart disease of about 19% compared to the control groups which is suggestive of some effect. Apart from this, the symptoms and signs of coronary heart disease can be reduced by regular moderate exercise (see 210 and 220). This is because heart rate and blood pressure are reduced at a particular exercise intensity which spares the heart through a reduction of cardiac work at the same cardiac output. In cardiac patients, cardiac output is also reduced after training which further reduces the work of the heart. The resulting increase in the effort tolerance and work capacity means that patients are better able to cope with their normal activities, as well as having the ability to deal safely with the occasional demands for vigorous brief effort that occur in daily life. The patient gains confidence in his ability to exercise safely and this reduces the depression that often follows a heart attack.

232/1   (1984)
Physical conditioning for patients with
coronary artery disease (Editorial)
Lancet **2,** 615-616
Review

232/2   **Adler, J.C., Mazzarella, N., Puzsier,
L. & Alba, A.**   (1987)
Treadmill training program for a
bilateral below-knee amputee patient
with cardiopulmonary disease
Arch Phys Med Rehabil **68,** 858-861
*Adult, Exercise programme, Handicap,
Intervention, Male, SECONDARY
PREVENTION*

232/3   **Alexander, L. & Schaal, S.**   (1982)
Effects of exercise on mitral valve
prolapse syndrome patients
Med Sci Sports Exerc **14,** 164
*Adult, Arrhythmia, Exercise programme,
Hazards, Intervention, Vigorous*

232/4   **Amundsen, L.R.**   (1979)
Establishing activity and training levels
for patients with ischemic heart disease
Phys Ther **59,** 754-758
Exercise programme, Review

232/5   **Andrew, G.M., Oldridge, N.B.,
Parker, J.O., Cunningham, D.A.,
Rechnitzer, P.A., Jones, N.L., Buck, C.,
Kavanagh, T., Shephard, R.J., Sutton,
J.R., & McDonald, W.**   (1981)
Reasons for drop-out from exercise
programs in post-coronary patients
Med Sci Sports Exerc **13,** 164-168
*Adult, Exercise programme, Longitudinal,
Male*

232/6   **Ben-Ari, E., Kellermann, J.J.,
Lapitod, C., Drory, Y., Fisman, E. &
Hayat, M.**   (1978)
Effect of prolonged intensive training on
cardiorespiratory response in patients
with angina pectoris
Br Heart J **40,** 1143-1148
*Adult, Angina, BLOOD PRESSURE,
CARDIAC PERFORMANCE, Exercise
programme, Intervention, Male,
RESPIRATORY FUNCTION, Vigorous*

232/7   **Ben-Ari, E., Kellerman, J.J.,
Rothbaum, D.A., Fisman, E. & Pines,
A.**   (1987)
Effects of prolonged intensive versus
moderate leg training on the untrained
arm exercise response in angina pectoris
Am J Cardiol **59,** 231-234
*Adult, Angina, BLOOD PRESSURE,
Comparative, Exercise
programme, Intervention, Male*

232/8   **Bengtsson, K.**   (1983)
Rehabilitation after myocardial
infarction
J Rehabil Med **15,** 1-9
Review

232/9   **Berg, A., Keul, J., Stippig, J. &
Stippig, L.**   (1981)
Effects of an outdoor exercise program
on cardiovascular and metabolic data in
patients with coronary heart disease
(CHD)
Int J Rehab Res **4,** 64-66
*Adult, BLOOD PRESSURE, CARDIAC
PERFORMANCE, Exercise programme,
Intervention, LIPIDS*

232/10   **Bjernulf, A., Boberg, J. & Froberg,
S.**   (1974)
Physical training after myocardial
infarction. Metabolic effects during short
and prolonged exercise before and after
physical training in male patients after
myocardial infarction
Scand J clin Lab Invest **33,** 173-185
*Adult, CARBOHYDRATE
TOLERANCE, Endocrine, Exercise
programme, Intervention, LIPIDS, Male*

232/11   Bjorntorp, P., Berchtold, P.,
Grimby, G., Lindholm, B.,Sanne, H.,
Tibblin, G. & Wilhelmsen, L.   (1972)
Effects of physical training on glucose
tolerance plasma insulin and lipids and
on body composition in men after
myocardial infarction
Acta Med Scand **192**, 439-443
Adult, Body composition,
CARBOHYDRATE TOLERANCE,
Exercise programme, Intervention,
LIPIDS, Male

232/12   Blumenthal, J.A., Rejeski, W.J.,
Walsh-Riddle, M., Emery, C.F., Miller,
H., Roark, S., Ribisl, P.M., Morris, P.B.,
Brubaker, P. & Williams, R.S.   (1988)
Comparison of high- and low-intensity
exercise training early after acute
myocardial infarction
Am J Cardiol **61**, 26-30
Adult, AEROBIC CAPACITY, BLOOD
PRESSURE, CARDIAC
PERFORMANCE, Exercise programme,
Intervention, LIPIDS, Male, Vigorous,
Weight

232/13   Brown, K.A., DeSanctis, R.W.,
DiCola, V., Boucher, C.A., Pohost, G.M.
& Okada, R.D.   (1986)
Long-term exercise and hemodynamic
follow-up in patients with previous right
ventricular myocardial infarction
Am Heart J **112**, 1321-1322
Adult, CARDIAC PERFORMANCE,
Leisure activity, Longitudinal

232/14   Bruce, E.H., Frederick, R., Bruce,
R.A. & Fisher,L.D.   (1976)
Comparison of active participants and
drop-outs in CAPRI cardiopulmonary
rehabilitation programmes
Am J Cardiol **37**, 53-60
Adult, AEROBIC CAPACITY, Exercise
programme, Female, Intervention, Male,
Recurrence

232/15   Bruce, R.A.   (1974)
Editorial: Marathon running after
myocardial infarction
J Am Med Ass **229**, 1637-1638
Review

232/16   Bruce, R.A., Kusumi, F. &
Frederick, R.   (1977)
Difference in cardiac function with
prolonged physical training for cardiac
rehabilitation
Am J Cardiol **40**, 597-603
Adult, AEROBIC CAPACITY,
CARDIAC PERFORMANCE, Exercise
programme, Longitudinal, Male

232/17   Brunner, D., Meshulam, N. &
Zeriekyer, F.   (1979)
Secondary prevention by physical
exercise in patients after myocardial
infarction (A controlled study in
randomized groups of exercising and
non-exercising patients) In: International
symposium state of prevention and
therapy in human arteriosclerosis and in
animal models (Eds) Hauss, W.H.
Westdeutscher Verlag **63**, 523-536
Adult, CARDIAC PERFORMANCE,
Exercise programme, Intervention, Male

232/18   Brunner, D., Meshulam, N. &
Zerikier, F.   (1977)
Physical exercise in the active
rehabilitation of patients suffering from
Ischemic Heart Disease
Med Sport **10**, 153-173
Adult, AEROBIC CAPACITY, Exercise
programme, Intervention,

232/19   Cardus, D., Fuentes, F. &
Srinivasin, R.   (1975)
Cardiac evaluation of a physical
rehabilitation program for patients with
ischemic heart disease
Arch Phys Med Rehabil **56**, 419-425
Adult, AEROBIC CAPACITY,. Exercise
programme, Intervention

232/20   Carson, P., Neophytou, M., Tucker, H. & Simpson, T.   (1973)
Exercise programme after myocardial infarction
Br Med J **2**, 213-216
Adult, Exercise programme, Intervention, Male, Recurrence

232/21   Carson, P., Phillips, R., LLoyd, M., Tucker, H., Neophytou, M., Buch, N.J., Gelson, A., Lawton, A. & Simpson, T.   (1982)
Exercise after myocardial infarction: a controlled trial
J Royal Coll Physicians **16**, 147-151
Adult, Cohort, Leisure activity, LIPIDS, Male, Recurrence, Weight

232/22   Ciske, P.E., Dressendorfer, R.H., Gordon, S. & Timmis, G.C.   (1986)
Attenuation of exercise training effects in patients taking beta blockers during early cardiac rehabilitation
Am Heart J **112**, 1016-1025
Adult, AEROBIC CAPACITY, Exercise programme, Intervention, PERCEIVED EXERTION, RESPIRATORY FUNCTION

232/23   Clausen, J.P.   (1976)
Circulatory adjustments to dynamic exercise and effect of physical training in normal subjects and in patients with coronary artery disease
Prog Cardiovasc Dis **18**, 459-495
CARDIAC PERFORMANCE, Review

232/24   Clausen, J.P., Larsen, O.A. & Trap-Jensen, J.   (1969)
Physical training in the management of coronary artery disease
Circulation **40**, 143-154
Adult, BLOOD PRESSURE, CARDIAC PERFORMANCE, Exercise programme, Intervention, Male

232/25   Clausen, J.P. & Trap-Jensen, J.   (1970)
Effects of training on the distribution of cardiac output in patients with coronary artery disease
Circulation **42**, 611-624
Adult, CARDIAC PERFORMANCE, Exercise programme, Intervention, Male, MUSCLE METABOLISM,

232/26   Clausen, J.P. & Trap-Jensen, J.   (1976)
Heart rate and arterial blood pressure during exercise in patients with angina pectoris. Effects of training and of nitroglycerin
Circulation **53**, 436-442
Acute exercise, Adult, Angina, BLOOD PRESSURE, Comparative, Exercise programme, Intervention, Male

232/27   Cobb, F.R., Williams, R.S., McEwan, P., Jones, R.H., Coleman, R.E. & Wallace, A.G.   (1982)
Effects of exercise training on ventricular function in patients with recent myocardial infarction
Circulation **66**, 100-108
Adult, AEROBIC CAPACITY, BLOOD PRESSURE, CARDIAC PERFORMANCE, Exercise programme, Intervention, LIPIDS

232/28   Conn, E.H., Williams, R.S. & Wallace, A.G.   (1982)
Exercise responses before and after physical conditioning in patients with severely depressed left ventricular function
Am J Cardiol **49**, 296-300
Adult, CARDIAC PERFORMANCE, Exercise programme, Intervention, Recurrence

232/29 **Conroy, R.M., Cahill, S., Mulcahy, R., Johnson, H., Graaham, I.M. & Hickey, N.** (1986)
The relation of social class to risk factors, rehabilitation, compliance and mortality in survivors of acute coronary heart disease
Scand J Soc Med **14**, 51-56
Adult, Cohort, Leisure activity, Male, Recurrence

232/30 **Cooksey, J.D., Reilly, P., Brown, S., Bomze, H. & Cryer, P.E.** (1978)
Exercise training and plasma catecholamines in patients with ischemic heart disease
Am J Cardiol **42**, 372-376
Adult, BLOOD PRESSURE, Endocrine, Exercise programme, HEART FUNCTION TEST, Intervention, Male

232/31 **Council on Scientific Affairs** (1981)
Physician supervised exercise programs in rehabilitation of patients with coronary heart disease
J Am Med Ass **245**, 1463-1466
Review

232/32 **Debusk, R.F.** (1977)
How to individualize rehabilitation after myocardial infarction
Geriatrics **32**, 77-79
Review

232/33 **Degré ,S., Degré-Coustry, C., Hoylaerts, M., Grevisse, M. & Denolin, H.** (1977)
Therapeutic effects of physical training in coronary heart disease
Cardiology **62**, 206-217
Review

232/34 **Degre, S., Lenaers, R., Messin, R., Vandermoten, P., Salhadin, Ph., Limage, M. & Denolin, H.** (1979)
Post-infarction exercise capacity after Lidoflazine treatment or physical training
Cardiology **64**, 35-47
Adult, AEROBIC CAPACITY, Exercise programme, Intervention, Male

232/35 **Dehn, M.M., Pansegrau, D.G. & Mitchell, J.H.** (1978)
Exercise training after acute myocardial infarction
Cardiovascular Clinics, F.A.Davis Company, Philadelphia **9**, 117-132
Review

232/36 **Dickstein, R.** (1986)
Stroke rehabilitation. Three exercise therapy approaches
Phys Ther **66**, 1233-1238
Adult, Exercise programme, Intervention, Stroke

232/37 **Drakonakis, A.C. & Ross, A.M.** (1978)
Comparative benefits of exercise training in grafted and ungrafted coronary patients
Am J Cardiol **41**, 432
Adult, AEROBIC CAPACITY, Comparative, Exercise programme, Intervention, Vigorous

232/38 **Dressendorfer, R.H., Smith, J.L., Amsterdam, E.A., & Mason, D.T.** (1982)
Reduction of submaximal exercise myocardial oxygen demand post-walk training program in coronary patients due to improved physical work efficiency
Am Heart J **103**, 358-362
Adult, AEROBIC CAPACITY, BLOOD PRESSURE, Exercise programme, Intervention, Male, PERCEIVED EXERTION

232/39 Ehsani, A.A., Biello, D.R., Schultz, J., Sobel, B.E. & Holloszy, J.O. (1986)
Improvement in left ventricular contractile function by exercise training in patients with coronary artery disease
Circulation **74**, 350-358
Acute exercise, Adult, AEROBIC CAPACITY, Angina, BLOOD PRESSURE, CARDIAC PERFORMANCE, Exercise programme, Female, Intervention, Male

232/40 Ehsani, A.A., Heath, G.W., Martin, W.H. 3rd, Hagberg, J.M. & Holloszy, J.O. (1984)
Effects of intense exercise training on plasma catecholamines in coronary patients
J Appl Physiol **57**, 154-159
Adult, AEROBIC CAPACITY, BLOOD PRESSURE, Endocrine, Exercise programme, HEART FUNCTION TEST, Intervention

232/41 Ehsani, A.A., Martin, W.H. 3rd, Heath, G.W. & Coyle, E.F. (1982)
Cardiac effects of prolonged and intense exercise training in patients with coronary artery disease
Am J Cardiol **50**, 246-254
Adult, AEROBIC CAPACITY, BLOOD PRESSURE, CARDIAC PERFORMANCE, Exercise programme, Intervention, Male, Vigorous

232/42 Erb, B.D., Fletcher, G.F., & Sheffield, T.L. (1979)
Standards for cardiovascular exercise treatment programs. American Heart Association subcommittee on rehabilitation target activity group
Circulation **59**, 1084A-1090A
Exercise programme, Review

232/43 Fagard, R., Reybrouck, T., Vanhees, L., Cattaert, A., Vanmeenen, T., Grauwels, R. & Amery, A. (1984)
The effects of beta blockers on exercise capacity and on training response in elderly subjects
Eur Heart J (SupplE) **5**, 117-120
Acute exercise, BLOOD PRESSURE, Elderly, Exercise programme, Intervention, PERCEIVED EXERTION, RESPIRATORY FUNCTION

232/44 Ferguson, R.J., Cote, P., Gauthier, P. & Bourassa, M.G. (1978)
Changes in exercise coronary sinus blood flow with training in patients with angina pectoris
Circulation **58**, 41-47
Adult, Angina, CARDIAC PERFORMANCE, Exercise programme, Intervention, Male

232/45 Fletcher, G.F. (1984)
Long-term exercise in coronary artery disease and other chronic disease states
Heart Lung **13**, 28-46
Review

232/46 Franklin, B.A., Besseghini, I .& Golden, L.H. (1978)
Low intensity physical conditioning:Effects on patients with coronary heart disease
Arch Phys Med Rehabil **59**, 276-280
Adult, Exercise programme, Intervention

232/47 Frick, M.H. & Katila, M. (1968)
Hemodynamic consequences of physical training after myocardial infarction
Circulation **37**, 192-202
Adult, CARDIAC PERFORMANCE, Exercise programme, Intervention, Male, RESPIRATORY FUNCTION

232/48 Froelicher, V., Battler, A. & McKirnan, M.D. (1980)
Physical activity and coronary heart disease
Cardiology **65**, 153-190
PRIMARY PREVENTION, Review

232/49   Froelicher, V., Jensen, D., Genter, F., Sullivan,M., McKirnan, M.D., Witztum, K., Scharf, J., Strong, M.L., & Ashburn, W.   (1984)
A randomized trial of exercise training in patients with coronary heart disease
J Am Med Ass **252,** 1291-1297
Adult, AEROBIC CAPACITY, CARDIAC PERFORMANCE, COLLATERALS, Exercise programme, Intervention, Male

232/50   Fu, F.H.   (1979)
The effects of two modes of training on post-myocardial infarction patients
J Sports Med **19,** 291-296
Adult, AEROBIC CAPACITY, Comparative, Exercise programme, Intervention,

232/51   Fuchs, P., Sevic, D., Fuchs, N., Carson, W. & Walter, J.   (1984)
The influence of coronary sport group training on the flexbility of joints, heart rate and blood pressure of coronary patients
J Sports Med **24,** 280
Adult, BLOOD PRESSURE, Exercise programme, Intervention, JOINTS

232/52   Goforth, D. & James, F.W.   (1985)
Exercise training in non-coronary heart disease. In: Exercise and the Heart, edition 2 (Ed.) Brest, A.N.
Cardiovascular Clinics, F.A.Davis Company Philadelphia **15,** 243-254

CARDIAC PERFORMANCE, Review

232/53   Gordon, N.F., Kruger, P.E. & Cilliers, J.F.   (1983)
Improved exercise ventilatory response after training in coronary heart disease during long term beta-adrenergic blockade
Am J Cardiol **51,** 755-758
Adult, AEROBIC CAPACITY, ANAEROBIC CAPACITY, Exercise programme, Intervention, Male

232/54   Gori, P., Pivotti, F., Masè, N., Zucconi, V. & Scardi, S.   (1984)
Compliance with cardiac rehabilitation in the elderly
Eur Heart J. (Suppl E) **5,** 109-111
AEROBIC CAPACITY, BLOOD PRESSURE, Elderly, Exercise programme, Intervention

232/55   Gottheiner, V.   (1968)
Long-range strenuous sports training for cardiac reconditioning and rehabilitation
Am J Cardiol **22,** 426-436
Adult, AEROBIC CAPACITY, Elderly, Exercise programme, Female, Intervention, Male, Vigorous

232/56   Greenberg, M.A., Arbeit, S. & Rubin, I.L.   (1979)
The role of physical training in patients with coronary artery disease
Am Heart J **97,** 527-533
Review

232/57   Grodzinski, E., Kreutz, E., Blümchen, G. & Borer, J.S.   (1983)
The behavior of the ejection fraction (EF) at rest and exercise in cardiac infarct patients before and after a 4-week training period. Comparison to a control group
Z Cardiol **72,** 105-118
Adult, CARDIAC PERFORMANCE, Exercise programme, Intervention

232/58   Hagberg, J.M., Ehsani, A.A. & Holloszy, J.O.   (1983)
Effect of 12 months of intense exercise training on stroke volume in patients with coronary artery disease
Circulation **67,** 1194-1199
Adult, AEROBIC CAPACITY, Blood pressure, CARDIAC PERFORMANCE, Exercise programme, Intervention, Male

232/59   Halfen, E.S., Zabialova, I.A., Ahvarts, I.L., Rumiantsev, B.L., Reshetniak, O.F., Khoroshenkova, M.F. & Belyaeva, A.E.   (1976)
Comparative evaluation of different programs of physical rehabilitation in acute myocardial infarction
Kardiologia **16**, 26-34
Adult, Comparative, Exercise programme, Intervention, Vigorous

232/60   Hansen, J.E., Sue, D.Y., Oren, A. & Wasserman, K.   (1987)
Relation of oxygen uptake to work rate in normal men and men with circulatory disorders
Am J Cardiol **59**, 669-674
Acute exercise, Adult, AEROBIC CAPACITY, BLOOD PRESSURE, Elderly, Male

232/61   Hartung, G.H. & Rangel, R.   (1981)
Exercise training in post-myocardial infarction patients: Comparisons of results with high risk coronary and post-by-pass patients
Arch Phys Med Rehabil **62**, 147-150
Adult, AEROBIC CAPACITY, Body composition, Exercise programme, Intervention, Male

232/62   Haskell, W.L.   (1974)
Physical activity after myocardial infarction
Am J Cardiol **33**, 776-783
Review

232/63   Haskell, W.L.   (1978)
Cardiovascular complications during exercise training of cardiac patients
Circulation **57**, 920-924
HAZARDS-CVS, Review

232/64   Haskell, W.L., Savin, W.M., Schroeder, J.S., Alderman, E.A., Ingles, N.B., Daughter, G.T. & Stinson, E.B.   (1981)
Cardiovascular responses to handgrip isometric exercise in patients following cardiac transplantation
Circulation Res (Suppl) **48**, I-156-I-161
Acute exercise, Adult, BLOOD PRESSURE, CARDIAC PERFORMANCE, Male, MUSCLE STRENGTH

232/65   Hellerstein, H.K.   (1977)
Limitations of marathon running in the rehabilitation of coronary patients: Anatomic and Physiologic determinants
Ann NY Acad Sci **301**, 484-494
Review

232/66   Hertanu, J.S., Davis. L. & Focseneanu, M.   (1986)
Cardiac rehabilation exercise program: Outcome assessment
Arch Phys Med Rehabil **67**, 431-435
Adult, AEROBIC CAPACITY, Elderly, Exercise programme, Intervention, Vigorous

232/67   Hoffman, A., Duba, J., Lengyel, M. & Majer, K.   (1987)
The effect of physical training on the physical work capacity of MI patients with left ventricular dysfunction
Eur Heart J (Suppl G) **8**, 43-40
Adult, Exercise programme, Intervention, Male, Recurrence

232/68   Hoiberg, A.   (1986)
Longitudinal Study of Cardiovascular Disease in U.S. Navy Pilots
Aviat Space Environ Med **57**, 438-442
Adult, Cohort, Male, Occupational activity, Recurrence

232/69   Jánosi, A., Hoffman, A. &
Hankóczy, J.   (1987)
Is exercise training harmful after
myocardial infarction?
Chest **92**, 933-934
Adult, Arrhythmia, Exercise programme,
Intervention, Male, Vigorous

232/70   Jensen, D., Atwood, J.E.,
Froelicher, V., McKirnan, M.D., Battler,
A., Ashburn, W. & Ross, J   (1980)
Improvement in ventricular function
during exercise studied with radionuclide
ventriculography after cardiac
rehabilitation
Am J Cardiol **46**, 770-777
Adult, AEROBIC CAPACITY, BLOOD
PRESSURE, CARDIAC
PERFORMANCE, Exercise programme,
Intervention, Vigorous

232/71   Kallio, V., Hämäläinen, H.,
Hakkila, J. & Luurila, O.J.   (1979)
Reduction in sudden death by a
multifactorial intervention programme
after acute myocardial infarction
Lancet **2**, 1091-1094
Adult, Exercise programme, Intervention,
LIPIDS, Recurrence

232/72   Kamyar, G.A. & Rokay, A.   (1975)
A study on the rehabilitation of ischemic
heart disease patients. The heart rate,
beta-receptor blocking agents and
strength-duration relationship of exercise
Jap Heart J **16**, 512-525
Acute exercise, Adult, MUSCLE
STRENGTH

232/73   Kavanagh, T.   (1983)
Exercise and the Heart
Ann Acad Med Singapore **12**, 331-337
Review

232/74   Kavanagh, T., Shephard, R.J. &
Pandit, V.   (1974)
Marathon running after myocardial
infarction
J Am Med Ass **229**, 1602-1605
Acute exercise, Adult, Male, Marathon,
Running

232/75   Kavanagh, T & Shephard,
R.J.   (1975)
Conditioning of post coronary patients:
comparison of continuous and interval
training
Arch Phys Med Rehabil **56**, 72-76
Adult, AEROBIC CAPACITY,
Comparative, Exercise programme,
HEART FUNCTION, Intervention,
Male, Running

232/76   Kavanagh, T. & Shephard,
R.J.   (1980)
Exercise for post-coronary patients: An
assessment of infrequent supervision
Arch Phys Med Rehabil **61**, 114-118
Adult, AEROBIC CAPACITY,
Intervention, Leisure activity

232/77   Kavanagh, T., Shephard, R.J.,
Chisholm,. A.W., Qureshi, S. & Kennedy,
J.   (1979)
Prognostic indexes for patients with
ischemic heart disease enrolled in an
exercise-centered rehabilitation program
Am J Cardiol **44**, 1230-1240
Adult, BLOOD PRESSURE, Body
composition, Exercise programme,
HEART FUNCTION TEST,
Intervention, LIPIDS, MALE,
Recurrence

232/78   Kavanagh, T., Shephard, R.J. &
Kennedy, J.   (1977)
Characteristics of postcoronary
marathon runners
Ann NY Acad Sci **301**, 455-465
Adult, AEROBIC CAPACITY, BLOOD
PRESSURE, Body composition,
Comparative, HEART FUNCTION,
PERSONALITY

232/79   Kavanagh, T., Shephard, R.J.,
Lindley, L.J. & Pieper, M.   (1983)
Influence of exercise and lifestyle
variables upon high density lipoprotein
cholesterol after myocardial infarction
Arteriosclerosis **3**, 249-259
Adult, Exercise programme, Intervention,
Leisure activity, LIPIDS, Male

232/80   Kavanagh, T., Yacoub, M.H., Mertens, D.J., Kennedy, J., Campbell, R.B. & Sawyer, P.   (1988)
Cardiorespiratory responses to exercise training after orthoptic cardiac transplantation
Circulation **77**, 162-171
Adult, AEROBIC CAPACITY, ANAEROBIC CAPACITY, BLOOD PRESSURE, Body composition, Exercise programme, Intervention, Male, PERCEIVED EXERTION, RESPIRATORY FUNCTION

232/81   Kellermann, J.J.   (1977)
Panel VI: Critical evaluation of studies concerning mortality and morbidity in coronary heart disease patients who have or have not participated in rehabilitation programmes
Biblthca Cardiol **36**, 150-154
Review

232/82   Kellermann, J.J., Ben-Ari, E., Fisman, E.   (1986)
Physical training in patients with ventricular impairment. Benefits/ limitations – open questions
Adv Cardiol **34**, 131-147
Review

232/83   Kentala, E.   (1972)
Physical fitness and feasibility of physical rehabilitation after myocardial infarction in men of working age
Ann Clin Res (Suppl 9) **4**,
Adult, Exercise programme, Intervention

232/84   Konig, K.   (1977)
Changes in physical capacity, heart size and function in patients after myocardial infarction who underwent a 4- to 6-week physical training program
Cardiology **62**, 232-246
Adult, AEROBIC CAPACITY, CARDIAC PERFORMANCE, Exercise programme, Intervention

232/85   Lazlett, L.J., Paumer, L., Scott-Baier, P. & Amsterdam, E.A.   (1982)
Efficacy of exercise training in patients with coronary artery disease who are taking propanolol
Circulation **68**, 1029-1034
Adult, Comparative, Exercise programme, Intervention

232/86   Lee, A.P., Ice, R., Blessey, R., & Sanmarco, M.E.   (1979)
Long-term effects of physical training on coronary patients with impaired ventricular function
Circulation **60**, 1519-1526
Adult, BLOOD PRESSURE, CARDIAC PERFORMANCE, Longitudinal

232/87   Leon, A.S. & Blackburn, H.   (1977)
Exercise rehabilitation of the coronary heart disease patient
Geriatrics **32**, 66-76
Review

232/88   Lerman, J., Bruce, R.A., Sivarajan, E., Petter, E. & Trimble, S.   (1976)
Low level dynamic exercises for earlier cardiac rehabilitation: aerobic and hemodynamic responses
Arch Phys Med Rehabil **57**, 355-360
Adult, CARDIAC PERFORMANCE, Exercise programme, Intervention

232/89   Letac, B., Cribier, A. & Desplanches, J.F.   (1977)
A study of left ventricular function in coronary patients before and after physical training
Circulation **56**, 375-378
Adult, BLOOD PRESSURE, CARDIAC PERFORMANCE, Exercise programme, Intervention, Male

232/90   Long, C. (Ed.)   (1980)
Prevention and rehabilitation in ischemic heart disease
Williams and Wilkins, Baltimore.
Review

232/91   **Markiewicz, W., Houston, N. & Debusk, R.**   (1979)
A comparison of static and dynamic exercise soon after myocardial infarction
Israel J Med Sci **15**, 894-897
Adult, Exercise programme, Intervention

232/92   **May, G.S., Eberlein, K.A., Furberg, C.D., Passamani, E.R. & DeMets, D.L.**   (1982)
Secondary prevention after myocardial infarction: A review of long-term trials
Prog Cardiovasc Dis **24**, 331-352
Recurrence, Review

232/93   **McCrimmon, D.R., Cunningham, D.A., Rechnitzer, P.A. & Griffiths, J.**   (1976)
Effect of training on plasma catecholamines in post-myocardial infarction patients
Med Sci Sports **8**, 152-156
Adult, Endocrine, Exercise programme, Intervention

232/94   **Miller, H.S.**   (1985)
Supervised versus non-supervised exercise rehabilitation of coronary patients. In: Exercise and the Heart, edition 2 (Ed.) Brest, A.N.
Cardiovascular Clinics, F.A.Davis Company, Philadelphia. **15**, 193-200
Review

232/95   **Musch, T.I., Moore, R.L., Leathers, D.J., Bruno, A. & Zelis, R.**   (1986)
Endurance training in rats with chronic heart failure induced by myocardial infarction
Circulation **74**, 431-441
Animal, AEROBIC CAPACITY, BLOOD PRESSURE, CARDIAC PERFORMANCE, Exercise programme, Intervention, MUSCLE METABOLISM

232/96   **Naksi, Y., Kataoka, Y., Bando, M., Hiasa, Y., Taki, H., Harada, M., Maeda, T. & Aikara, T.**   (1987)
Effects of physical exercise training on cardiac function and graft patency after coronary artery by-pass grafting
J Thorac Cardiovasc Surg **93**, 65-72
Adult, BLOOD PRESSURE, CARDIAC PERFORMANCE, Exercise programme, Female, Intervention, Male

232/97   **Naughton, J.**   (1978)
The National Exercise and Heart Disease Project. The pre-randomization exercise program
Cardiology **63**, 352-367
Adult, Body composition, BLOOD PRESSURE, Cohort, Exercise programme, LIPIDS, Male, MOOD

232/98   **Naughton, J.**   (1979)
Exercise and myocardial infarction: The National Exercise and Heart Disease Project: An overview. Proceedings of the Workshop on Physical Conditioning and Rehabilitation
US DHSS PIH NIH
Review

232/99   **Naughton, J.**   (1985)
Cardiac rehabilitation: current status and future possibilities. In: Exercise and the Heart, edition 2 (Ed.) Brest, A.N.
Cardiovascular Clinics , F.A.Davis Company, Philadelphia **15**, 185-192
Review

232/100   **Newell, J.P., Kappagoda, C.T., Stoker, J.B., Deverall, P.B., Watson, D.A. & Linden, R.J.**   (1980)
Physical training after heart valve replacement
Br Heart J **44**, 638-649
Adult, Exercise programme, Intervention

232/101   **Noakes, T.D.**   (1979)
Prescribing exercise for the cardiac patient
S A Med J **55**, 969-970
Review

232/102   Noakes, T.D.   (1982)
Criticisms of exercise after heart attack –
variations on an old theme
S A Med J **62**, 238-240
Review

**232/103   Nye, E.R. & Poulsen,
W.T.**   (1974)
An activity programme for coronary
patients: a review of morbidity, mortality
and adherence after 5 years
N Z Med J **79**, 1010-1013
*Adult, Exercise programme, Intervention,
Recurrence*

**232/104   Obma, R.T., Wilson, P.K., Goebel,
M.E. & Campbell, D.E.**   (1979)
Effect of a conditioning program in
patients taking propanolol for angina
pectoris
Cardiology **64**, 365
*Adult, Angina, Exercise programme,
Intervention*

232/105   Oldridge, N.B.   (1982)
Compliance and exercise in primary and
secondary prevention of coronary heart
disease: A Review
Prev Med **11**, 56-70
PRIMARY PREVENTION, Review

**232/106   Oldridge, N.B. & Jones,
N.L.**   (1986)
Preventive use of exercise rehabilitation
and myocardial infarction
Acta Med Scand (Suppl 711) **220**, 123-
129
Review

**232/107   Oldridge, N.B., LasDalle, D. &
Jones, N.L.**   (1980)
Exercise rehabilitation of female patients
with coronary heart disease
Am Heart J **100**, 755-757
Female, Review

**232/108   Oldridge, N.B., Nagle, F.J., Balke,
B., Carliss, R.J. & Kahn, D.R.**   (1978)
Effects of surgery and 32 months of
physical conditioning on treadmill
performance
Arch Phys Med Rehabil **59**, 268-275
*Adult, AEROBIC CAPACITY, Exercise
programme, Longitudinal, Male*

**232/109   Oldridge, N.B., Wicks, J.R.,
Hanley, C., Sutton, J.R. & Jones,
N.L.**   (1978)
Non-compliance in an exercise
rehabilitation program for men who have
suffered a myocardial infarction
Can Med Ass J **118**, 361-364
*Adult, Body composition, Cohort,
Comparative, Exercise programme,
Leisure activity, Male, PERSONALITY,
Recurrence*

**232/110   Opasich, C., Cobelli, F., Assandri,
J., Calsamiglia, G., Febo, M.T., Larovere,
M.T., Pozzoli, M., Tramarin, R.,
Traversi, E. & Specchia, G.**   (1984)
Is old age a contraindiction to cardiac
rehabilitation after acute myocardial
infarction?
Eur Heart J. (Suppl E) **5**, 105-107
*AEROBIC CAPACITY, Elderly,
Exercise programme, Intervention, Male*

**232/111   Paffenbarger, R.S. & Hyde,
R.T.**   (1984)
Exercise in the prevention of coronary
heart disease
Prev Med **13**, 3-22
*EPIDEMIOLOGY-CHD, PRIMARY
PREVENTION, Review*

232/112   Palatsi, I.   (1976)
Feasibility of physical training after
myocardial infarction and its effect on
return to work, morbidity and mortality
Acta Med Scand (Suppl 599) **201**, 1-84
Adult, Exercise programme, Intervention

232/113   **Pollock, M.L.** (1985)
Exercise regimens after myocardial
revascularisation surgery: rationale and
results. In: Exercise and the Heart,
edition 2 (Ed.) Brest, A.N.
*Cardiovascular Clinics, F.A.Davis
Company, Philadelphia.* **15,** 159-174
Review

232/114   **Pollock, M.L. & Pels,
A.E.** (1984)
Exercise prescription for the cardiac
patient: an update
Clin Sports Med **3,** 425-469
Exercise programme, Review

232/115   **Pratt, C.M., Welton, D.E.,
Squires, W.G., Kirby, T.E. Hartung, G.H.
& Miller, R.R.** (1981)
Demonstration of training effect during
chronic beta-adrenergic blockade in
patients with coronary artery disease
Circulation **64,** 1125-1129
*Adult, AEROBIC CAPACITY, BLOOD
PRESSURE, CARDIAC
PERFORMANCE, Exercise programme,
Intervention, Male*

232/116   **Pyfer, H.R., Mead, W.F.,
Frederick, R.C. & Docne, B.L.** (1976)
Exercise rehabilitation in coronary heart
disease: community group programs
Arch Phys Med Rehabil **57,** 335-342
Adult, Intervention, Leisure activity

232/117   **Raffo, J.A., Luksic, I.Y.,
Kappagoda, C.T., Mary, D.A.S.G.,
Whitaker, W. & Lindern, R.J.** (1980)
Effects of physical training on
myocardial ischaemia in patients with
coronary artery disease
Br Heart J **43,** 262-269
*Adult, BLOOD PRESSURE, Exercise
programme, HEART FUNCTION
TEST, Intervention*

232/118   **Rechnitzer, P.A., Cunningham,
D.A., Andrew, G.M., Buck, C.W., Jones,
N.L., Kavanagh, T., Oldridge, N.B.,
Parker, J.O., Shephard, R.J., Sutton,
J.R. & Donner, A.P.** (1983)
Relation of exercise to the recurrence rate
of myocardial infarction in men
Am J Cardiol **51,** 65-69
*Adult, Cohort, Exercise programme,
Male, Recurrence, Vigorous,*

232/119   **Rechnitzer, P.A., Pickard, H.A.,
Paivio, A.U., Yuhasz, M.S. &
Cunningham, D.A.** (1972)
Long-term follow-up study of survival
and recurrence rate following myocardial
infarction in exercising and control
subjects
Circulation **45,** 853-857
*Adult, Exercise programme, Longitudinal,
Male, Recurrence*

232/120   **Rechnitzer, P.A., Sangal, S.,
Cunningham, D.A., Andrew, G., Buck, C.,
Jones, N.L., Kavanagh, T., Parker, J.O.,
Shephard, R.J. & Yuhasz, M.S.** (1975)
A controlled prospective study of the
effect of endurance training on the
recurrence rate of myocardial infarction.
A description of the experimental design
Am J Epidemiol **102,** 358-365
*Adult, Cohort, Exercise programme,
Male, Recurrence, Vigorous*

232/121   **Redwood, D.R., Rosing, D.R. &
Epstein, S.E.** (1972)
Circulatory and symptomatic effects of
physical training in patients with
coronary artery disease and angina
pectoris
N Eng J Med **286,** 959-965
*Adult, Angina, CARDIAC
PERFORMANCE, COAGULATION,
Exercise programme, Intervention*

232/122 **Roland, J.M., Banks, D.C., Edwards, B. & Fentem, P.H.** (1986)
The relationship of arrhythmias to walking activity during mobilization after myocardial infarction
Postgrad Med J **62**, 255-258
Adult, Customary activity, HAZARDS-CVS, HEART FUNCTION TEST

232/123 **Rossi, P., Giordano, A., Tamiz, A., Schiavo, B. & Minuco, G.** (1979)
Effects of training and of verapamil on exercise capacity in patients recovering from myocardial infarction
Cardiology **64**, 372-385
Adult, AEROBIC CAPACITY, CARDIAC PERFORMANCE, Comparative, Exercise programme, Intervention

232/124 **Sanne, H.** (1973)
Exercise tolerance and physical training of non-selected patients after myocardial infarction
Acta Med Scand (Suppl 551) **194**, 1-124
Adult, AEROBIC CAPACITY, Exercise programme, Female, Intervention, Male

232/125 **Sanne, H.** (1986)
Rehabilitation after a myocardial infarction
Acta Med Scand (Suppl 712) **220**, 72-78
Review

232/126 **Sargeant, A.J., Crawley, M.A. & Davies, C.T.M.** (1979)
Physiologic responses to exercise in myocardial infarction patients following residential rehabilitation
Arch Phys Med Rehabil **60**, 121-125
Acute exercise, Adult, AEROBIC CAPACITY

232/127 **Saunamaki, K.I.** (1978)
Feasibility and effect of physical training with maximum intensity in men after acute myocardial infarction
Scand J Rehabil Med **10**, 155-162
Adult, AEROBIC CAPACITY, Exercise programme, Intervention, Male, Vigorous

232/128 **Shaw, L.W.** (1981)
Effects of a prescribed supervised exercise program on mortality and cardiovascular morbidity in patients after a myocardial infarction
Am J Cardiol **48**, 39-46
Adult, Cohort, Exercise programme, Recurrence,

232/129 **Shephard, R.J.** (1980)
Exercise and recurrence of myocardial infarction
Am Heart J **100**, 404-405
Review

232/130 **Shephard, R.J.** (1985)
Exercise regimens after myocardial infarction: rationale and results. In: Exercise and the Heart, edition 2 (Ed.) Brest, A.N.,
Cardiovascular Clinics, F.A.Davis Company, Philadelphia **15**, 145-158
Review

232/131 **Shephard, R.J., Corey, P. & Kavanagh, T.** (1981)
Exercise compliance and the prevention of a recurrence of myocardial infarction
Med Sci Sports Exerc **13**, 1-5
Adult, Cohort, Exercise programme, HEART FUNCTION TEST, Male, Recurrence

232/132 **Shephard, R.J., Kavanagh, R.T. & Tuck, J.** (1983)
Marathon jogging in post-myocardial infarction patients
J Cardiac Rehab **3**, 321-329
Adult, Exercise programme, Intervention, Male, Marathon, Running

232/133 **Sim, D.N. & Neill, W.A.** (1974)
Investigation of the physiological bases for increased exercise threshold for angina pectoris after physical conditioning
J Clin Invest **54**, 763-770
Adult, Angina, BLOOD PRESSURE, COLLATERALS, Exercise programme, HEART FUNCTION TEST, Intervention

232/134   **Stein, R.A.**   (1977)
The effect of exercise training on heart
rate during coitus in the post-myocardial
infarction patient
Circulation **55**, 738-740
Adult, AEROBIC CAPACITY, Exercise
programme, Intervention, Male

232/135   **Tavazzi, L. & Ignone, G.**   (1987)
Rehabilitation: Effect on exercise
arrhythmias
Eur Heart J (Suppl D) **8**, 83-90
Arrhythmia, Review, SECONDARY
PREVENTION

232/136   **Tavazzi, L., Kellermann, J.J. &**
Denolin, H. (Eds)   (1988)
International workshop on physical
training and ventricular dysfunction
Eur Heart J **9**, 1-78
Review

232/137   **Teo, K. & Horgan, J.**   (1986)
Exercise response and resting left
ventricular function after cessation of
training in myocardial infarction and
coronary artery by-pass patients
Ir Med J **79**, 342-6
Adult, AEROBIC CAPACITY, Exercise
programme, HEART FUNCTION
TEST, Intervention

232/138   **Ungerman-deMent, P. & Bemis,**
A.   (1986)
Exercise program for patients after
cardiac surgery
Arch Phys Med Rehabil **67**, 463-466
Adult, CARDIAC PERFORMANCE,
Exercise programme, Intervention,
JOINTS

232/139   **Van der Hauwaert, L.**   (1986)
Exercise and sports in congenital heart
disease. In: Sports cardiology exercise in
health and cardiovascular disease (Eds.)
Fagard, R.H. & Bekaert, I.E.
Martinus Nijhoff 205-213
Adult, Children, Exercise programme,
Review

232/140   **Vanhees, L., Fagard, R. & Amery,**
A.   (1982)
Influence of beta adrenergic blockade on
effects of physical training in patients
with ischaemic heart disease
Br Heart J **48**, 33-38
Adult, AEROBIC CAPACITY,
Comparative, Exercise programme,
Intervention, Male, RESPIRATORY
FUNCTION

232/141   **Varnauskas, E., Bergman, H.,**
Houk, P. & Bjorntorp,P.   (1966)
Hemodynamic effects of physical
training in coronary patients
Lancet **2**, 8-12
Adult, CARDIAC PERFORMANCE,
Exercise programme, Intervention,
LIPIDS

232/142   **Weiner, D.A.**   (1985)
Predischarge exercise testing after
myocardial infarction: prognostic and
therapeutic features In: Exercise and the
Heart, edition 2 (Ed.) Brest, A.N.
Cardiovascular Clinics, F.A.Davis
Company, Philadelphia **15**, 95-104
Review

232/143   **Wenger, N.K.**   (1977)
Critical evaluation of cardiac
rehabilitation
Chest **71**, 317-318
Review

232/144   **West, R.R. & Evans, D.A.**   (1986)
Lifestyle changes in long term survivors
of acute myocardial infarction
J Epidemiol Community Health **40**, 103-
109
Adult, Cohort, Leisure activity,

232/145   **Wilhelmson, L., Sanne, H.,
Elmfeldt, D., Grimby, G., Tibblin, G. &
Wedel, H.**   (1975)
A controlled trial of physical training
after myocardial infarction. Effects on
risk factors, non-fatal re-infarction, and
death
Prev Med **4**, 491-508
*Adult, AEROBIC CAPACITY, BLOOD
PRESSURE, Exercise programme,
Intervention, LIPIDS, Recurrence,
Vigorous*

232/146   **Williams, M.A., Maresh, C.M.,
Aronow, W.S., Esterbrooks, D.J.,
Mohiuddin, S.M. & Sketch,
M.H.**   (1984)
The value of early out-patient cardiac
exercise programmes for the elderly in
comparison with other selected age
groups
Eur Heart J (Suppl E) **5**, 113-115
*Adult, BLOOD PRESSURE, Body
composition, Comparative, Elderly,
Exercise programme, Intervention, Male,
PERCEIVED EXERTION, Weight*

232/147   **Williams, R.S.**   (1985)
Exercise training of patients with
ventricular dysfunction and heart failure.
In: Exercise and the Heart, edition 2
(Ed.) Brest, A.N.
*Cardiovascular Clinics, F.A.Davis
Company, Philadelphia* **15**, 219-232
Review

232/148   **Williams, R.S., McKinnis, R.A.,
Cobb, F.R., Higgenbotham, M.B.,
Wallace, A.G., Coleman, R.E. & Califf,
R.M.**   (1984)
Effects of physical conditioning on left
ventricular ejection fraction in patients
with coronary artery disease
Circulation **70**, 69 -75
*Adult, CARDIAC PERFORMANCE,
Exercise programme, HEART
FUNCTION, Intervention*

232/149   **Woodhouse, S.P., Hathirat, S.,
Jensen, E., Johnson, A.L. & Klassen,
G.A.**   (1976)
Effect of physical training on
haemodynamic performance following
myocardial infarction: a controlled
study
Can Med Ass J **115**, 239-244
*Adult, CARDIAC PERFORMANCE,
Exercise programme, Intervention, Male,
RESPIRATORY FUNCTION*

KEYWORDS are listed in the appendix in addition the following specific keywords have been used in this section:

Angina
Arrhythmia
Cardiac abnormalities
Case reports (cardiovascular incidents related to exercise reported in detail)
CHD-morbidity
CHD-mortality
Coronary heart disease
Hypertrophy
Myocardial infarction
Sudden cardiac death

Summary of evidence: exercise ameliorates existing hazards

THE PROBLEM

Individuals may be reluctant to take up exercise because they are more aware of the risks than of the benefits. There is an apparent contradiction between the accumulated evidence which shows that increased physical activity confers several health benefits including reduction in the risk of a heart attack, and the cardiac deaths which occur occasionally during vigorous exercise.

SCOPE

This section contains references reporting sudden death during athletic activities and epidemiological studies of the incidence of untoward cardiac events during exercise testing under laboratory conditions. There are also epidemiological references describing death rates related to activity particular in joggers, squash players and the military. The studies are mainly of men. (See section 410 for orthopaedic hazards.)

METHODOLOGICAL DIFFICULTIES

Sudden death during exercise has to be examined by retrospective epidemiological methods and are hampered by the unreliability of reports of exercise and the difficulty of finding suitable controls of known customary activity level.

EVIDENCE

Exercise is safe unless it is too strenuous for the individual concerned, unless it is performed erratically, or if warning symptoms are ignored. Regular exercise decreases the risk of a heart attack, but it does not confer immunity to this multifactorial condition. Many middle-aged people have some degree of undeclared damage to their coronary arteries. Thus, some individuals, even those engaged in a sensible exercise regime, will die of a heart attack while exercising. Their death should be attributed to disease and not to the exercise. Young apparently healthy people sometimes die on the sports field; in this situation an unsuspected abnormality is often found at autopsy. A small increased cardiac risk during strenuous exercise in middle age must be judged against the greatly reduced overall risk of a heart attack gained by regular vigorous exercise. This risk is more than two and a half times greater in sedentary individuals than in their more active peers.

233/1   **Abdon, N.J., Landin, K. & Johansson, B.W.**   (1984)
Athlete's bradycardia as an embolising disorder? Symptomatic arrhythmias in patients aged less than 50 years.
Br Heart J **52,** 660-666
Adult, Arrhythmia, Athlete, Cardiac abnormalities, Leisure activity, Vigorous

233/2   Areskog, N.H.   (1987)
Exercise induced arrhythmias in valvular
heart disease
Eur Heart J (Suppl D) **8**, 43-45
*Acute exercise, Adult, Arrhythmia, Case
reports*

233/3   Bharati, S., Dreifus, L.S., Chopskie,
E. & Lev, M.   (1988)
Conduction system in a trained jogger
with sudden death
Chest **93**, 348-351
*Adult, Autopsy, Cardiac abnormalities,
Case reports, Leisure activity, Male,
Running, Sudden cardiac death*

233/4   Billman, G.E., Schwartz, P.J. &
Stone, H.L.   (1984)
The effect of daily exercise on
susceptibility to sudden cardiac death
Circulation **69**, 1182-1189
*Animal, Arrhythmia, BLOOD
PRESSURE, CARDIAC
PERFORMANCE, Customary activity,
Sudden cardiac death*

233/5   Bjuro, T., Vedin, A., Werko, L. &
Wilhelmsson, C.   (1975)
Cardiovascular diseases and sudden
death in connection with physical exercise
and competitions
Lakartidningen, **72**, 335-338
*Adult, Athlete, Case reports, CHD-
morbidity, Leisure activity, Sudden
cardiac death*

233/6   Bove, A.A.   (1985)
Effects of strenuous exercise on
myocardial blood flow
Med Sci Sports Exerc **17**, 517-521
COLLATERALS, Review

233/7   Cantwell, J.D. & Fletcher,
G.F.   (1969)
Cardiac complications while jogging
J Am Med Ass **210**, 130-132
*Adult, Case reports, Coronary Heart
Disease, Exercise programme, Male*

233/8   Cobb, L.A. & Weaver, W.D.   (1986)
Exercise: a risk for sudden death in
patients with coronary heart disease
J Am Coll Cardiol **7**, 215-219
*Arrhythmia, Review, SECONDARY
PREVENTION, Sudden cardiac death*

233/9   Coplan, N.L., Gleim, G.W. &
Nicholas, J.A.   (1988)
Exercise and sudden cardiac death
Am Heart J **115**, 207-212
*Cardiac abnormalities, CHD-mortality,
Review, Sudden cardiac death*

233/10   DeMaria, A.N., Vera, Z.,
Amsterdam, E.A., Mason, D.T. &
Massumi, R.A.   (1974)
Disturbances of cardiac rhythm and
conduction induced by exercise.
Diagnostic, prognostic and therapeutic
implications
Am J Cardiol **33,**. 732-736
*Arrhythmia, HEART FUNCTION
TEST, Review*

233/11   Dressendorfer, R.H., Wade, C.E. &
Scaff, J.H.   (1985)
Increases morning heart rate in runners:
A valid sign of overtraining?
Phys Sportsmed **13**, 77-86
*Adult, Athlete, BLOOD PRESSURE,
CARBOHYDRATE TOLERANCE,
CARDIAC PERFORMANCE,
Endocrine, Leisure activity, Male,
Marathon, Running, Vigorous*

233/12   Ector, H., Verlinden, M., Eynde,
E.V., Bourgois, J., Hermans, L., Fagard,
R. & De Geest, H.   (1984)
Bradycardia, ventricular pauses,
syncope, and sports
Lancet **8403**, 591-594
*Adult, Arrhythmia, Athlete, CARDIAC
PERFORMANCE, Female, Leisure
activity, Male*

233/13   **Ekblom, B., Hartley, L.H. & Day, W.C.**   (1979)
Occurrence and reproducibility of exercise induced ventricular ectopy in normal subjects
Am J Cardiol **43**, 35-40
Acute exercise, Adult, Arrhythmia, Leisure activity, SECONDARY PREVENTION

233/14   **Ellestad, M.H.**   (1985)
Exercise-induced arrhythmias and hypotensions: significance and clinical management. In: Exercise and the Heart, edition 2 (Ed) Brest, A.N.
Cardiovascular Clinics, F.A. Davis Company, Philadelphia. **15**, 125-132
Review

233/15   **Epstein, S.E. & Maron, B.J.**   (1986)
Sudden death and the competitive athlete: perspectives on pre-participation screening studies
J Am Coll Cardiol **7**, 220-230
Review

233/16   **Fletcher, G.F. & Cantwell, J.D.**   (1977)
Ventricular fibrillation in a medically supervised cardiac exercise program
J Am Med Ass **238**, 2627-2629
Adult, Angina, Arrhythmia, Case reports, Exercise programme, Intervention, SECONDARY PREVENTION

233/17   **Freeman, Z.**   (1985)
Exercise and sudden cardiac death
Med J Australia **142**, 383-384
Review

233/18   **Furlanello, F., Bettini, R. & Cozzi, F.**   (1984)
Ventricular arrhythmias and sudden death in athletes. In: Clinical aspects of life-threatening arrhythmias (Eds.) Greenberg, H.M., Kulbertus, H.E., Moss, A.J. & Schwartz, P.J.
Ann NY Acad Sci **427**, 253-279
Review

233/19   **Gibbons, L.W., Cooper, K.H., Meyer, B.M. & Ellison, R.L.**   (1980)
The acute cardiac risk of strenuous exercise
J Am Med Ass **244**, 1799-1801
Adult, Exercise programme, Female, Longitudinal, Male

233/20   **Green, L.H., Cohen, S.I. & Kurland, G.**   (1976)
Fatal myocardial infarction in marathon racing
Ann Intern Med **84**, 704-706
Acute exercise, Adult, Autopsy, Case reports, Leisure activity, Male, Marathon, Myocardial Infarction, Running

233/21   **Gutgesell, H.P., Gessner, I.H., Vetter, V.L., Yabek, S.M. & Norton, J.B**   (1986)
Recreational and occupational recommendations for young patients with heart disease. A Statement for Physicians by the Committee on Congenital Caridac Defects for the Council on Cardiovascular Disease in the Young American Heart Association
Circulation **74**, 1195A-1198A
Review

233/22   **Handler, J.B., Asay, R.W., Warren, S.E. & Shea, P.M.**   (1982)
Symptomatic coronary artery disease in a marathon runner
J Am Med Ass **248**, 717-719
Adult, Case reports, Coronary heart disease, Leisure activity, LIPIDS, Male, Marathon, Running

233/23   **Hanzlick, R. & Stivers, R. R.**   (1983)
Sudden death in a marathon runner with origin of the right coronary artery from the left sinus of Valsalva
Am J Cardiol **51**, 1467
Adult, Autopsy, Case Reports, Hypertrophy, Male, Marathon, Sudden cardiac death,

233/24   **Haskell, W.L.**   (1982)
Sudden cardiac death during vigorous
exercise
Int J Sports Med **3**, 45-48
Review

233/25   **Hayashi, K.D. & Lewis,
E.R.**   (1980)
Sudden death in a marathon runner with
widely patent coronary arteries
Clin Cardiol **3**, 288
*Adult, Autopsy, Case reports, Male,
Sudden cardiac death*

233/26   **Hellerstein, H.K. & Moir,
T.W.**   (1985)
Distance running in the 1980s:
cardiovascular benefits and risks. In:
Exercise and the Heart, edition 2 (Ed.)
Brest, A.N.
*Cardiovascular Clinics, F.A. Davis
Company, Philadelphia.* **15** , 75-86
Review

233/27   **Hossack, K.F. & Hartwig,
R.**   (1982)
Cardiac arrest associated with supervised
cardiac rehabilitation
J Cardiac Rehab **2**, 402
*Adult, SECONDARY PREVENTION,
Sudden cardiac death*

233/28   **Izeki, T.**   (1973)
Statistical observation on sudden deaths
in sport
Br J Sports Med **7**, 172-176
*Autopsy, Cardiac abnormalities, Case
reports, Children, Female, Hazards,
Leisure activity, Male,*

233/29   **Jackson, R.T., Beaglehole, R. &
Sharpe, N.**   (1983)
Sudden death in runners
N Z Med J **96**, 289-292
*Adult, Autopsy, Case reports, CHD-
morbidity, Leisure activity, Myocardial
infarction, Running, Sudden cardiac death*

233/30   **Kark, J.A., Posey, D.M.,
Schumacher, H.R. & Ruehle,
C.J.**   (1987)
Sickle-cell trait as a risk factor for sudden
death in physical training
N Eng J Med **317**, 781-787
*Adult, Comparative, Intervention, Male,
Occupational Activity, Sudden cardiac
death*

233/31   **Kennedy, H.L., Caralis, D.G.,
Poblete, F. & Pescarmona, J.E.**   (1977)
Ventricular arrhythmia 24 hours before
and after maximal treadmill testing
Am Heart J **94**, 718-724
*Acute exercise, Adult, Arrhythmia,
HEART FUNCTION TEST,
SECONDARY PREVENTION*

233/32   **Koplan, J.P.**   (1979)
Cardiovascular deaths while running
J Am Med Ass **242**, 2578-2579
EPIDEMIOLOGY-CHD, Review

233/33   **Koplan, J.P., Siscovick, D.S. &
Goldbaum, G.M.**   (1985)
The risks of exercise: a public view of
injuries and hazards
Public Health Reports **100**, 189-194
Review

233/34   **Koskenvuo, K.**   (1976)
Sudden death among Finnish conscripts
Br Med J **2**, 1413-1415
*Adult, Coronary Heart Disease, Male,
Occupational activity, Sudden cardiac
death*

233/35   **Kramer, M.R., Driori, Y. & Lev,
M.**   (1988)
Sudden death in young soldiers. High
incidence of syncope prior to death
Chest **93**, 345-347
*Adult, Autopsy, Cardiac abnormalities,
Case reports, Hypertrophy, Occupational
activity, Sudden cardiac death*

233/36   **Kraus, J.F. & Conroy, C.**   (1984)
Mortality and morbidity from injury in
sport and recreation
Ann Rev Publ Health **5**, 163-192
Review

233/37   Leach, J.R., Charles, N., Sands, M.J. Jr., Lochman, A.S. & Skinner, W.   (1982)
Cardiac arrest during exercise training after myocardial infarction
Conn Med **46**, 239-243
Adult, Exercise programme, Intervention, SECONDARY PREVENTION, Sudden cardiac death

233/38   Maron, B.J., Epstein, S.E. & Roberts, W.C.   (1986)
Causes of sudden death in competitive athletes
J Am Coll Cardiol **7**, 204-214
Adult, Athlete, Cardiac abnormalities, Leisure activity, Sudden cardiac death, Vigorous

233/39   Maron, B.J., Roberts, W.C., McAllister, H.A Jr., Rosing, D.R. & Epstein, S.E.   (1980)
Sudden death in young athletes
Circulation **62**, 218-229
Adult, Athlete, Autopsy, Case reports, Children, HEART FUNCTION TEST, Hypertrophy, Sudden cardiac death

233/40   Mead, W.F., Pyfer, H.R., Thrombold, J.C. & Frederick, R.C.   (1976)
Successful resuscitation of two near simultaneous cases of cardiac arrest with a review of fifteen cases occurring during exercise
Circulation **53**, 187-189
Adult, Arrhythmia, Case Reports, Exercise programme, HEART FUNCTION TEST, Male, SECONDARY PREVENTION, Sudden cardiac death,

233/41   Moncur, J.   (1973)
A study of fatalities during sport in Scotland (1969)
Br J Sports Med **7**, 162-163
Adult, Cardiac abnormalities, CHD-mortality, Female, Hazards, Leisure activity, Male,

233/42   Morales, A.R., Romanelli, R. & Boucek, R.J.   (1980)
The mural left anterior descending coronary artery, strenuous exercise and sudden death
Circulation **62**, 230
Adult, Autopsy, Case reports, Female, Leisure activity, Male, Running, Sudden cardiac death, Swimming

233/43   Moritz, A.R. & Zamchek, N.   (1946)
Sudden and unexpected deaths of young soldiers
Arch Pathol **42**, 459-494
Adult, Case reports, Male, Occupational activity

233/44   Noakes, T.D., Higginson, L. & Opie, L.H.   (1983)
Physical training increases ventricular fibrillation thresholds of isolated rats hearts during normoxia, hypoxia and regional ischaemia
Circulation **67**, 24-30
Animal, Arrhythmia, Exercise programme, Intervention,

233/45   Noakes, T.D., Opie, L. H. & Rose, A.G.   (1984)
Marathon running and immunity to coronary heart disease: Fact versus fiction
Clin Sports Med **3**, 527-543
Adult, Autopsy, Case reports, Coronary heart disease, Leisure activity, Male, Marathon, Running, Sudden cardiac death, Vigorous

233/46   Noakes, T.D., Opie, L.H., Rose, A.G. & Kleynhans, P.H.T.   (1979)
Autopsy-proved coronary atherosclerosis in marathon runners
N Eng J Med **301**, 86-89
Adult, Autopsy, Case reports, Coronary heart disease, Leisure activity, Male, Marathon

233/47   Noakes, T.D., Rose, A.G. & Opie,
L.H.   (1979)
Hypertrophic cardiomyopathy
associated with sudden death during
marathon racing
Br Heart J **41**, 624-627
Adult, Autopsy, Case reports, CARDIAC
PERFORMANCE, Hypertrophy,
Leisure activity, Male, Marathon,
Running, Sudden Cardiac Death

233/48   Noakes, T.D., Opie, L.H., Beck,
W., McKechnie, J., Benchimol, A. &
Desser, K.   (1977)
Coronary heart disease in marathon
runners
Ann N Y Acad Sci **301**, 593-619
Review

233/49   Northcote, R.J., Flannigan, C. &
Ballantyne, D.   (1986)
Sudden death and vigorous exercise – a
study of 60 deaths associated with squash
Br Heart J **55**, 198-203
Adult, Autopsy, Case reports, Coronary
heart disease, Female, Leisure activity,
Male, Sudden cardiac death, Vigorous

233/50   Northcote, R.J. & Ballantyne,
D.   (1984)
Reducing the prevalence of exercise
related cardiac death
Br J Sports Med **18**, 288-292
Review

233/51   Northcote, R.J., Evans, A.D.B. &
Ballantyne, D.   (1984)
Sudden death in squash players
Lancet **1**, 148-151
Adult, Arrhythmia, Autopsy, Case reports,
Coronary Heart Disease, Female,
Hypertrophy, Leisure activity, Male,
Sudden cardiac death

233/52   Opie, L.H.   (1975)
Sudden death and sport
Lancet **1**, 263-266
Adult, Autopsy, Case reports, Coronary
heart disease, Leisure activity, LIPIDS,
Male, Sudden cardiac death

233/53   Pantano, J.A. & Oriel,
R.J.   (1982)
Prevalence and nature of cardiac
arrhythmias in apparently normal well
trained runners
Am Heart J **104**, 762-768
Acute exercise, Adult, Arrhythmia,
Leisure activity

233/54   Pedoe, D.T.   (1983)
Cardiological problems in sport
Br J Hosp Med **29**, 213-220
Hypertrophy, Review, Sudden cardiac
death

233/55   Pedoe, D.T.   (1984)
Marathon medicine
Br Med J **288**, 1322-1323
JOINTS, Marathon, Review

233/56   Pedoe, D.T.   (1984)
Popular marathons, half marathons, and
other long distance runs:
recommendations for medical support
Br Med J **288**, 1355-1359
JOINTS, Marathon, Review

233/57   Poole-Wilson, P.A.   (1984)
Potassium and the heart
Clin Endocrinol Metab **13**, 249-263
Arrhythmia, HEART FUNCTION
TEST, Review

233/58   Rasmussen, V., Hauso, S. &
Skagen, K   (1978)
Cerebral attacks due to excessive vagal
tone in heavily trained persons
Acta Med Scand **204**, 401-405
Adult, Arrhythmia, Athlete, Leisure
activity, Male, Vigorous

233/59   Robertson, H.K.   (1977)
Heart disease in life-long cyclists (Letter)
Br Med J **2**, 1635-1636.
Adult, Coronary Heart Disease, Elderly,
EPIDEMIOLOGY-CHD, Leisure
activity, Male

233/60   Schwartz, P.J., Billman, G.E. &
Stone, H.L.   (1984)
Autonomic mechanisms in ventricular
fibrillation induced by myocardial
ischemia during exercise in dogs with
healed myocarcardial infarction. An
experimental preparation for sudden
cardiac death
Circulation **69,** 790-800
*Acute exercise, Animal, Arrhythmia,
Sudden cardiac death*

233/61   Shephard, R.J.   (1984)
Identification of individuals at high risk.
In: Proceedings of symposium on
exercise, health and medicine (Ed.) J. N.
Morris
London: UK Sports Council 49-51
Review

233/62   Shephard, R.J.   (1977)
Do risks of exercise justify costly caution?
Phys Sports Med **5,** 58-65
Review

233/63   Shephard, R.J. & Kavanagh,
T.   (1978)
Predicting the exercise catastrophe in the
post-coronary patient
Can Fam Phys **24,** 614-618
*Adult, Arrhythmia, Exercise programme,
Intervention, Running, SECONDARY
PREVENTION*

233/64   Shephard, R.J.   (1984)
Can we identify those for who exercise is
hazardous?
Sports Med **1,** 75-86
Review

233/65   Siegel, R.J., French, W.J. &
Roberts, W.C.   (1982)
Spontaneous exercise testing. Running as
an early unmasker of underlying cardiac
amyloidosis
Arch Intern Med **142,** 345
*Adult, Case reports, Female, Leisure
activity, Male, Running*

233/66   Siscovick, D.S., Laporte, R.E. &
Newman, J.M.   (1985)
The disease specific benefits and risks of
physical activity and exercise
Public Health Reports **100,** 180-188
Review

233/67   Siscovick, D.S., Weiss, N.S.,
Fletcher, R.H. & Lasky, T.   (1984)
The incidence of primary cardiac arrest
during vigorous exercise
N Eng J Med **311,** 874-877
*Adult, Case-control, Coronary heart
disease, EPIDEMIOLOGY-CHD,
Leisure activity, Male, Sudden cardiac
death, Vigorous*

233/68   Thompson, P.D.   (1982)
Cardiovascular hazards of physical
activity
Exerc Sport Sci Rev **10,** 208-235
Review

233/69   Thompson, P.D., Funk, E.J.,
Carleton, R.A. & Sturner, W.Q.   (1980)
Incidence of death during jogging in
Rhode island from 1975 through 1980
J Am Med Ass **247,** 2535-2538
*Adult, Autopsy, Case reports,
EPIDEMIOLOGY-CHD, Leisure
activity, Male, Running, Sudden cardiac
death*

233/70   Thompson, P.D. & Mitchell,
J.H.   (1984)
Exercise and sudden cardiac death:
protection or provocation
N Eng J Med **311,** 914-915.
Review

233/71   Thompson, P.D., Stern, M.P.,
Williams, P., Duncan, K., Haskell, W.L.
& Wood, P.D.   (1979)
Death during jogging or running: a study
of 18 cases
J Am Med Ass **242,** 1265-1267
*Adult, Autopsy, Case reports, Coronary
heart disease, Leisure activity, Running,
Sudden cardiac death*

233/72   Tsung, S.H., Huang, T.Y. & Chang,
H.H.   (1982)
Sudden death in young athletes
Arch Pathol Lab Med **106**, 168-170
Athlete, Autopsy, Case reports, Children,
Hypertrophy, Leisure activity, Male,
Sudden cardiac death

233/73   Vander, L., Franklin, B.A. &
Rubenfire, M.   (1982)
Cardiovascular complications of
recreational physical activity: a
retrospective survey
Med Sci Sports Exerc **14**, 115
Adult, Coronary Heart Disease, Leisure
activity, Sudden Cardiac Death

233/74   Viitasalo, M.T., Kala, R., Eisalo, A.
& Halonen, P.I.   (1979)
Ventricular arrhythmias during exercise
testing, jogging and sedentary life
Chest **76**, 21-26
Adult, Arrhythmia, HEART FUNCTION
TEST, Leisure activity, Male, Running,
SECONDARY PREVENTION

233/75   Virmani, R., Robinowitz, M. &
McAllister, H.A.   (1982)
Non-traumatic death in joggers: a series
of 30 patients at autopsy
Am J Med **72**, 874-882
ADULT, Autopsy, Case reports,
Coronary heart disease, Hypertrophy,
Leisure activity, Male, Running, Sudden
cardiac death

233/76   Virmani, R., Robinowitz, M. &
McAllister, H. Jr.   (1985)
Exercise and the heart: a review of cardiac
pathology associated with physical
activity
Pathol Annual **20**, 431-462
Review

233/77   Vuori, I.   (1986)
The cardiovascular risks of physical
activity
Acta Med Scand (Suppl) **711**, 205-214
Review

233/78   Vuori, I., Makarainen, M. &
Jaaskelainen, A.   (1978)
Sudden death and physical activity
Cardiology **63**, 287-304
Review

233/79   Vuori, I., Suurnakki, L. &
Suurnakki, T.   (1982)
Risk of sudden cardiovascular death
(SCVD) in exercise
Med Sci Sports Exerc **14**, 114-115
Adult, Autopsy, Leisure activity, Male,
Sudden cardiac death

233/80   Waller, B.F.   (1985)
Exercise-related sudden death in young
(age 30 years) and old (age 30 years)
conditioned subjects: In, Exercise and the
Heart, edition 2 (Ed.) Brest, A.N.
Cardiovascular Clinics, F.A.Davis
Company, Philadelphia. **15**, 9-74
Adult, Athlete, Autopsy, Cardiac
abnormalities, Case reports, Children,
Female, Hypertrophy, Leisure activity,
Male, Sudden cardiac death

233/81   Waller, B.F., Csere, R.S., Baker,
W.P. & Roberts, W.C.   (1981)
Running to death
Chest **79**, 346-349
Adult, Autopsy, Case reports, Coronary
heart disease, Leisure activity, LIPIDS,
Male, Running, Sudden cardiac death

233/82   Waller, B.F. & Roberts,
W.C.   (1980)
Sudden death while running in
conditioned runners aged 40 years or over
Am J Cardiol **45**, 1292-1300
Adult, Autopsy, Case reports, Coronary
heart disease, Leisure activity, Male,
Running, Sudden cardiac death

233/83   Waters, D.D., Chaitman, B.R.,
Dupras, G., Theroux, P. & Mizgala,
H.F.   (1979)
Coronary artery spasm during exercise in
patients with variant angina
Circulation **59**, 580-585
Acute exercise, Adult, Angina, Case
reports, HEART FUNCTION TEST

233/84   **Wiedermann, C.J, Becker, A.E.,**
Hopferwieser, T., Mühlberger, V. &
Knapp, E.   (1987)
Sudden death in a young competitive
athlete with Wolff-Parkinson-White
syndrome
Eur Heart J **8**, 651-655
Arrhythmia, Athlete, Autopsy,
CARDIAC PERFORMANCE, Case
reports, Children, Hypertrophy, Male,
Sudden cardiac death

233/85   **Williams, R.S., Schocken, D.D.,**
Morey, M. & Koisch, F.P.   (1981)
Medical aspects of competitive distance
running
Postgraduate Med **70**, 41-50
Review

233/86   **Wren, C.**   (1987)
Arrhythmias in children: influence of
exercise and the role of exercise testing
Eur Heart J (Suppl D) **8**, 25-28
Arrhythmia, Cardiac abnormalities,
Children, Review

KEYWORDS are listed in the appendix in addition the following specific keywords have been used in this section:

Angina
Arrhythmia
Cardiac pacing
Cardiac abnormalities
CHD-morbidity
CHD-mortality
Coronary by-pass surgery
Diagnosis
Early post myocardial test
ECG
Heart failure
Hypertrophy
Maximal test
Prognosis
Safety
ST Segment depression
Submaximal Test

Summary of evidence: exercise ameliorates low exercise capacity following myocardial infarction and bedrest

THE PROBLEM

Cardiac patients and those caring for them are often frightened of the effects of exercise. Rehabilitation may be expedited by strategic use of a controlled test of heart function during exercise in a protected medical environment.

SCOPE

This section contains references dealing primarily with acute changes produced in the heart by exercise under controlled laboratory conditions and mainly in cardiac patients. There are also references on suitable exercise prescriptions for specified groups.

METHODOLOGICAL DIFFICULTIES

The prognostic interpretation of ECG information is still open to debate. It will probably remain a blunt but non-invasive method. More information can be obtained by visualizing the coronary arterial tree using angiography but this is invasive and carries some risk in itself.

EVIDENCE

It is clear that exercise testing under laboratory conditions can provide useful diagnostic information, guidelines for rehabilitation and encouragement for the safe progression of an exercise programme.

234/1 **Ameisen, O., Okin, P.M., Devereux, R.B., Hochreiter, C., Miller, D.H., Zullo, M.A., Borer, S.J. & Kligfield, P.** (1985) Predictive value and limitations of the ST/HR slope.
Br Heart J **53**, 547-551
Adult, Angina, Comparative, CORONARY ARTERIES, Diagnosis, Prognosis, S-T segment depression

234/2 **American College of Sports Medicine** (1986) Guidelines for graded exercise testing and exercise prescription
Ed 3, Philadelphia, Lea & Febiger
Acute exercise, Exercise programme, Review

234/3 **Amsterdam, E.A. & Mason, D.T.** (1977) Exercise testing and indirect assessment of myocardial oxygen consumption in evaluation of angina pectoris
Cardiology **62**, 174-189
Angina, CORONARY ARTERIES, Review, SECONDARY PREVENTION

234/4 **Attinà, D.A., Falorni, P.L., Pieri, A., Iannizzotto, C. & De Saint Pierre, G.** (1980)
The electrocardiogram of the middle-aged men who practice physical activity outside of their normal work-time. In: Sports Cardiology International conference (Eds.) Lubich, T. & Venerando, A.
Aulo Gaggi, Bologna 257-261
Adult, Comparative, Cycling, ECG, Leisure activity, Male

234/5 **Atwood, J.E., Kawanishi, S., Myers, J. & Froelicher, V.F.** (1988)
Exercise testing in patients with aortic stenosis
Chest **93**, 1083-1087
Adult, Diagnosis, Hazards-CVS, Male, Safety

234/6 **Barton, C.W., Katz, B., Schork, M.A. & Rosenthal, A.** (1983)
Value of treadmill exercise test in pre- and post-operative children with valvular aortic stenosis
Clin Cardiol **6**, 473-477
Acute exercise, Children, Cardiac abnormalities, Review

234/7 **Blackburn, H., Taylor, H.L., Hamrell, B., Buskirk, E., Nicholas, W.C. & Thorsen, R.D.** (1973)
Premature ventricular complexes induced by stress testing
Am J Cardiol **31**, 441-449
Adult, Arrhythmia, Prognosis

234/8 **Bruce, R.A. & DeRouen, T.A.** (1978)
Exercise testing as a predictor of heart disease and sudden death
Hospital Practice **13**, 69-75
CHD-morbidity, CORONARY ARTERIES, Longitudinal, Prognosis, Review, Sudden cardiac death

234/9 **Bruce, R.A., DeRouen, T.A. & Hossack, K.F.** (1980)
Value of maximal exercise tests in risk assessment of primary coronary heart disease events in healthy men
Am J Cardiol **46**, 371-378
Acute exercise, Adult, CHD-morbidity, Longitudinal, Male, Maximal test, PRIMARY PREVENTION

234/10 **Bruce, R.A., DeRouen, T.A. & Hossack, K.F.** (1980)
Pilot study examining the motivational effects of maximal exercise testing to modify risk factors and health habits
Cardiology **66**, 111-119
Acute exercise, Adult, PRIMARY PREVENTION

234/11 **Bruce, R.A., DeRouen, T., Peterson, T., Irving, J.B., Chinn, N., Blake, B. & Hofer, V.** (1977)
Non-invasive predictors of sudden cardiac death in men with coronary heart disease. Predictive value of maximal stress testing
Am J Cardiol **39**, 833-840
Adult, CARDIAC PERFORMANCE, CORONARY ARTERIES, Longitudinal, Male, Prognosis, SECONDARY PREVENTION, Sudden cardiac death

234/12 **Bruce, R.A., Fisher, L.D. & Hossack, K.F.** (1985)
Validation of exercise-enhanced risk assessment of coronary heart disease events: Longitudinal changes in incidence in Seattle community practice
J Am Coll Cardiol **5**, 875-881
Adult, CHD-mortality, Coronary by-pass surgery, Male, Intervention, PRIMARY PREVENTION, Prognosis, SECONDARY PREVENTION

234/13 **Bruce, R.A., Gey, G.O., Cooper, E.N., Fisher, L.D. & Peterson, R.R.** (1974)
Seattle Heart Watch: Initial clinical, circulatory and electrocardiographic responses to maximal exercise
Am J Cardiol **33**, 459-469
Acute exercise, Adult, BLOOD PRESSURE, CHD-morbidity, Leisure activity, Longitudinal, Maximal test, PRIMARY PREVENTION, SECONDARY PREVENTION

234/14 **Calvert, A.F., Bernstein, L. & Bailey, I.K.** (1977)
Physiological responses to maximal exercise in a normal Australian population – comparative values in patients with anatomically defined coronary artery disease
Aust N Z J Med **7**, 497-506
Acute exercise, Adult, BLOOD PRESSURE, Comparative, ECG, Female, Male, Maximal test, S-T segment depression

234/15 **Camm, A.J., Evans, K.E., Ward, D.E. & Martin, A.** (1980)
The rhythm of the heart in active elderly subjects
Am Heart J **99**, 598-603
Arrhythmia, Elderly

234/16 **Chaing, B.N., Alexander, E.R., Bruce, R.A., Thompson, D.J. & Ting, N.** (1969)
Factors relating to S-T segment depression after exercise in middle-aged Chinese men
Circulation **40**, 315-325.
Adult, Male, S-T segment depression

234/17 **Chalmers, R.J., Johnson, R.H., Al Bradan, R.H. & Williams, B.O.** (1976)
Metabolic changes during exercise testing of patients with ischaemic heart disease
Eur J Physiol **35**, 578-581
Acute exercise, Adult, Endocrine

234/18 **Cohn, J.N. (Ed)** (1987)
Quantitative exercise testing for the cardiac patient: The value of monitoring gas exchange
Circulation (Suppl 6 Pt. II) **76**, VI 1-VI 58
Review

234/19 **Coplan, N.L., Gleim, G.W. & Nicholas, J.A.** (1986)
Principles of exercise prescription for patients with coronary artery disease
Am Heart J **112**, 145-149
CORONARY ARTERIES, Exercise programme, Review, SECONDARY PREVENTION

234/20 **Coumel, P. & Cokkinos, D.V.** (1987)
Symposium on exercise in the diagnosis and evaluation of treatment of arrhythmias
Eur Heart J (Suppl D) **8**, 1-161
Arrhythmia, Review

234/21 **Cumming, G.R., Samm, J., Borysyk, L. & Kich, L.** (1975)
Electrocardiographic changes during exercise in asymptomatic men: 3 year follow-up
Can Med Ass J **112**, 578-581
Acute exercise, Adult, CHD-morbidity, ECG, Longitudinal, Male, Maximal test

234/22 **Davies, B., Ashton, W.D. & Rowlands, D.J.** (1986)
Exertional risk factors in apparently healthy males: an interim report. In: Sports Cardiology Exercise in health and cardiovascular disease. (Eds.) Fagard, R.H. & Bekaert, I.E.
Martinus Nijhoff 151-160
Adult, Cohort, CORONARY ARTERIES, ECG, HAZARDS-CVS, Leisure activity, Male

234/23 **DeBusk, R.F., Valdez, R., Houston, N. & Haskell, W.** (1978)
Cardiovascular responses to dynamic and static effort soon after myocardial infarction. Application to occupational work assessment
Circulation **58**, 368-375
Adult, Arrhythmia, BLOOD PRESSURE, HEART FUNCTION TEST, Male, Maximal test, Prognosis, SECONDARY PREVENTION

234/24 **Deckers, J.W., Fioretti, P. & Browere, R.W.** (1987)
Prediction of 1-year outcome after complicated and uncomplicated myocardial infarction: Bayesian analysis of predischarge exercise test results in 300 patients
Am Heart J **113**, 90-95
Acute exercise, Adult, CHD-mortality, ECG, Prognosis, SECONDARY PREVENTION

234/25 **Detry, J.M. & Bruce, R.A.** (1979)
Effects of physical training on exertional S-T segment depression in coronary heart disease
Circulation **44**, 335-45
Adult, Exercise programme, Intervention, S-T segment depression, SECONDARY PREVENTION

234/26 **Elamin, M.S., Boyle, R., Kardash, M.M., Smith, D.R., Stoker, J.B., Whitaker, W., Mary, D.A.S.G. & Linden, R.J.** (1982)
Accurate detection of coronary heart disease by new exercise test
Br Heart J **48**, 311-320
Adult, Angina, CORONARY ARTERIES, Diagnosis, SECONDARY PREVENTION, S-T segment depression

234/27 **Ellestad, M.H. & Wan, M.K.C.** (1975)
Predictive implications of stress testing. Follow-up of 2,700 subjects after maximum treadmill stress testing
Circulation **51**, 363-369
Adult, Maximal test, Prognosis,

234/28 **Ewart, C.K., Taylor, C.B., Reese, L.B. & Debusk, R.F.** (1983)
Effects of early post-myocardial infarction exercise testing on self-perception and subsequent physical activity
Am J Cardiol **51**, 1076-1080
Adult, Customary activity, Early post-myocardial test, MOOD, SECONDARY PREVENTION

234/29 **Fadayomi, M.O. & Akinroye, K.K.** (1987)
Implications of positive treadmill exercise tests in asymptomatic adult African blacks
Eur Heart J **8**, 611-617
Acute exercise, Adult, CORONARY ARTERIES, Female, Male, Prognosis, S-T segment depression

234/30 **Ferro, G., Romano, M., Carella, G., Cotecchia, M.R., Di Maro, T., Chiariello, M. & Condorelli, M.** (1986)
Relation between QT and QS2 intervals during exercise and recovery. Response in patient with coronary artery disease and age-matched control subjects
Chest **90**, 558-561
Adult, Comparative, CORONARY ARTERIES, ECG, HAZARDS-CVS, Male, SECONDARY PREVENTION, Sudden cardiac death

234/31 **Fioretti, P., Deckers, J.W., Brower, R.W., Simoons, M.L., Beelen, J.A.J.M. & Hugenholtz, P.G.** (1984)
Predischarge stress test after myocardial infarction in the old age: Results and prognositic value
Eur Heart J (Suppl E) **5**, 101-104
Adult, BLOOD PRESSURE, CHD-mortality, Elderly, Early post-myocardial test, Prognosis, SECONDARY PREVENTION

234/32   Foster, C., Lemberger, K.,
Thompson, N.N., Sennett, S.M., Hare, J.,
Pollock, M.L., Pels, A.E. & Schmidt,
D.H.   (1986)
Functional translation of exercise
responses from graded exercise testing to
exercise training
Am Heart J **112**, 1309-1316
Adult, AEROBIC CAPACITY, Exercise
programme, Intervention

234/33   Fox, K.M.   (1982)
Exercise heart rate/ST segment relation.
Perfect predictor of coronary disease?
Br Heart J **48**, 309-310
Angina, CHD-morbidity, CORONARY
ARTERIES, Diagnosis, Review, S-T
segment depression

234/34   Fox, K.M.   (1982)
Exercise testing in the diagnosis of
ischaemic heart disease
Brit Med J **284**, 611-612
Angina, CHD-morbidity, CORONARY
ARTERIES, Diagnosis, Review, S-T
segment depression, SECONDARY
PREVENTION

234/35   Froelicher, V.F., Thomas, M.M.,
Pillow, C. & Lancaster, M.C.   (1974)
Epidemiologic study of asymptomatic
men screened by maximal treadmill
testing for latent coronary artery disease
Am J Cardiol **34**, 770-776
Acute exercise, Adult, CHD-morbidity,
Male, Maximal test, S-T segment
depression

234/36   Gaul, G.   (1984)
Stress testing in persons above the age of
65 years: applicability and diagnostic
value of a standardized maximal
symptom-limited testing protocol
Eur Heart J (Suppl.E) **5**, 51-53
Diagnosis, Elderly, Female, Male,
Maximal test

234/37   Glover, D.R., Robinson, C.S. &
Murray, R.G.   (1984)
Diagnostic exercise testing in 104 patients
over 65 years of age
Eur Heart J (Suppl E) **5**, 59-61
Diagnosis, Elderly, Maximal test,
Prognosis

234/38   Gohlke, H., Betz, P. & Roskamm,
H.   (1987)
Prognostic importance of exercise-
induced ST-segment depression in
patients with documented coronary
artery disease
Eur Heart J (Suppl G) **8**, 109-114
Acute exercise, Adult, Longitudinal,
Prognosis, S-T segment depression,

234/39   Goldshlager, N., Cake, D. & Cohn,
K.   (1973)
Exercise-induced ventricular
arrhythmias in patients with coronary
artery disease. Their relation to
angiographic findings
Am J Cardiol **31**, 434-440
Adult, Arrhythmia, CORONARY
ARTERIES, SECONDARY
PREVENTION

234/40   Hamm, L.F., Stull, G.A. & Crow,
R.S.   (1986)
Exercise testing after myocardial
infarction: historic perspective and
current uses
Prog Cardiovasc Dis **28**, 463-476
Early post-myocardial test, Prognosis,
Review, SECONDARY PREVENTION

234/41   Handler, C.E.   (1986)
Exercise testing after myocardial
infarction
Cardiology in Practice 30-34
Early post-myocardial test, Prognosis,
Review, SECONDARY PREVENTION

234/42   Hellerstein, H.K. & Franklin,
B.A.   (1983)
Exercise testing and prescription In:
Rehabilitation of the Coronary Patient
John Wiley & Sons, New York
Acute exercise, Review

234/43   Hetherinton, M., Haennel, R., Teo, K.K. & Kappagoda, T.   (1986)
Importance of considering ventricular function when prescribing exercise after acute myocardial infarction
Am J Cardiol **58**, 891-895
Adult, CARDIAC PERFORMANCE, Comparative, SECONDARY PREVENTION

234/44   Hossack, K., Eldridge, J., Wolfel, E. Leddy, C. & Berger, N.   (1987)
Aerobic responses to low level exercise testing following an acute myocardial infarction
Am Heart J **113**, 694-699
Acute exercise, Adult, Early post-myocardial test, Prognosis, SECONDARY PREVENTION

234/45   Jamnes, F.W., Schwartz, D.C., Kaplan, S. & Spilkin, S.P.   (1982)
Exercise electrocardiogram, blood pressure and working capacity in young patients with valvular or discrete subvalvular aortic stenosis
Am J Cardiol **50**, 769-775
Acute exercise, BLOOD PRESSURE, Children, Cardiac abnormalities, Diagnosis, S-T segment depression

234/46   Jones, N.L. & Campbell, E.J.M.   (1982)
Clinical exercise testing (2nd edition)
W B Saunders Co, Philadelphia
Review

234/47   Kanarek, D.J. & Hand, R.W.   (1984)
The response of cardiac and pulmonary disease to exercise testing
Clin Chest Med **5**, 181
RESPIRATORY FUNCTION, SECONDARY FUNCTION, Review

234/48   Kardash, M., Boyle, R., Elamin, M.S., Stoker, J.B., Mary, D.A.S.G. & Linden, R.J.   (1982)
Detection of severity of coronary artery disease by the ST segment/heart rate relationship in patients on beta-blocker therapy
Cardiovasc Res **16**, 508-515
Adult, Angina, CORONARY ARTERIES, Diagnosis, SECONDARY PREVENTION, S-T segment depression

234/49   Kavanagh, T. & Shephard, R.J.   (1976)
Maximum exercise tests on 'postcoronary' patients
J Appl Physiol **40**, 611-618
Adult, AEROBIC CAPACITY, HAZARDS-CVS, Maximal test, SECONDARY PREVENTION

234/50   Kellermann, J.J., Hayet, M. & Fishman, E.   (1986)
Exercise testing: Intercenter variabilities, prognostic value, work and training prescription
Adv Cardiol **33**, 64-73
Exercise programme, Prognosis, Review

234/51   Kerber, R.E., Miller, R.A. & Najjar, S.M.   (1975)
Myocardial ischemic effects of isometric, dynamic and combined exercise in coronary artery disease
Chest **67**, 388
Acute exercise, Adult, BLOOD PRESSURE, CHD-morbidity, SECONDARY PREVENTION, S-T segment depression

234/52   Kozlowski, J.H. & Ellestad, M.H.   (1984)
The exercise test as a guide to management and prognosis. In: Clinics in Sports Medicine. Symposium on cardiac rehabilitation (Eds.) Franklin, B.A. & Rubenfire, M.
W.B. Saunders Company **3**, 395-416
Prognosis, Review

234/53   **Kveselin, D.A., Rocchini, A.P., Rosenthal, A., Crowley, D.C., Dick, M. & Snider, A.R.**   (1985)
Hemodynamic determinants of exercise-induced ST-segment depression in children with valvular aortic stenosis
Am J Cardiol **87**, 725-730
Acute exercise, Children, Cardiac abnormalities, CARDIAC PERFORMANCE, S-T segment depression

234/54   **Landin, R.J., Linnemeier, T.J., Rothbaum, D.A., Chappelear, J. & Noble, R.J.**   (1985)
Exercise testing and training of the elderly patient. In: Exercise and the Heart, edition 2 (Ed.) Brest, A.N.
Cardiovascular Clinics, F.A.Davis Company, Philadelphia **15**, 201-218
Elderly, Review, SECONDARY PREVENTION

234/55   **Linden, R.J. & Mary, D.A.S.G.**   (1982)
Limitations and reliability of exercise electrocardiography in coronary heart disease
Cardiovasc Res **16**, 675-710
Angina, CORONARY ARTERIES, Diagnosis, Review, S-T segment depression, SECONDARY PREVENTION

234/56   **Linderholm, H., Osterman, G. & Teien, D.**   (1985)
Detection of coronary artery disease by means of exercise ECG patients with aortic stenosis
Acta Med Scand **218**, 181-188
Acute exercise, Adult, Diagnosis, ECG

234/57   **Lipkin, D.P., Scriven, A.J., Crake, T. & Poole-Wilson, P.A.**   (1986)
Six minute walking test for assessing exercise capacity in chronic heart failure
Br Med J **292**, 653-655
Acute exercise, Adult, AEROBIC CAPACITY, Heart failure

234/58   **Lozner, E.C. & Morganroth, J.**   (1977)
New criteria to enhance the predictability of coronary artery disease by exercise testing in asymptomatic subjects
Circulation **56**, 799-802
Acute exercise, Adult, CHD-morbidity, ECG, Female, Male, Maximal test, S-T segment depression

234/59   **Lutz, J.F. & Wenger, N.K.**   (1985)
Use of exercise testing in non-coronary heart disease, In: Exercise and the Heart, edition 2 (Ed.) Brest, A.N.
Cardiovascular Clinics, F.A.Davis Company, Philadelphia **15**, 233-242
Review

234/60   **Magder, S., Linnarsson, D. & Gullstrand, L.**   (1981)
The effect of swimming on patients with ischemic heart disease
Circulation **63**, 979-986
Adult, Male, Maximal test, Prognosis, Safety, SECONDARY PREVENTION, Swimming,

234/61   **McHenry, P.L.**   (1977)
Risks of graded exercise testing
Am J Cardiol **39**, 935-937
Acute exercise, HAZARDS-CVS, Review

234/62   **McNeer, J.F., Margolis, J.R., Lee, K.L., Kisslo, J.A., Peter, R.H., Kong, Y., Behar, V.S., Wallace, A.G., McCants, C.B. & Rosati, C.B.**   (1978)
The role of the exercise test in the evaluation of patients for ischemic heart disease
Circulation **57**, 64-70
Acute exercise, Adult, ECG, Maximal test, Prognosis, SECONDARY PREVENTION, S-T segment depression

234/63   Meizlich, J.L., Berger, H.J. &
Zaret, B.L.   (1985)
Exercise nuclear imaging for the
evaluation of coronary heart disease. In:
Exercise and the Heart, edition 2 (Ed.)
Brest, A.N.
*Cardiovascular Clinics, F.A.Davis
Company, Philadelphia.* **15**, 105-124
Review

234/64   Mocellin, R.   (1986)
Exercise testing in children with
congenital heart disease
Pediatrician **13**, 18-25
Cardiac abnormalities, Children

234/65   Myers, J., Ahnve, S., Froelicher, V.,
Sullivan, M. & Friis, R.   (1987)
Influence of exercise training on spatial
R-wave amplitude in patients with
coronary artery disease
J Appl Physiol **62**, 1231-1235
Adult, Exercise programme, Intervention

234/66   Nicklin, D. & Balaban,
D.J.   (1984)
Exercise EKG in asymptomatic
normotensive subjects (Letter)
N Eng J Med **310**, 852-853
Acute exercise, Adult, Diagnosis, ECG

234/67   Niemela, K.O., Ikaheima, M.J.,
Linnaluoto, M.L. & Takkunen, J.
T.   (1983)
Functional limitation in aortic valve
disease: superiority of bicycle test to
symptom rated appraisal
Ann Clin Res **15**, 113-118
Adult, Comparative, Submaximal test

234/68   Nudel, D., Gootman, N., Brunson,
S., Stenzler, A., Shenker, R.I. & Gauthier,
B.G.   (1980)
Exercise performance of hypertensive
adolescents
Pediatrics **65**, 1073-1078
*BLOOD PRESSURE, Children,
Comparative, Diagnosis, Maximal test*

234/69   Nylander, E., Ekman, I., Marklund,
T., Sinnerstad, B., Karlsson, E. & Wranne,
B.   (1986)
Severe aortic stenosis in elderly patients
Br Heart J **55**, 480-487
Acute exercise, Diagnosis, Elderly

234/70   Oakley, D.G. & Oakley,
C.M.   (1982)
Significance of abnormal
electrocardiograms in highly trained
athletes
Am J Cardiol **50**, 985-989
*Adult, Athlete, CARDIAC
PERFORMANCE, ECG, HAZARDS-
CVS, Hypertrophy, Leisure activity,
Male, Vigorous*

234/71   Okin, P.M., Kligfield, P., Ameisen,
O. & Goldberg, H.L.   (1985)
Improved accuracy of the
electrocardiogram: identification of
three-vessel coronary disease in stable
angina pectoris by analysis of peak rate
related changes in ST segments
Am J Cardiol **55**, 271-276
*Acute exercise, Adult, Angina, ECG,
SECONDARY PREVENTION, S-T
segment depression*

234/72   Padmanabhan, V.T. & Gulotta,
S.J.   (1977)
Submaximal treadmill exercise testing of
patients with coronary artery disease
Postgraduate Med **61**, 215-227
Acute exercise, Diagnosis, Review

234/73   Papouchado, M. & Pitcher,
D.W.   (1986)
Ventricular pacing improves exercise
tolerance in patients with chronic heart
block
Br Heart J **56**, 366-371
*Adult, AEROBIC CAPACITY,
Arrhythmia, Cardiac pacing*

234/74   Patterson, R., Horowitz. S., Eng, C., Rudin, A., Meller, J., Halgashs, D.A., Pichard, A.D., Goldsmith, S.D., Herman, M.V. & Gorlin, R.   (1982)
Can exercise electrocardiography and thallium-201 myocardial imaging exclude the diagnosis of coronary artery disease?
Am J Cardiol **49**, 1127-1135
Acute exercise, Adult, CHD-morbidity, ECG

234/75   Piovano, G., Caselli, G. & Pozzilli, P.   (1980)
Frequency of ECG abnormalities in athletes. A study of 12,000 ECGs. In: Sports Cardiology International conference (Eds.) Lubich, T. & Venerando, A.
Aulo Gaggi, Bologna 625-630
Adult, Athlete, Arrhythmia, ECG, Leisure activity, Vigorous

234/76   Podczeck, A., Frohner, K., Föderler, G., Meisl, K., Unger, G. & Steinbach, K.   (1984)
Exercise test in patients over 65 years of age after the first myocardial infarction
Eur Heart J (Suppl E) **5**, 89-92
Arrhythmia, Elderly, Early post-myocardial test, Female, Male, Prognosis, SECONDARY PREVENTION, S-T segment depression,Submaximal test

234/77   Pool, J., Scheffer, M.G., Simoons, M.L. & Parijn, M.   (1984)
Clinical value of exercise testing in elderly patients
Eur Heart J (Suppl E) **5**, 47-50
Diagnosis, Elderly, Maximal test

234/78   Powles, A.C.P., Sutton, J.R., Wicks, J.R., Oldridge, N.B. & Jones, N.L.   (1979)
Reduced heart rate response to exercise in ischemic heart disease: The fallacy of the target heart rate in exercise testing
Med Sci Sports **11**, 227-233
Acute exercise, Adult, ECG, Prognosis, Male, SECONDARY PREVENTION

234/79   Rauscha, F., Glogar, D., Weber, H., Niederberger, M. & Kaindl, F.   (1984)
Diagnostic value of exercise testing versus long-term ECG in evaluation of arrhythmias in old age
Eur Heart J (Suppl E) **5**, 79-83
Arrhythmia, Diagnosis, ECG, Elderly, Maximal test, S-T segment depression

234/80   Rochmis, P. & Blackburn, H.   (1971)
Exercise tests. A survey of procedures, safety, litigation experience in approximately 170,000 tests
J Am Med Ass **217**, 1061-1066
Acute exercise, Adult, CHD-mortality

234/81   Samek, L., Betz, F. & Schnellbacher, K.   (1984)
Exercise testing in elderly patients with coronary artery disease
Eur Heart J (Suppl E) **5**, 69-73
BLOOD PRESSURE, Elderly, Male, SECONDARY PREVENTION, Submaximal test

234/82   Sandric, S.   (1980)
Echocardiography in sports medicine: Clinical diagnostic possibilities and its limitations. In: Sports Cardiology International conference (Eds.) Lubich, T. & Venerando, A.
Aulo Gaggi Bologna 6707-6716
Adult, Athlete, Arrhythmia, CARDIAC PERFORMANCE, Diagnosis, ECG, Hypertrophy, Leisure activity, Vigorous

234/83   Saunamäki, K.I.   (1984)
Early post-myocardial infarction exercise testing in subjects 70 years or more of age. Functional and prognostic evaluation
Eur Heart J (Suppl E) **5**, 93-96
AEROBIC CAPACITY, Elderly, Early post-myocardial test, Maximal test, Prognosis, SECONDARY PREVENTION

234/84   **Savin, W.M., Haskell, W.L., Schroeder, J.S. & Stinson, E.B.**   (1980)
Cardiorespiratory responses of cardiac transplant patients to graded, symptom-limited exercise
Circulation **62**, 55-60
Adult, CARDIAC PERFORMANCE, Comparative, Male, RESPIRATORY FUNCTION, SECONDARY PREVENTION

234/85   **Sheffield, L.T., Maloof, J.A., Sawyer, J.A. & Roitman, D.**   (1978)
Maximal heart rate and treadmill performance of healthy women in relation to age
Circulation **57**, 79-84
Acute exercise, Adult, Comparative, ECG, Female, Leisure activity, Maximal test, S-T segment depression

234/86   **Shephard, R.J.**   (1982)
Prognostic value of exercise testing for ischaemic heart disease
Brit J Sports Med **16**, 220-229
CHD-morbidity, Prognosis, Review, SECONDARY PREVENTION

234/87   **Specchia, G., La Rovere, M.T., Falcone, C., Campara, C., Traversi, E., Caizzi, V. & DeServi, S.**   (1986)
Cardiac arrhythmias during exercise-induced myocardial ischaemia in patients with coronary artery disease
Eur Heart J (Suppl A) **7**, 45-52
Acute exercise. Adult, Arrhythmia, ECG, SECONDARY PREVENTION, S-T segment depression

234/88   **Spiro, S.G.**   (1977)
Exercise testing in clinical medicine
Br J Dis Chest **71**, 145-172
Review

234/89   **Tzivoni, D., Gottlieb, S. & Klein, J.**   (1986)
Identification of low risk post infarction patients
Cardiologia **31**, 635-639
Acute exercise, Prognosis, Review

234/90   **Wasserman, K., Hansen, J.E., Sue, D.Y. & Whipp, B.J.**   (1987)
Principles of exercise testing and interpretation
Lea and Febiger, Philadelphia,
Acute exercise, Diagnosis, Prognosis, Maximal testing, Review

234/91   **Wenger, N.K.**   (1985)
Cardiovascular drugs: effects on exercise testing and exercise training of the coronary patient. In: Exercise and the Heart, edition 2 (Ed.) Brest, A.N.
Cardiovascular Clinics, F.A.Davis Company, Philadelphia. **15**, 133-144
Review, SECONDARY PREVENTION

234/92   **Whitmer, J.T., James, F.W., Kaplan, S., Schwartz, D.C. & Knight, M.J.S.**   (1981)
Exercise testing in children before and after surgical treatment of aortic stenosis
Circulation **63**, 254-263
Acute exercise, Children, Cardiac abnormalities, Diagnosis, Prognosis, S-T segment depression

234/93   **Zohman, L.R., Young, J.L. & Kattus, A.A.**   (1983)
Treadmill walking protocol for the diagnostic evaluation and exercise programming of cardiac patients
Am J Cardiol **51**, 1081-1086
Acute exercise, Adult, Diagnosis, Exercise programme, SECONDARY PREVENTION

240 ARTERIES OTHER THAN CORONARY

KEYWORDS are listed in the appendix in addition the following specific keywords have been used in this section:

Intermittent claudication
Viscosity
Walking distance (used as a measure of improvement)

Summary of evidence: exercise does not cure the disease but the general benefits have an ameliorating effect

THE PROBLEM

Occlusion of the major arteries of the legs is a painful and disabling condition which impairs walking capacity (intermittent claudication). Graded exercise programmes based upon walking can be shown to reduce symptoms and increase walking capacity. The general effects of the exercise will include favourable changes in skeletal muscle enzyme levels which facilitate local energy production and an improved capillarity. Can the exercise also promote the development of collateral arteries or reverse or cure the obliterative disease?

SCOPE

This section contains references dealing primarily with changes produced by exercise in intermittent claudication. There are also background references on blood flow (rheology).

METHODOLOGICAL DIFFICULTIES

Reliable measurement of muscle blood flow by non-invasive methods is impossible during walking. The natural course of the disease is erratic. Periods of remission may therefore be easily confused with a putative effect of exercise on symptoms.

EVIDENCE

There is no clear evidence that exercise produces improvements in the natural history of obliterative disease of the lower limb arteries or that it promotes the development of collateral vessels. However such patients can still benefit from exercise in other ways (see sections in 100) and there is no evidence that exercise such as walking within their tolerance of pain does harm.

240/1   **Boyd, C.E.**   (1984)
Pain free physical training in intermittent claudication
J Sports Med Phys Fitness **24**, 112-122
Adult, Exercise programme, Intermittent claudication, Intervention

240/2   **Buchwalsky, R., Blümchen, G., Battke, K., Barmeyer, J. & Reindell, H.**   (1974)
Psychosomatic aspects involved in a long term training programme for patients with peripheral occlusive artery disease
Rehabilitation **13**, 144-150
Adult, Customary activity, Exercise programme, Intermittent claudication, Intervention, Walking distance

240/3   **Cachovan, M., Marees, H. & Kunitsch, G.**   (1976)
Influence of interval training on the physical capacity and peripheral circulation in patients with intermittent claudication
Z Kardiol **65**, 54-67
Adult, Customary activity, Exercise programme, Intermittent claudication, Intervention, Walking distance

240/4   Clifford, P.C., Davies, P.W., Hayne, J.A. & Baird, R.N.   (1980)
Intermittent claudication: Is supervised exercise class worth while?
Br Med J **1**, 1503-1505
Adult, Customary activity, Exercise programme, Intermittent claudication, Intervention, Walking distance

240/5   Clyne, C.A.C., Mears, H., Weller, R.O. & O'Donnell, T.F.   (1985)
Calf muscle adaptation to peripheral vascular disease
Cardiovascular Res **19**, 507-512
Adult, Intermittent claudication, MUSCLE METABOLISM

240/6   Cox, J. M.   (1987)
Exercise and smoking habits in patients with and without low back pain and leg pain
J Manipulative Phys Ther **10**, 239-245
Adult, Comparative, JOINTS

240/7   Dahllof, A.-G., Holm, J. & Schersten, T.   (1983)
Exercise training of patients with intermittent claudication
Scand J Rehabil Med (Suppl 9) **15**, 20-26
Adult, Customary activity, Exercise programme, Longitudinal, MUSCLE METABOLISM, Intermittent claudication, Walking distance

240/8   Dahllof, A.-G., Holm, J., Schersten, T. & Sivertsson, R.   (1976)
Peripheral arterial insufficiency. Effect of physical training on walking tolerance, calf blood flow, and blood flow resistance
Scand J Rehabil Med **8**, 19-26
Adult, Customary activity, Exercise programme, Intermittent claudication, Intervention, Viscosity, Walking distance

240/9   Dälhof, A.-G., Björntorp, P., Holm, J. & Schersten, T.   (1974)
Metabolic activity of skeletal muscle in patients with peripheral arterial insufficiency
Eur J Clin Invest **4**, 9
Acute exercise, Adult, Intermittent claudication, MUSCLE METABOLISM

240/10   Edlund, A.   (1987)
Leg exercise increases prostacyclin synthesis without activating platelets in both healthy and athersclerotic humans
Adv Prostaglandin Thromboxane Leukotriene Res **17A**, 447-449
Acute exercise , Adult

240/11   Ekroth, R., Dahllöf, A.-G., Gundevall, B., Holm, J. & Schersten, T.   (1978)
Physical training of patients with intermittent claudication: Indications, methods, and results
Surgery **48**, 640-643
Adult, Customary activity, Exercise programme, Intermittent claudication, Intervention, Walking distance

240/12   Ericsson, B., Haeger, K. & Lindell, S.E.   (1970)
Effect of physical training on intermittent claudication
Angiology **21**, 188-192
Adult, Customary activity, Exercise programme, Intermittent claudication, Intervention, Male, Walking distance

240/13   Ernst, E.E.   (1987)
Influence of regular physical activity on blood rheology
Eur Heart J (Suppl G) **8**, 59-62
Adult, Athlete, Comparative, Leisure activity, Male, Viscosity, Vigorous

240/14   Ernst, E.E.   (1987)
Physical exercise for peripheral vascular disease – a review
Vasa **16**, 227-231
Review

240/15   **Ernst, E.E., Aschenbrenner, E. & Matrai, A.**   (1986)
Blood rheology in athletes
J Sports Med Phys Fitness **4**, 207
Adult, Athlete, Viscosity

240/16   **Ernst, E.E. & Matrai, A.**   (1985)
Relationship between fitness and blood rheology
Clin Hemorheol **5**, 507
Adult, AEROBIC CAPACITY, Athlete, Exercise programme, Intervention, Vigorous, Viscosity

240/17   **Ernst, E.E. & Matrai, A.**   (1987)
Intermittent claudication, exercise, and blood rheology
Circulation **76**, 1110-1114
Adult, BLOOD PRESSURE, CARBOHYDRATE TOLERANCE, Customary activity, Exercise programme, Intermittent claudication, Intervention, Viscosity, Walking distance

240/18   **Eugene, M., Vandewalle, H., Bertholon, J.F. & Teillac, A.**   (1986)
Arterial elasticity and physical working capacity in young men
J Appl Physiol **61**, 1720-1723
Acute exercise, Adult, BLOOD PRESSURE, Male

240/19   **Franco, A.**   (1981)
Treatment of intermittent claudication by physical atraining. Techniques and place of re-education
J Mal Vasc **6**, 6-7
Adult, Customary activity, Exercise programme, Intermittent claudication, Intervention, Walking distance

240/20   **Gerdle, B., Hedberg, B., Angquist, K.-A. & Fugl-Meyer, A.R.**   (1986)
Isokinetic strength and endurance in peripheral arterial insufficiency with intermittent claudication
Scand J Rehabil Med **18**, 9-15
Acute exercise, Adult, Comparative, Intermittent claudication, MUSCLE STRENGTH, Male

240/21   **Holdich, T.A.H., Reddy, P.J., Walker, R.T. & Dormandy, J.A.**   (1986)
Transcutaneous oxygen tension during exercise in patients with claudication
Br Med J **292**, 1625-1628
Acute exercise, Adult, Intermittent claudication

240/22   **Holm, J., Dahllöf, A.-G., Björntorp, P. & Scherstén, T.**   (1973)
Enzyme studies in muscles of patients with intermittent claudication. Effect of training
Scand J clin Lab Invest (Suppl 128) **31**, 201-205
Adult, Customary activity, Exercise programme, Intermittent claudication, Intervention, MUSCLE METABOLISM, Walking distance

240/23   **Housley, E.**   (1988)
Treating claudication in five words
Br Med J **296**, 1483
Intermittent claudication, Review

240/24   **Hovind, H., Holm, A.B., Holstein, P. & Nielsen, S.L.**   (1976)
Walking exercise in intermittent claudication
Ugeskr Laeger **138**, 90-93
Adult, Customary activity, Exercise programme, Intermittent claudication, Intervention, Walking distance

240/25   **Jonason, T., Jonzon, B., Ringqvist,I. & Oman-Rydberg, A.**   (1979)
Effect of physical training on different categories of patient with intermittent claudication
Acta Med Scand **206**, 253-258
Adult, Customary activity, Exercise programme, Intervention, Intermittent claudication, Walking distance

240/26   Jonason, T. & Ringqvist, I.   (1987)
Prediction of the effect of training on the
walking tolerance in patients with
intermittent claudication
Scand J Rehabil Med **19**, 47-50
Adult, Customary activity, Exercise
programme, Intervention, Intermittent
claudication, Walking distance

240/27   Jonason, T., Ringqvist, I. & Oman-
Rydberg, A.   (1981)
Home training of patients with
intermittent claudication
Scand J Rehabil Med **13**, 137-141
Customary activity, Elderly, Exercise
programme, Intervention, Intermittent
claudication, Walking distance

240/28   Jonason, T. & Ringqvist, I.   (1987)
Effect of training on the post-exercise
ankle blood pressure reaction in patients
with intermittent claudicatioon
Clin Physiol **7**, 63-69
Adult, Exercise programme, Intermittent
claudication, Intervention

240/29   Kiesewetter, H.   (1987)
Training by walking and drug therapy of
peripheral arterial occlusive disease
Vasa (Suppl) **20**, 384-387
Adult, Exercise Programme, Intermittent
claudication, Intervention

240/30   Kiesewetter, H., Jung, F. & Blume,
J.   (1986)
Conservative drug therapy and walking
exercise in stage IIb peripheral arterial
occlusion disease
Klin Wochenschr **15**, 1061-1069
Adult, Customary activity, Exercise
programme, Intermittent claudication,
Intervention

240/31   Kroese, A.   (1982)
Physical activity and the peripheral
circulation
Scand J Soc Med (Suppl) **29**, 47-49
Intermittent claudication, MUSCLE
METABOLISM, Review

240/32   Larsen, O.A. & Lassen,
N.A.   (1966)
Effect of daily muscular exercise in
patients with intermittent claudication
Lancet, **2**, 1093-1096.
Adult, Customary activity, Exercise
programme, Intermittent claudication,
Intervention, Walking distance

240/33   Lepäntalo, M., Sundberg, S. &
Gordin, A.   (1984)
The effects of physical training and
flunarizine on walking capacity in
intermittent claudication
Scand J Rehabil Med **16**, 159-162
Adult, Customary activity, Exercise
programme, Intermittent claudication,
Intervention, Viscosity, Walking distance

240/34   Loubet, J.M.   (1974)
Physical treatment of circulatory
disorders of the lower limbs
Phlebologie **27**, 65-67.
Adult, Exercise programme, Intervention

240/35   Maas, U.   (1982)
Effect of interval training for length of
walk, hemodynamics and ventilation in
patients with intermittent claudication. I.
Change in length of walk
Vasa **11**, 91-96
Adult, Customary activity, Exercise
programme, Intermittent claudication,
Intervention, Walking distance

240/36   Myhre, K. & Sørlie, D.G.   (1982)
Physical activity and peripheral
atherosclerosis
Scand J Soc Med (Suppl) **29**, 195-201
Intermittent claudication, Review

240/37   Puls, A. & Thadani, U.   (1986)
Rupture of abdominal aortic aneurysm
during exercise. Gated blood pool
studies
Am J Med **81**, 887-889
Acute exercise, Adult, Hazards, Male

240/38   Ruckley, C.V.   (1986)
Claudication
Br Med J **292**, 970-971
Intermittent claudication, Review

240/39   **Ruell, P.A., Imperial, E.S., Bonar, F.J., Thursby, P.F. & Gass, G.C.**   (1984)
Intermittent claudication. The effect of physical training on walking tolerance and venous lactate concentration
Eur J Appl Physiol **52**, 420-425
Adult, Customary activity, Exercise programme, Elderly, Intermittent claudication, Intervention, LIPIDS, Walking distance

240/40   **Schneider, S.H.**   (1986)
Atherosclerosis and physical activity
Diabetes Metab Rev **1**, 513-553
Review

240/41   **Schoop, W.**   (1973)
Mechanism of beneficial action of daily walking training of patients with intermittent claudication
Scand J clin Lab Invest (Suppl 128) **31**, 201-205
Adult, Customary activity, Exercise programme, Intermittent claudication, Intervention, Walking distance

240/42   **Skinner, J.S. & Strandness, D.E.**   (1967)
Exercise and intermittent claudication. II.Effect of physical training
Circulation **36**, 23-29
Adult, Customary activity, Exercise programme, Intermittent claudication, Intervention, Male, Walking distance

240/43   **Sørlie, D.G., Myhre, K. & Mjøs, O.D.**   (1978)
Exercise- and post-exercise metabolism of the lower leg in patients with peripheral arterial insuffciency
Scand J clin Lab Invest **38**, 635-642
Acute exercise, Adult

240/44   **Thulesius, O.**   (1978)
Systemic and ankle blood pressure before and after exercise in patients with arterial insufficiency
Angiology **29**, 374-378
Acute exercise, Adult, BLOOD PRESSURE, CARDIAC PERFORMANCE, Intermittent claudication

240/45   **Zetterquist, S.**   (1970)
Effect of daily training on the nutritive blood flow in exercising ischemic legs
Scand J clin Lab Invest **25**, 101-111
Adult, Customary activity, Exercise programme, Intermittent claudication, Intervention, Male

KEYWORDS are listed in the appendix in addition the following specific keywords have been used in this section:

Intermittent claudication
Varicose veins
Vasoregulatory asthenia

Summary of evidence: exercise ameliorates problems associated with varicose veins and helps prevent deep vein thrombosis

THE PROBLEM

Varicose veins are common, especially in women, and become worse after pregnancy; they are at best disfiguring, sometimes painful and at worst can lead to varicose ulcers. Walking exercise is often prescribed, what are its effects?

SCOPE

This section contains references dealing with changes produced by exercise in patients with varicose veins, phlebitis, and deep vein thrombosis. References dealing with the effect of exercise on vasoregulatory asthenia is included here but varicose veins are only one of the possible causes of this condition.

EVIDENCE

There is evidence that the discomfort caused by varicose veins in the legs is relieved and that the convalescence of patients with varicose ulcer is shortened by including exercise among the measures directed towards the reduction of the local venous pressure. The pumping action of the leg muscles during rhythmic activity such as walking is of value in maintaining venous flow, reducing venous back pressure and pooling. There is also evidence that leg exercise reduces the incidence of deep vein thrombosis.

250/1   (1977)
Exercise for deep venous thrombosis (Editorial)
Lancet **2**, 963
Review

250/2   **Ali, M.S.**   (1984)
Deep vein thrombosis in a jogger
Am J Sports Med **12**, 169
Adult, HAZARDS-CVS, Leisure activity, Running

250/3   **Borg, G. & Linderholm, H.**   (1970)
Exercise performance and perceived exertion in patients with coronary insufficiency, arterial hypertension and vasoregulatory asthenia
Acta Med Scand **187**, 17-26
Acute exercise, Adult, BLOOD PRESSURE, SECONDARY PREVENTION, Vasoregulatory asthenia

250/4   **Clayton, M.L. & Thompson, T.R.**   (1987)
Activity, air boots and aspirin as thromboembolism prophylaxis in knee arthroplasty
Orthopedics **10**, 1525-1527
Adult, Exercise programme

250/5   **Corson, S.L.**   (1984)
Prophylaxis against thromboembolism in gynecologic patients
J Reproduc Med **29**, 845-862
Review

250/6   **Grimby, G., Nilsson, N.J. & Sanne, H.**   (1964)
Cardiac output during exercise in patients with varicose veins
Scand J clin Lab Invest **16**, 21-30
Acute exercise, Adult, CARDIAC PERFORMANCE, Female, Varicose veins

250/7   Holmgren, A., Jonsson, B., Levander, M., Linderholm, H., Mossfeldt, F., Sjostrand, T. & Strom, G.   (1959)
Physical training involving large muscle groups in a successful treatment for vasoregulatory asthenia
Acta Med Scand **165**, 89-103
Adult, Exercise programme, Female, Intervention, Male, Vasoregulatory asthenia

250/8   Holmgren, A., Jonsson, B., Levander, M., Linderholm, H., Sjöstrand, T.& Ström, G.   (1959)
E.C.G. changes in vasoregulatory asthenia and the effect of physical training
Acta Med Scand **165**, 259-271
Adult, Exercise programme, HEART FUNCTION TEST, Intervention, Vasoregulatory asthenia

250/9   Holmgren, A., Jonsson, B., Levander-Lindgren, M., Linderholm, H., Mossfeldt, F., Sjostrand, T. & Strom, G.   (1959)
Blood lactate concentration in relation to absolute and relative work load in normal men and in mitral stenosis, atrial septal defect and vasoregulatory asthenia
Acta Med Scand **163**, 186-193
Acute exercise, Adult, Comparative, Male, Vasoregulatory asthenia

250/10   Holmgren, A. & Ström, G.   (1959)
Vasoregulatory asthenia in a female athlete and Da Costa's syndrome in a male athlete successfully treated by physical training
Acta Med Scand **164**, 113-118
Adult, Athlete, Exercise programme, Female, Hazards, Intervention, Male, Vasoregulatory asthenia

250/11   Kenney, W.L. & Armstrong, C.G.   (1987)
The effect of aerobic conditioning on venous pooling in the foot
Med Sci Sports Exerc **19**, 474-479
Adult, AEROBIC CAPACITY, Exercise programme, Intervention, Male

250/12   Marmasse, J.   (1975)
Physical methods in the treatment and prevention of deep phlebitis of the leg
Phlebologie **28**, 47-64
Review

250/13   Quarfordt, P.G., Eklølf, B., Ohlin, P., Plate, G. & Saltin, B.   (1984)
Intramuscular pressure, blood flow and skeletal muscle metabolism in patients with venous claudication
Surgery **95**, 191-195
Adult, Intermittent claudication, MUSCLE METABOLISM

250/14   Raven, P.B., Young, D.R., Varas, T.S. & Overn, S.P.   (1983)
Fitness related alteration in leg venous compliance
Med Sci Sports Exerc **15**, 250
Adult, AEROBIC CAPACITY, Comparative, Male

KEYWORDS are listed in the appendix in addition the following specific keywords have been used in this section:

Airway calibre
Asthma
Bronchitis
COPD (Chronic obstructive pulmonary disease)
Cystic fibrosis
Endorphins
Gas transfer
LFT (Lung function test)
MVV (Maximum ventilatory volume)
Respiratory muscle
Tuberculosis
Ventilatory control

Summary of evidence: exercise ameliorates respiratory diseases by improving exercise tolerance

THE PROBLEM

Exercise is not limited by ventilatory capacity in those who are young and healthy. However, is a very sedentary lifestyle or bedrest associated with diminished respiratory muscle capability? Although exercise is not thought to change lung function as such, does it influence ventilatory dimensions in children? In those with diseased lungs, does it ameliorate their disease? Exercise will induce bronchospasm in asthmatics and atopic individuals. Is exercise therefore harmful in asthma?

SCOPE

This section contains references dealing primarily with changes produced by exercise on ventilatory capacity, lung function and physical capabilities in respiratory patients. There are studies of all age groups, of men and women, of sedentary and athletic groups, of growth in children, of normal subjects and patients (see keywords for diseases). Many studies concerning the mechanism of exercise-induced asthma are included. There are studies of the acute effects of exercise especially on patients. There are no animal studies.

METHODOLOGICAL DIFFICULTIES

A fundamental difficulty in assessing effect on any variable on the growth of children is their unpredictable growth curve. Asthma is by definition characterised by profound variations in airway resistance so that a baseline is difficult to define.

EVIDENCE

It is clear that exercise can be undertaken safely in the presence of respiratory diseases provided proper medical advice and necessary medication are sought. It is beneficial for such patients because well-trained leg muscles put less strain on disordered lungs (see section 120 and 140). In asthma the disability induced by inactivity is of more serious consequence for the physical capacity of the asthmatic than exercise induced bronchospasm which can be avoided by the prophylactic use of bronchodilator aerosol. There is no evidence for a permanent effect on ventilatory capacities of exercise during growth and adolescence (see section 430). There is only tentative evidence for an increase in the strength of respiratory muscles through exercise in sedentary individuals. Like the heart, respiratory muscles are continually active and therefore do not deteriorate from lack of activity in the way peripheral skeletal muscles can. The lack of any exercise effect on lung function as such is confirmed.

300/5   Andréasson, B., Jonson, B., Kornfält, R., Nordmark, E. & Sandström, S.   (1987)
Long-term effects of physical exercise on working capacity and pulmonary function in cystic fibrosis
Acta Paediatr Scand **76**, 70-75
AEROBIC CAPACITY, Children, Cystic fibrosis, Exercise programme, Female, Gas transfer, Handicap, Intervention, LFT, Male

300/1   **Aarseth, H.P.**   (1982)
The effect of regular physical activity on the organs of ventilation
Scand J Soc Med (Suppl) **29**, 51-53
Asthma, Gas transfer, Handicap, Lung volume, Review

300/6   **Andrew, G.M., Becklake, M., Guleria, J.S. & Bates, D.**   (1972)
Heart and lung functions in swimmers and non-athletes during growth
J Appl Physiol **32**, 245-251
Athlete, Children, Comparative, Female, Gas transfer, GROWTH, Heart function tests, Leisure activity, LFT, Longitudinal, Male, Swimming, Vigorous

300/2   **Adams, L., Frankel, H., Garlick, J., Guz, A., Murphy, K. & Semple, S.J.**   (1984)
The role of spinal cord transmission in the ventilatory response to exercise in man
J Physiol **355**, 85-97
Acute exercise, Adult, Handicap, LFT, Ventilatory control

300/7   **Araujo, I., Schrijen, F. & Peslin, R.**   (1986)
Pulmonary haemodynamic response to two-stage exercise in patients with chronic bronchitis
Eur J Respir Dis **69**, 270-275
Acute exercise, Adult, CARDIAC PERFORMANCE, COPD

300/3   **Alison, J.A., Samios, R. & Anderson, S.D.**   (1981)
Evaluation of exercise training in patients with chronic airway obstruction
Phys Ther **61**, 1273-1277
Adult, COPD, Exercise programme, Intervention, LFT

300/8   **Arborelius, M. Jr. & Svenonius, E.**   (1984)
Decrease of exercise induced asthma after physical training
Eur J Respir Dis (Suppl) **65**, 25
Asthma, Children, Exercise programme, Handicap, Intervention, LFT, Swimming

300/4   **Alpert, J.S., Bass, H., Szucs, M.M., Banas, J.S., Dalen, J.E. & Dexter, L.**   (1974)
Effects of physical training on hemodynamics and pulmonary function at rest and during exercise in patients with chronic obstructive pulmonary disease
Chest **66**, 647-651
Adult, CARDIAC PERFORMANCE, COPD, Exercise programme, Gas transfer, Handicap, Intervention, LFT, MVV, Respiratory muscle,

300/9   **Bar-Yishay, E., Gur, I., Inbar, O., Neuman, I., Dlin, R.A. & Godfrey, S.**   (1982)
Differences between swimming and running as stimuli for exercise-induced asthma
Eur J Appl Physiol **48**, 387-397
Acute exercise, Asthma, Children, Comparative, Handicap, LFT, Running, Swimming

300/10   **Belman, M.J.**   (1986)
Exercise in chronic obstructive
pulmonary disease
Clin Chest Med **7**, 585-597
COPD, Review

300/11   **Belman, M.J. & Gaesser,
G.A.**   (1988)
Ventilatory muscle training in the elderly
J Appl Physiol **64**, 899-905
***AEROBIC CAPACITY, Elderly,
Exercise programme, Gas transfer,
Intervention, LFT, MVV, PERCEIVED
EXERTION, Respiratory muscle***

300/12   **Belman, M.J. & Kendregan,
B.A.**   (1981)
Exercise training fails to increase skeletal
muscle enzymes in patients with chronic
obstructive pulmonary disease
Am Rev Respir Dis **123**, 256-261
***Adult, COPD, Handicap, Intervention,
LFT, MUSCLE METABOLISM***

300/13   **Belman, M.J. & Kendregan,
B.A.**   (1982)
Physical training fails to improve
ventilatory muscle endurance in patients
with chronic obstructive pulmonary
disease
Chest **81**, 440-443
***Adult, COPD, Exercise programme,
Intervention, LFT, MVV, Respiratory
muscle***

300/14   **Belman, M.J. & Sieck,
G.C.**   (1982)
The ventilatory muscles – fatigue,
endurance and training
Chest **82**, 761-766
Respiratory muscle, Review

300/15   **Bense, L., Wiman, L.-G. &
Hedenstierna, G.**   (1987)
Onset of symptoms in spontaneous
pneumothorax: correlations to physical
activity
Eur J Resir Dis **71**, 181-186
Acute exercise, Adult

300/16   **Berglund, E.**   (1979)
Limiting factors during exercise in
patients with lung disease
Bull Europ Physiopath Resp **15**, 15-23
Review

300/17   **Biersteker, M.W.A. & Biersteker,
P.A.**   (1985)
Vital capacity in trained and untrained
health young adults in the Netherlands
Eur J Appl Physiol **54**, 46-53
***Adult, Body composition, Comparative,
Female, Leisure activity, LFT, Male,***

300/18   **Blomquist, M., Freyschuss, U.,
Wiman, L-G. & Strandvik, B.**   (1986)
Physical activity and self treatment in
cystic fibrosis
Arch Dis Child **61**, 362-367
***Children, Cystic fibrosis, Exercise
programme, Gas transfer, Handicap,
Intervention, LFT, Vigorous***

300/19   **Bolton, J.W., Weinman, D.S.,
Haynes, J.L., Hornung, C.A., Olsen, G.N.
& Almond, C.H.**   (1987)
Stair climbing as an indicator of
pulmonary function
Chest **92**, 783-788
***Acute exercise, Adult, Customary activity,
LFT, Male***

300/20   **Braun, S.R., Fregosi, R. & Reddan,
W.G.**   (1982)
Exercise training in patients with COPD
Postgraduate Med **71**, 163-173
***COPD, Exercise programme,
Intervention, Review***

300/21   **Brischetto, M.J., Millman, R.P.,
Peterson, D.D., Silage, D.A. & Pack,
A.I.**   (1984)
Effect of aging on ventilatory response to
exercise and CO2
J Appl Physiol **56**, 1143-1150
***Acute exercise, Adult, Comparative,
Elderly, Gas transfer, LFT, Ventilatory
control***

300/22   **Bundgaard, A.**   (1985)
Exercise and the asthmatic
Sports Med **2,** 254-266
Asthma, Handicap, Review

300/23   **Bundgaard, A., Inglemann-Hansen, T., Halkjaer-Kristensen, J., Schmidt, A., Bloch, I. & Anderson, P.K.**   (1983)
Short term physical training in bronchial asthma
Br J Dis Chest **77,** 147-152
Adult, AEROBIC CAPACITY, Asthma, Exercise programme, Female, Intervention, LFT, Male, Weight

300/24   **Bundgaard, A., Inglemann-Hansen, T., Schmidt, A. & Halkjaer-Kristensen, J.**   (1982)
Effect of physical training on peak oxygen consumption rate and exercise-induced asthma in adult asthmatics
Scand J clin Lab Invest **42,** 9-13
Adult, AEROBIC CAPACITY, Asthma, Exercise programme, Female, Handicap, Intervention, LFT, Male, Vigorous

300/25   **Cahory, J.E.**   (1975)
Symposium: Exercise and Asthma – Seattle, Washington
Pediatrics (Suppl 2) **56,** 844-846
Asthma, Review

300/26   **Carter, R., Nicotra, B., Clark, L., Zinkgraf, S., Williams, J., Peavler, M., Fields, S. & Berry, J.**   (1988)
Exercise conditioning in the rehabilitation of patients with chronic obstructive pulmonary disease
Arch Phys Med Rehabil **69,** 118-122
Adult, AEROBIC CAPACITY, COPD, Exercise programme, Gas transfer, Intervention, LFT, MVV

300/27   **Carter, R., Peavler, M., Zinkgraf, S., Williams, J. & Fields, S.**   (1987)
Predicting maximal exercise ventilation in patients with chronic obstructive pulmonary disease
Chest **92,** 253-259
Adult, COPD, Handicap, LFT, MVV

300/28   **Casaburi, R., Storer, T.W. & Wasserman, K.**   (1986)
Endurance training reduces ventilatory demand during heavy exercise
Am Rev Respir Dis (Suppl) **133,** A45
Adult, AEROBIC CAPACITY, ANAEROBIC CAPACITY, Exercise programme, Gas transfer, Intervention, Ventilatory control

300/29   **Casaburi, R. & Wasserman, K.**   (1986)
Exercise training in pulmonary rehabilitation (Editorial)
N Engl J Med **314,** 1509-1511
ANAEROBIC CAPACITY, COPD, Handicap, Review

300/30   **Casaburi, R., Storer, T.W. & Wasserman, K.**   (1987)
Mediation of reduced ventilatory response to exercise after endurance training
J Appl Physiol **63,** 1533-1538
Acute exercise, Adult, AEROBIC CAPACITY, ANAEROBIC CAPACITY, Exercise programme, Intervention, LFT, Ventilatory control

300/31   **Celli, B.R., Rassulo, J. & Make, B.J.**   (1986)
Dyssynchronous breathing during arm but not leg exercise in patients with chronic airflow obstruction
N Engl J Med **314,** 1485-1490
Acute exercise, Adult, Comparative, COPD, Handicap, Respiratory muscle

300/32   **Cerny, F.J.**   (1987)
Breathing patterns during exercise in young black and Caucasian subjects
J Appl Physiol **62,** 2220-2223
Acute exercise, Adult, Children, Comparative, LFT

300/33 **Cerny, F.J., Pullano, T.P. & Cropp, G.J.** (1982)
Cardiorespiratory adaptations to exercise in cystic fibrosis
Am Rev Respir Dis **126**, 217-220
Acute exercise, BLOOD PRESSURE, Children, Comparative, Cystic fibrosis, Handicap, Intervention, Leisure activity, LFT, MVV, Respiratory muscle

300/34 **Clanton, T.L., Dixon, G.F., Drake, J. & Gadek, J.E.** (1987)
Effects of swim training on lung volumes and inspiratory muscle conditioning
J Appl Physiol **62**, 39-46
Adult, Athlete, Female, Intervention, Leisure activity, LFT, MVV, Respiratory muscle, Swimming

300/35 **Dantzker, D.R. & D'Alonzo, G.E.** (1986)
The effect of exercise on pulmonary gas exchange in patients with severe chronic obstructive pulmonary disease
Am Rev Respir Dis **134**, 1135-1139
Acute exercise, Adult, COPD, Gas transfer, Handicap, LFT, Ventilatory control

300/36 **Dean, M., Bell, E., Kershaw, C.R., Guyer, B.M. & Hide, D.W.** (1988)
A short exercise and living course for asthmatics
Br J Dis Chest **82**, 155-161
Asthma, Children, Handicap, Intervention, Leisure activity

300/37 **Degre, S., Sergysels, R., Messin, R., Vandermoten, P., Salhadin, P., Denolin, H. & De Coster, A.** (1974)
Hemodynamic responses to physical training in patients with chronic lung disease
Am Rev Respir Dis **110**, 395-402
Adult, AEROBIC CAPACITY, CARDIAC PERFORMANCE, Exercise programme, Gas transfer, Handicap, Intervention, LFT, Male

300/38 **Dillard, T.A.** (1987)
Ventilatory limitation of exercise. Prediction in COPD (Editorial)
Chest **92**, 195-196
Acute exercise, COPD, Handicap, LFT, MVV, Review

300/39 **Eiken, O., Lind, F. & Bjurstedt, H.** (1986)
Effects of blood volume ditribution on ventilatory variables at rest and during exercise
Acta Physiol Scand **127**, 507-512
Acute exercise, Adult, LFT, Male, MUSCLE METABOLISM, Ventilatory control

300/40 **Estrup, C.** (1986)
Effect of respiratory muscle training in patients with neuromuscular diseases and in normals
Respiration **50**, 36-43
Adult, Comparative, Exercise programme, Handicap, Intervention, Respiratory muscle

300/41 **Fanta, C.H., Leith, D.E. & Brown, R.** (1983)
Maximal shortening of inspiratory muscles: effect of training
J Appl Physiol **54**, 1618-1623
Adult, Exercise programme, Female, Intervention, LFT, Male, Respiratory muscles

300/42 **Fitch, K.D.** (1986)
The effects of running training on exercise-induced asthma
Ann Allergy **57**, 90-94
Asthma, Children, Exercise programme, Handicap, Intervention

300/43 **Fitch, K.D., Morton, A.R. & Blanksby, B.A.** (1976)
Effects of swimming training on children with asthma
Arch Dis Child **51**, 190-194
Asthma, Body composition, Children, Handicap, Intervention, Leisure activity, Swimming

300/44   Goldstein, S.A. & Askanazi, J.(1986)
Exercise, diet, and the rehabilitation of lung patients
Curr Concepts Nutr **15**, 183-201
COPD, Review

300/45   Goldstein, S.A., Weissman, C., Askanazi, J., Rothkopf, M., Milic-Emili, J. & Kinney, J.M.   (1987)
Metabolic and ventilatory responses during very low level exercise
Clin Sci **73**, 417-424
Acute exercise, Adult, Comparative, Female, Gas transfer, LFT, Male, Ventilatory control

300/46   Graff-Lonnevig, V., Bevegård, S., Eriksson, B.O., Kraepelien, S. & Saltin, B.   (1980)
Two years' follow-up of asthmatic boys participating in a physical activity programme
Acta Paediatr Scand **69**, 347-352
AEROBIC CAPACITY, Asthma, Children, Exercise programme, Handicap. Intervention, LFT, Male

300/47   Graff-Lonnevig, V., Bevegård, S., Eriksson, B.O., Kreapelien, S. & Saltin, B.   (1978)
Effect of a physical education program on the cardiopulmonary function and the exercise capacity of boys with bronchial asthma. In: Children and Exercise IX (Eds.) Berg, K. & Eriksson, B.O.
University Park Press, Baltimore
AEROBIC CAPACITY, Asthma, CARDIAC PERFORMANCE, Children, Exercise programme, Handicap, Intervention, LFT, Male

300/48   Grassino, A., Gross, D., Macklem, P.T., Roussos, C.H.. & Zagelbaum, G.   (1979)
Inspiratory muscle fatigue as a factor limiting exercise
Bull Europ Physiopath Resp **15**, 105-111
Acute exercise, Adult, Exercise programme, Handicap, Intervention, Respiratory muscles

300/49   Gross, D., Ladd, H.W., Riley, E.J.. Macklem, P.T. & Grassino, A.   (1980)
The effect of training on strength and endurance of the diaphragm in quadriplegia
Am J Med **68**, 27-35
Adult, Exercise programme, Female, Handicap, Intervention, Male, Respiratory muscle

300/50   Haas, F., Pasierski, S., Levine, N., Bishop, M., Axen, K., Pineda, H. & Haas. A.   (1987)
Effect of aerobic training on forced expiratory airflow in exercising asthmatic humans
J Appl Physiol **63**, 1230-1235
Adult, Asthma, Exercise programme, Handicap, Intervention, LFT, MVV

300/51   Hale, T., Spriggs, J. & Hamley, E.J.   (1976)
Effectiveness of an exercise regime on the rehabilitation of chronic obstructive lung disease patients using heart-rate as the parameter
Br J Sports Med **10**, 71-75
Adult, CARDIAC PERFORMANCE, COPD, Exercise programme, Intervention, Male

300/52   Hedlin, G., Graff-Lonnevig, V. & Freyschuss, U.   (1986)
Working capacity and pulmonary gas exchange in children with exercise-induced asthma
Acta Paediatr Scand **75**, 947-954
Acute exercise, Asthma, Children, Gas transfer, Handicap, LFT

300/53   Henriksen, J.M. & Nielsen, T.T.   (1983)
Effect of physical training on exercise-induced bronchoconstriction
Acta Paediatr Scand **72**, 31-36
Asthma, Children, Exercise programme, Handicap, Intervention, LFT

300/54   Henriksen, J.M., Toftegaard
Nielsen, T. & Dahl, R.   (1981)
Effects of physical training on plasma
citrate and exercise-induced asthma
Scand J clin Lab Invest **41**, 225-229
Airway calibre, Asthma, Children,
Exercise programme, Intervention, LFT

300/55   Jagodzinski,J., Baj, K., Buczek, W.,
Bronz, Z., Jaworski, A., Wozniakowska,
U., Wyzewski, Z., Bogulawska, E. &
Kosecki, K.   (1975)
Physical fitness in tuberculosis patients
having undergone general exercise
therapy
Gruzlica **43**, 727-735
Adult, Exercise programme, Intervention,
MUSCLE STRENGTH, Tuberculosis

300/56   Kanstrup, I.-L. & Ekblom,
B.   (1978)
Influence of age and physical activity on
central hemodynamics and lung function
in active adults
J Appl Physiol **45**, 709-717
Adult, AEROBIC CAPACITY,
CARDIAC PERFORMANCE, Female,
Gas transfer, Inactivity, LFT,
Longitudinal, Male

300/57   Keens, T.   (1979)
Exercise training programs for pediatric
patients with chronic lung disease
Ped Clin N Am **26**, 517-524
Children, Exercise programme,
Intervention, Review

300/58   Keens, T.G., Krastins, I.R.B.,
Wannamaker, E.M., Levison, H., Crozier,
D.N. & Bryan, A.C.   (1977)
Ventilatory muscle endurance training in
normal subjects and patients with cystic
fibrosis
Am Rev Respir Dis **116**, 853-860
Adult, Children, Comparative, Cystic
fibrosis, Exercise programme, Handicap,
Intervention, Leisure activity, LFT, MVV,
Respiratory muscle,

300/59   Leisti, S., Finnila, M. & Kiuru,
E.   (1979)
Effects of physical training on hormonal
responses to exercise in asthmatic
children
Arch Dis Child **54**, 524-528
Asthma, Children, Endocrine, Exercise
programme, GROWTH, Handicap,
Intervention, LFT

300/60   Leith, D.E. & Bradley, M.   (1976)
Ventilatory muscle strength and
endurance training
J Appl Physiol **41**, 508-516
Adult, Intervention, LFT, MVV,
Respiratory muscle

300/61   Levine, S., Weiser, P. & Gillen,
J.   (1986)
Evaluation of a ventilatory muscle
endurance training program in the
rehabilitation of patients with chronic
obstructive pulmonary disease
Am Rev Respir Dis **133**, 400-406
Adult, COPD, Customary activity, Gas
transfer, Handicap, Intervention, LFT,
Male, MOOD, MVV, Respiratory muscle

300/62   Loke, J., Mahler, D.A. & Virgulto,
J.A.   (1982)
Respiratory muscle fatigue after
marathon running
J Appl Physiol **52**, 821-824
Acute exercise, Adult, Leisure activity,
LFT, Male, Marathon, MVV,
Respiratory muscle

300/63   Ludwick, S.K., Jones, J.W., Jones,
T.K., Fukuhara, J. & Strunk,
R.C.   (1986)
Normalization of cardiopulmonary
endurance in severely asthmatic children
after bicycle ergometry therapy
J Pediatr **109** 446-451
AEROBIC CAPACITY, Asthma,
Children, Exercise programme, Handicap,
Intervention, LFT

300/64   **Mallinson, B.M., Cockroft, C., Burgess, D.A. & Spicak, V.** (1981)
Exercise training for children with asthma
Physiotherapy **67**, 106-108
Asthma, Children, Exercise programme, Intervention

300/65   **Martin, A.J.** (1986)
Respiratory muscle training in Duchenne muscular dystrophy
Dev Med Child Neurol **28**, 314-318
Children, Exercise programme, Handicap, Intervention, LFT, Respiratory muscle

300/66   **McFadden, E.R. Jr.** (1987)
Exercise and asthma (Editorial)
N Engl J Med **317**, 502-504
Asthma, Handicap, Review

300/67   **McGavin, C.R., Gupta, S.P., Lloyd, E.L. & McHardy, G.J.R.** (1977)
Physical rehabilitation for the chronic bronchitic; results of a controlled trial of exercises in the home
Thorax **32**, 307-311
Adult, COPD, Customary activity, Handicap, Intervention, LFT

300/68   **McKenzie, D.K. & Gandevia, S.C.** (1986)
Strength and endurance of inspiratory, expiratory and limb muscles in asthma
Am Rev Respir Dis **134**, 999-1004
Acute exercise, Adult, Asthma, Comparative, Female, Handicap, Male, MUSCLE STRENGTH, Respiratory muscle

300/69   **McKeon, J.L., Turner, J., Kelly, C., Dent, A. & Zimmerman, P.V.** (1986)
The effect of inspiratory resistive training on exercise capacity in optimally treated patients with severe chronic airflow limitation
Aust NZ J Med **16**, 648-652
Acute exercise, Adult, Intervention, LFT, Respiratory Muscle

300/70   **Mertens, D.J., Shephard, R.J. & Kavanagh, T.** (1978)
Long-term exercise therapy for chronic obstructive lung disease
Respiration **35**, 96-107
Adult, BLOOD PRESSURE, Body composition, COPD, Exercise programme, Intervention, LFT, Male, MUSCLE STRENGTH, MVV, Perceived exertion

300/71   **Morton, A.R., Fitch K.D. & Davis, T.** (1979)
The effect of 'warm up' on exercise-induced asthma
Ann Allergy **42**, 257-260
Acute exercise, Adult, Asthma, Comparative, Handicap, LFT

300/72   **Neary, P.J.** (1985)
The effects of prior exercise on the lactate and ventilatory thresholds
J Sports Sci **3**, 189-195
Acute exercise, Adult, LFT

300/73   **Nickerson, B.G., Bautista, D.B., Namey, M. A., Richards, W. & Keens, T.G.** (1983)
Distance running improves fitness in asthmatic children without pulmonary complications or changes in exercise-induced bronchospasm
Pediatrics **71**, 147-152
Asthma, Children, Intervention, Leisure activity, LFT, Respiratory muscle, Running

300/74   **O'Neill, P.A., Dodds, M., Phillips, B., Poole, J. & Webb, A.K.** (1987)
Regular exercise and reduction of breathlessness in patients with cystic fibrosis
Br J Dis Chest **81**, 62-69
Adult, AEROBIC CAPACITY, Cystic fibrosis, Exercise programme, Handicap, Intervention, LFT

300/75   Orenstein, D.M., Franklin, B.A., Doershuk, C.F., Hellersteinf, H.K., Germann, K.J., Horowitz, J.G. & Stern, R.C.   (1981)
Exercise conditioning and cardiopulmonary fitness in cystic fibrosis: The effects of a three-month supervised running program
Chest **80**, 392-398
Adult, Children, Cystic fibrosis, Exercise programme, Handicap, Intervention, LFT, Respiratory muscle, Running

300/76   Orenstein, D.M., Henke, K.G. & Cerny, F.J.   (1983)
Exercise and cystic fibrosis
Phys Sports Med **11**, 57-63
Cystic fibrosis, Handicap, Review

300/77   Orenstein, D.M., Reed, M.E., Grogan, F.T. & Crawford, L.V.   (1985)
Exercise conditioning in children with asthma
J Pediatr **106**, 556-560
AEROBIC CAPACITY, Asthma, Children, Exercise programme, Handicap, Intervention, LFT, MVV

300/78   Oseid, S. & Edwards, A.M. (Eds)   (1983)
The asthmatic child in play and sport
Pitman Medical Books, London
Asthma, Handicap, Review

300/79   Osterback, L. & Qvarnberg, Y.   (1987)
A prospective study of respiratory infections in 12-year-old children actively engaged in sports
Acta Paediatr Scand **76**, 944-949
Children, Comparative, Female, GENERAL HEALTH, Leisure activity, Male

300/80   Rasmussen, B. R., Klausen, K., Clausen, J. P. & Trap-Jensen, J.   (1975)
Pulmonary ventilation, blood gases, and blood pH after training of the arms or the legs
J Appl Physiol **38**, 250-256
Adult, CARDIAC PERFORMANCE, Exercise programme, Gas transfer, Intervention, LFT, Male

300/81   Robinson, E.P. & Kjeldgaard, J.M.   (1982)
Improvement in ventilatory muscle function with running
J Appl Physiol **52**, 1400-1406
Adult, Exercise programme, Intervention, LFT, MVV, Respiratory muscle, Running

300/82   Schneider, M.R., Melton, B.H. & Reisch, J.S.   (1980)
Effects of a progressive exercise program on absenteeism among school children with asthma
J School Health **50**, 92-95
Asthma, Children, Exercise programme, Intervention

300/83   Sergysels, R., DeCoster, A., Degre, S. & Denolin, H.   (1979)
Functional evaluation of a physical rehabilitation program including breathing exercises and bicycle training in chronic obstructive lung disease
Respiration **38**, 105-111
Adult, COPD, Exercise programme, Intervention, LFT, Respiratory muscle

300/84   Shayevitz, M.B. & Shayevitz, B.R.   (1986)
Athletic training in chronic obstructive pulmonary disease
Clin Sports Med **5**, 471-491
COPD, Handicap, Review

300/85   Shephard, R.J.   (1982)
Training and the respiratory system – Therapy for asthma and other obstructive diseases
Ann Clin Res (Suppl 34) **14**, 191-198
Asthma, COPD, Handicap, Review

300/86   **Sheppard, D.**   (1987)
What does exercise have to do with
'exercise induced' asthma? (Editorial)
Am Rev Respir Dis **136**, 547-549
Asthma, Handicap, Review

300/87   **Sinclair, D.J.M. & Ingram,
C.G.**   (1980)
Controlled trial of supervised exercise
training in chronic bronchitis
Br Med J **1**, 519-521
*Adult, Bronchitis, Customary activity,
Handicap, Intervention, LFT, MUSCLE
STRENGTH*

300/88   **Sprynarova, S. & Parizkova,
J.**   (1969)
Comparison of the functional circulatory
and respiratory capacity in girl gymnasts
and swimmers
J Sports Med **9**, 165-172
*AEROBIC CAPACITY, Body
composition, Children, Comparative,
Female, Leisure activity, LFT, MVV,
Swimming*

300/89   **Stanghelle, J.K. & Skyberg,
D.**   (1983)
The successful completion of the Oslo
Marathon by a patient with cystic fibrosis
Acta Paediatr Scand **72**, 935-938
*Acute exercise, AEROBIC CAPACITY,
Children, Cystic fibrosis, Handicap,
Leisure activity, Marathon, LFT,
LIPIDS, Running*

300/90   **Stewart, R.I.**   (1985)
Exercise in paitents with chronic
obstructive pulmonary disease
S A Med J **67**, 87-89
COPD, Handicap, Review

300/91   **Strauss, G.D., Osher, A., Wang, C.-
I., Goodrich, E., Gold, F., Colman, W.,
Stabile, M., Dobrenchuk, A. & Kenns,
T.G.**   (1987)
Variable weight training in cystic fibrosis
Chest **92**, 273-276
*Children, Cystic fibrosis, Exercise
programme, Handicap, Intervention, LFT,
MVV, MUSCLE STRENGTH, Weight*

300/92   **Svenonius, E., Kautto, R. &
Arborelius, M. Jr.**   (1983)
Improvement after training of children
with exercise-induced asthma
Acta Paediatr Scand **72**, 23-30
*Asthma, Children, Exercise programme,
Handicap, Intervention, LFT, Swimming*

300/93   **Tal, A., Pasterkamp, H. &
Chernick, V.**   (1985)
Endogenous opiates and response to
exercise in asthmatic children and
adolescents
Pediatr Pulmonol **1**, 46-51
*Acute exercise, Asthma, Children,
Endorphins*

300/94   **Walker, J. & Cooney, M.**   (1987)
Improved respiratory function in
quadreplegics after pulmonary therapy
and arm ergometry (Letter)
N Engl J Med **316**, 486-487
*Adult, Handicap, Intervention, LFT,
MUSCLE STRENGTH, Respiratory
muscle*

300/95   **Warren, J.B., Keynes, R.J., Brown,
M.J., Jenner, D.A. & McNicol,
M.W.**   (1982)
Blunted sympatho-adrenal response to
exercise in asthmatic subjects
Br J Dis Chest **76**, 147-149
*Acute exercise, Adult, Asthma, Endocrine,
Handicap*

300/96   **Weg, J.G.**   (1985)
Therapeutic exercise in patients with
chronic obstructive pulmonary disease.
In: Exercise and the Heart, edition 2
(Ed.) Brest, A.N.
*Cardiovascular Clinics, F.A.Davis
Company, Philadelphia.* **15**, 261-276
COPD, Exercise programme, Review

300/97 **Weissman, C., Askanazi, J., Rosenbaum, S.H., Hyman, A.I., Milic-Emili, J. & Kinney, J.M.** (1986)
The effects of posture on the metabolic and ventilatory response to low level steady state exercise
Clin Sci **71**, 553-558
Acute exercise, Adult, Comparative, LFT, Male, Ventilatory control

300/98 **Witten, M.L. & Wilkerson, J.E.** (1986)
An association between aerobic fitness and lung closing volume
Int J Sports Med **7**, 271-275
Acute exercise, Adult, LFT

300/99 **Yamamoto, Y., Mutoh, Y., Koboyashi, H. & Miyashita, M.** (1987)
Effects of reduced frequency breathing on arterial hypoxemia during exercise
Eur J Appl Physiol **56**, 522-527
Acute exercise, Adult, Gas transfer

300/100 **Yerg, J.E. 2nd, Seals, D.R., Hagberg, J.M. & Holloszy, J.O.** (1985)
Effect of endurance exercise training on ventilatory function in older individuals
J Appl Physiol **58**, 791-794
Adult, AEROBIC CAPACITY, Athlete, Comparative, Exercise programme, Gas transfer, Intervention, Leisure activity, LFT, Male, MVV, Ventilatory control

300/101 **Zach, M.S., Oberwaldner, B. & Haüsler, F.** (1982)
Cystic fibrosis: physical exercise versus chest physiotherapy
Arch Dis Child **57**, 587-589
Children, Cystic fibrosis, Handicap, Intervention, Leisure activity, LFT, Vigorous

300/102 **Zach, M.S., Purrer, B. & Oberwaldner, B.** (1981)
Effect of swimming on forced expiration and sputum clearance in cystic fibrosis
Lancet **ii**, 1201-1203
Children, Cystic fibrosis, Exercise programme, Handicap, Intervention, LFT, Swimming

KEYWORDS are listed in the appendix in addition the following specific keywords have been used in this section:

Arthritis
Back
E. stimulation
Joint range
O. arthritis
R. arthritis
Stiffness

Summary of evidence: exercise ameliorates osteo- and rheumatoid arthritis and cures or prevents loss of joint range due to inactivity

THE PROBLEM

When joints have become stiff and their range of movement has deteriorated, can suitable exercise reverse these disabilities? Does exercise prevent the deterioration in joint function with age or arthritis?

SCOPE

This section contains references dealing primarily with changes produced by exercise on joint stiffness and range of joint movement. The exercise consists of repeated brief efforts to extend the joint to the full extent of its range. There are references on both sedentary and athletic groups, on arthritis (both rheumatoid and osteo-arthritis), the hazards of over-use and on rehabilitation after immobilisation due to injury. Few studies have been reported dealing with these areas and the quality of the references is therefore variable.

METHODOLOGICAL DIFFICULTIES

Joint range is often assessed crudely in clinical settings and valid measurements are not made. The epidemiological studies are hampered by unreliable reporting of relevant customary activity either retrospectively or prospectively and also by the long time course of osteoarthritis. Rheumatoid arthritis has an erratic time course with periods of remission and exacerbation which confuse the attempt to mount controlled trials.

EVIDENCE

It is clear that reduced range of movement and stiffness which is due to lack of use can be reversed by gentle stretching exercises even in the elderly and those with arthritis. A deliberate effort to maintain function is needed in these groups. If the effort to increase joint range is restricted to that which can be produced by the individual's own muscles then there is no risk of injury. Hyperextensible joints are not desirable as they are more prone to dislocation. Yoga exercises are of benefit but should be approached cautiously. In arthritis, exercise appears to have beneficial effects by providing joint lubrication and maintaining range despite pain. This may reduce the need for medication. Exercise must be avoided during the acute inflammatory phases of osteo or rheumatoid arthritis. Repetitive impact loading may exacerbate pre-existing tendencies to develop osteo-arthritis but moderate exercise taken on resilient surfaces is not associated with an increase in arthritis in later life. Overuse can produce inflammation of tendons which takes time to heal. During the healing phase frequent movement but avoidance of tendon loading is needed.

410/1 Acheson, R.M. & Ginsberg, G.N. (1973)
New Haven survey of joint diseases XVI. Impairment disability and arthritis
Br J Prev **27**, 168-176
Arthritis, Review

410/2 Adams, I.D. (1979)
Osteoarthrosis and sport
J Roy Soc Med **72**, 185-187
O. arthritis, Review

410/3 Adrian, M.J. (1981)
Flexibility in the aging adult. In: Exercise and Aging. The scientific basis (Eds.) Smith, E.L. & Serfass, R.C.
Enslow Publishers, Hillside NJ.
Review

410/4 Allander, E. , Bjornsson, O.J., Olafsson, O., Sigfusson, N. & Thorsteinsson, J. (1974)
Normal range of joint movements in shoulder, hip, wrist and thumb with special reference to side; a comparison between two populations
Internl J Epidemiol **3**, 253-261 Adult, Comparative, Joint range

410/5 Andersson, G. (1986)
Occurrence of athletic injuries in voluntary participants in a 1-year extensive newspaper exercise campaign
Int J Sports Med **7**, 222-225
Adult, Hazards, Leisure activity

410/6 Barrack, R.L., Skinner, H.B., Brunet, M.E. & Cook, S.D. (1984)
Joint kinesthesia in the highly trained knee
J Sports Med Phys Fitness **24**, 18
Adult, Comparative, Female, Leisure activity, Male, Vigorous

410/7 Basmajian, J.V. (1987)
Therapeutic exercise in the management of rheumatic diseases
J Rheumatol (Suppl) **15**, 22-25
Arthritis, Review

410/8 Bell, R.D. & Hoshizaki, T.B. (1981)
Relationships of age and sex with range of motion of seventeen joint actions in humans
Can J Appl Sports Sci **6**, 202-206
Adult, Comparative, Elderly. Female, Joint range, Male

410/9 Bergström, G., Aniansson, A., Bjelle, A., Grimby, G., Lundgren-Lindquist, B. & Svanborg, A. (1985)
Functional consequences of joint impairment at age 79
Scand J Rehabil Med **17**, 183-190
Customary activity, Elderly, Joint range

410/10 Bergström, G., Bjelle, A., Sorensen, L.B., Sundh, V. & Svanborg, A. (1985)
Prevalence of symptoms and signs of joint impairment at age 79
Scand J Rehabil Med **17**, 173-182
Elderly, Joint range

410/11 Beyer, R.F. (1981)
Regulation of connective tissue metabolism in aging and exercise: a review. In: Frontiers of Exercise Biology. Symposium.
Review

410/12 Booth, F.W. & Gould, E.W. (1975)
Effects of training and disuse on connective tissue
Exerc Sports Sci Rev **3**, 83-112
BONES, MUSCLE STRENGTH, Review

410/13 Brodelius,A. (1961)
Osteoarthrosis of the talar joints in footballers and ballet dancers
Acta Orthop Scand **30**, 309-314.
Adult, Hazards, Leisure activity, Vigorous

410/14 **Brody, D.M.** (1980)
Running injuries
Clinical Symposia **32**
Hazards, Review

410/15 **Burke, M.J., Fear, E.C. & Wright,
V.** (1977)
Bone and joint changes in pneumatic
drillers
Ann Rheum Dis **36**, 276-279
*Adult, Hazards, Male, Occupational
activity, O. arthritis*

410/16 **Burry, H.C.** (1987)
Sport, exercise and arthritis
Br J Rheumatol **26**, 386-388
Arthritis, Review

410/17 **Chapman, E.A., de Vries, H.A. &
Swezey, R.** (1972)
Joint stiffness: Effects of exercise on
young and old men
J Gerontol **27**, 218-221
*Adult, Elderly, Exercise programme,
Intervention, Male, MUSCLE
STRENGTH, Stiffness*

410/18 **Clarke, H.H.** (1975)
Joint and body range of movement
Phys Fitness Res Dig **5**, 1
Joint range, Review

410/19 **Cotten, D.J. & Waters,
J.S.** (1970)
Immediate effect of four types of warm-
up activities upon static flexibility of four
selected joints
Am Correct Ther J **24**, 133-136
Adult, Intervention, Joint range

410/20 **de Vries, H.A.** (1962)
Evaluation of static stretching for
improvement
Res Quart **32**, 222-239
*Adult, Exercise programme, Intervention,
Male*

410/21 **DeHaven, K.E.** (1986)
Athletic injuries: comparison by age,
sport and gender
Am J Sports Med **14**, 218-224
Hazards, Review

410/22 **Ekblom, B.** (1982)
Short and long-term physical training in
patients with rheumatoid arthritis
Ann Clin Res (Suppl 34) **14**, 109-110
*Adult, Exercise programme, Intervention,
R. arthritis*

410/23 **Ekblom, B., Lovgren, O., Alderin,
M., Fridstrom, M. & Satterstrom,
G.** (1975)
Effect of short-term physical training on
patients with rheumatoid arthritis
Scand J Rheumatol **4**, 80-91
*Adult, Exercise programme, Intervention,
R. arthritis*

410/24 **Enwemeka, C.S.** (1986)
Radiographic verification of knee
goniometry
Scand J Rehabil Med **18**, 47-49
Adult, Joint range

410/25 **Frank, C., Akeson, W.H., Woo,
S.L., Amiel, D. & Coutts, R.D.** (1984)
Physiology and therapeutic value of
passive joint motion
Clin Orthop **185**, 113-125
Intervention, Joint range, Review

410/26 **Frekany, G.A. & Leslie,
D.K.** (1975)
Effects of an exercise programme on
selected flexibility measurements of
senior citizens
The Gerontologist **April**, 182-183
*Elderly, Exercise programme,
Intervention, Joint range*

410/27 **Garrick, J.G.** (1986)
The epidemiology of aerobic dance
injuries
Am J Sports Med **14**, 67-72
Hazards, Review

410/28 **Garrick, J.G. & Requa,
R.K.** (1978)
Injuries in high school sports
Pediatrics **61**, 465-469
Athlete, Children, Comparative, Hazards

410/29   **Germain, N.W. & Blair, S. N.**   (1983)
Variability of shoulder flexion in age, activity and sex
Amer Corr Ther J **37**, 156-160
Adult, Customary activity, Exercise programme, Female, Intervention, Joint range, Male

410/30   **Grobaker, M.R. & Stull, G.A.**   (1975)
Thermal applications as a determinant of joint flexibility
Amer Corr Ther J **29**,
Adult, Intervention, Joint range, Male

410/31   **Hall, S.J.**   (1985)
Mechanical contribution to lumbar stress in female gymnasts
Med Sci Sports **18**, 599
Adult, Athlete, Female, Hazards

410/32   **Hardy, L. & Jones, D.**   (1986)
Dynamic flexibility and proprocetive neuromuscular facilitation
Res Quart **57**, 150-153
Adult, Female, Intervention

410/33   **Harris, M.L.**   (1968)
Flexibility : a Review of the literature
Phy Ther **49**, 591-601
Joint range, Review

410/34   **Haywood, K.M., Clark, B.A. & Mayhew, J.L.**   (1986)
Differential effects of age-group gymnastics and swimming on body composition, strength, and flexibility
J Sports Med Phys Fitness **26**, 416-420
Athlete, Body composition, Children, Comparative, Female, Joint range, MUSCLE STRENGTH

410/35   **Heck, C.V., Hendryson, I.E. & Rowe, C.R.**   (1965)
Joint Motion – method of measuring and recording
American Academy of Orthopaedic Surgeons
Review

410/36   **Hortobagyi, T., Faludi, J., Tihanyi, J. & Merkely, B.**   (1985)
Effects of intense 'stretching'-flexibility training on the mechanical profile of the knee extensors and on the range of motion of the hip joint
Int J Sports Med **6**, 317-321
Adult, Joint range

410/37   **Hoshizaki, T.B. & Bell, R.D.**   (1984)
Factor analysis of 17 joint flexibility measures
J Sports Sci **2**, 97-103
Adult, Joint range

410/38   **Jackson, A.W.**   (1986)
The relationship of the sit and reach test to criterion measures of hamstring and back flexibility in young females
Res Quart **57**, 183-186
Children, Female, Joint range

410/39   **Jackson, A.W., Wiltse, L. & Cirincione, R.**   (1976)
Spondylolysis in the female gymnast
Clin Orthop **117**, 68-73
Adult, Back pain, Comparative, Female, Hazards

410/40   **Johns, R.J. & Wright, V.**   (1962)
Relative importance of various tissues in joint stiffness
J Appl Physiol **17**, 824-828
Animal, E. stimulation, Stiffness

410/41   **Jurvelin, J.**   (1986)
Effect of physical exercise on indentation stiffness of articular cartilage in the canine knee
Int J Sports Med **7**, 106-110
Animal, Stiffness

410/42   **Koplan, J.P., Powell, K.E., Sikes, R.K., Shirley, R.W. & Campbell, C.C.**   (1982)
An epidemiologic study of the benefits and risks of running
J Am Med Ass **248**, 3118-3121
Review

410/43   **Kraus, J.F. & Conroy, C.**   (1984)
Mortality and morbidity from injury in
sports and recreation
Ann Rev Publ Hlth **5**, 163-192
Hazards, Review

410/44   **Lane, N.E., Bloch, D.A., Wood,
P.D. & Fries, J.F.**   (1987)
Aging,long-distance running, and the
development of musculoskeletal
disability
Am J Med **82**, 772-780
*BLOOD PRESSURE, Comparative,
Elderly, Hazards, Leisure activity,
Occupational activity, O. arthritis*

410/45   **Marcinik, E.J.**   (1986)
Sprain and strain injuries in the Navy: the
possible role of physical fitness in their
prevention
Aviat Space Environ Med **57**, 800-804
Adult, Back pain, Hazards, Male

410/46   **Mayerson, N.H. & Milano,
R.A.**   (1984)
Goniometric measurement reliability in
physical medicine
Arch Phys Med Rehabil **65**, 92-94
Joint range

410/47   **McCain, G.A.**   (1986)
Role of physical fitness training in the
fibrosis/fibromyalgia syndrome
Am J Med (Suppl 3A) **81**, 73-77
*Adult, Comparative, Exercise programme,
Intervention, Pain*

410/48   **Micheli, L.J.**   (1986)
Lower extremity overuse injuries
Acta Med Scand **Suppl. 711**, 171-177
Hazards, Review

410/49   **Micheli, L.J.**   (1986)
Pediatric and adolescent sports injuries:
recent trends
Exerc Sport Sci Rev **14**, 359-374
Children, Hazards, Review

410/50   **Muckle, D.S.**   (1987)
Cartilage and joint limitations on
exercise. In: Exercise: Benefits, Limits
and Adaptations (Eds.) Macleod, D.,
Maughan, R., Nimmo, M., Reilly, T. &
Williams, C.
E. & F. Spon, London 220-238
Review

410/51   **Munroe, R.A. & Romance,
T.J.**   (1975)
Use of the Leighton Flexometer in the
development of a short flexibility test
battery
Amer Corr Ther J **29**, 22-25
Joint range

410/52   **Murray, R.O. & Duncan,
C.**   (1971)
Athletic activity in adolescence as an
etiological factor in degenerative hip
disease
J Bone Joint Surg **53B**, 406-419
Athlete, Children, Hazards, Male

410/53   **Murray-Leslie, C.F., Lintott, D.J.
& Wright, V.**   (1977)
The knees and ankles in sport and veteran
military parachutists
Ann Rheum Dis **36**, 327-331
Adult, Leisure activity, Male, O.arthritis

410/54   **Nicholas, J.**   (1970)
Injuries to knee ligaments – relationship
to looseness and tightness
J Am Med Ass **212**, 2236-2239
*Adult, Athlete, Comparative, Hazards,
Joint range, Male*

410/55   **Nordemar, R., Ekblom., B.
Zachrisson, L. & Lundqvist, K.**   (1981)
Physical training in rheumatoid arthritis:
a controlled long-term study
Scand J Rheumatol **10**, 17-23
*Adult, Exercise programme, Intervention,
R. arthritis*

410/56   **Panush, R.S. & Brown,
D.G.**   (1987)
Exercise and arthritis
Sports Med **4**, 54-64
Review

410/57   **Panush, R.S., Schmidt, C., Caldwell, J.R., Edwards, N.L., Longley, S., Yonker, R., Webster, E., Nauman, J., Stork, J. & Pettersson, H.**   (1986)
Is running associated with degenerative joint disease?
J Am Med Ass **255,** 1152-1154
Adult, Athlete, Comparative, Male, O. arthritis, Running

410/58   **Pollock, M.L., Gettman, L.R., Milesis, C.A. Bah, M.D., Durstine, L. & Johnson, R.B.**   (1977)
Effects of frequency and duration of training on attrition and incidence of injury
Med Sci Sports **9,** 31-36
Adult, AEROBIC CAPACITY, Body composition, Exercise programme, Hazards, Intervention, Male

410/59   **Powell, K.E., Kohl, H.W., Casperson, C.J. & Blair, S.N.**   (1986)
An epidemiological perspective on the causes of running injuries
Phys & Sportsmed **14,** 100
Hazards, Review

410/60   **Puranen, J., Ala-Ketola, L., Peltokallio, P. & Saarela, J.**   (1975)
Running and primary osteoarthritis of the hip
Br Med J **2,** 424-425.
Adult, Hazards, Leisure activity, O. arthritis, Running

410/61   **Reid, D.C., Burnham, R.S., Saboe, L.A. & Kushner, S.F.**   (1987)
Lower extremity flexibility patterns in classical ballet dancers and their correlation to lateral hip and knee injuries
Am J Sports Med **15,** 347-352
Adult, Joint range, Leisure activity, Vigorous

410/62   **Rikli, R. & Busch, S.**   (1986)
Motor performance in women as a function of age and physical activity level
J Gerontol **41,** 645-649
Adult, Comparative, Customary activity, Female, MUSCLE STRENGTH

410/63   **Rutherford, G.W., Miles, R.B., Brown, V.R. & MacDonald, B.**   (1981)
Overview of sports related injuries to persons 5-14 years of age
U.S.Consumer Product Safety Commission, Washington, DC.
Hazards, Review

410/64   **Schank, J.A., Herdman, S.J. & Bloyer, R.G.**   (1986)
Physical therapy in the multidisciplinary assessment and management of osteoarthritis
Clin Ther (Suppl B) **9,** 14-23
O. arthritis, Review

410/65   **Sheehan, G.A.**   (1977)
An overview of overuse syndromes in distance runners
Ann NY Acad Sci **301,**
Review

410/66   **Skinner, H.B.**   (1986)
Exercise-related knee joint laxity
Am J Sports Med **14,** 30-34
Joint range

410/67   **Sohn, R.S. & Micheli, L.J.**   (1985)
The effect of running on the pathogenesis of osteoarthritis of the hips and knees
Clin Orthop **(198)** 106-109
Adult, Leisure activity, O. arthritis, Running, Swimming

410/68   **Solgaard, S., Carlsen, A., Kramhøft, M. & Petersen, V.**   (1986)
Reproducibility of goniometry of the wrist
Scand J Rehabil Med **18,** 5-7
Adult, Joint range

410/69   **Solomon, L.**   (1976)
Patterns of osteoarthritis of the hip
J Bone Joint Surg **58B,** 176-183
O. arthritis, Review

410/70   **Song, T.M.K.**   (1983)
Effects of seasonal training on
anthropometry, flexibility, strength and
cardiorespiratory function in junior
female track and field athletes
J Sports Med **23**, 168-177
*AEROBIC CAPACITY, ANAEROBIC
CAPACITY, Athlete, Body composition,
Children, Female, Joint range*

410/71   **Sullivan, J.A.**   (1984)
Recurring pain in the pediatric athlete
Pediatr Clin North Am **31**, 1097-112
Athlete, Children, Hazards, Review

410/72   **Suominen, H., Heikkinen, E. &
Parkatti, T.**   (1977)
Effect of eight weeks' physical training on
muscle and connective tissue of the M.
Vastus Lateralis in 69-year-old men and
women
J Gerontol **32**, 33-37
*Elderly, Exercise programme,
Intervention, MUSCLE
METABOLISM, MUSCLE
STRENGTH,*

410/73   **Suwalski, M.**   (1982)
Importance of physical training of
rheumatic patients
Ann Clin Res **14**, 107-109
*Adult, Exercise programme, Intervention,
R. arthritis*

410/74   **Tegner, Y.**   (1986)
Strengthening exercises for old cruciate
ligament tears
Acta Orthop Scand **57**, 130-134
Adult, Exercise programme, Intervention

410/75   **Tipton, C.M., Matthes R.D.,
Maynard, J.A. & Carey, R.**   (1975)
The influence of physical activity on
ligaments and tendons
Med Sci Sports **7**, 165-175
Animal, Review

410/76   **Tipton, C.M., Vailas, A.C. &
Matthes, R.D.**   (1986)
Experimental studies on the influences of
physical activity on ligaments, tendons,
and joints: a brief review
Acta Med Scand (Suppl) **711**, 157-168
Review

410/77   **Vailas, A.C., Pedrini, V.A., Pedrini-
Mille, A. & Holloszy, J.O.**   (1985)
Patellar tendon matrix changes
associated with aging and voluntary
exercise
J Appl Physiol **58**, 1572-1576
*Animal, Exercise programme,
Intervention, Male*

410/78   **Vailas, A.C., Tipton, C.M.,
Laughlin, H.L., Tcheng, T.K. & Matthes,
R.D.**   (1978)
Physical activity and hypophysectomy on
the aerobic capacity of ligaments and
tendons
J Appl Physiol **44**, 542-546
*Animal, Comparative, Exercise
programme, Intervention*

410/79   **Vandor, E., Jorza, L., Joz, S.A. &
Balint, B.J.**   (1982)
The lactate dehydrogenase activity
isoenzyme in normal and hypokinetic
tendons
Eur J Appl Physiol **49**, 63-68
Autopsy, Customary activity

410/80   **Wallin, D., Ekblom, B., Grahn, R &
Nordenborg, T.**   (1985)
Improvement of muscle flexibility, A
comparison between two techniques
Am J Sports Med **13**, 263-268
Adult, Intervention, Joint range

410/81   **Wright, V. & Johns, R.J.**   (1960)
Observations on the measurement of
joint stiffness
Arthritis and Rheumatism **3**, 328-340
Review, Stiffness

KEYWORDS are listed in the appendix in addition the following specific keywords have been used in this section:

Amenorrhea
Femur (bones being measured for density or mass)
Menopause
Osteoporosis
Radius (bones being measured for density or mass)
Vertebrae (bones being measured for density or mass)

Summary of evidence: exercise ameliorates or cures low bone density due to lack of bone loading which in turn helps to prevent osteoporotic fracture in older women

THE PROBLEM

In some women bones become fragile through loss of substance and bone density falls so low in later life that they suffer osteoporotic fractures of the radius, the femur or the vertebrae. These fractures constitute a large burden of misery for the individual and expense for the NHS. Can exercise increase bone density in young to middle-aged adults and thereby offset the loss which occurs in later life? Can exercise reduce the rate of loss in peri-menopausal women which is rapid due to changes in hormonal status? Can exercise reverse the loss once it has occurred in older women?

SCOPE

This section contains references dealing primarily with changes produced by exercise on bone density. The exercise consists of repetitive, brief but substantial loading of the bone, through the effect of gravity on body mass or applied muscle force. There are references dealing with all ages and both sexes. The emphasis is on studies of middle-aged women but there are a number of studies of female athletes with amenorrhea. There are some background references on methodology, osteoporosis and fracture, some animal studies and studies of the effects of inactivity and over-use.

METHODOLOGICAL DIFFICULTIES

Methods of assessing bone density are of limited sensitivity and cannot all be applied to the bones of most interest. The effects of exercise are likely to be specific to the bone being loaded. Any selective effects on cortical or trabecular bone, and on the balance of osteoblastic and osteoclastic activity can only be determined, if at all, from bone biopsies. These considerations affect the strength of bone in resisting fracture.

EVIDENCE

It is clear that improvements in bone density of 5-10% can be obtained at all ages. One brief bout of exercise such as climbing a flight of stairs may have a prolonged stimulating effect on osteoblasts. Such exercise, regularly taken from childhood onwards, may ensure a high adult bone mass which can offset the inevitable menopausal loss. There is no clear evidence as yet that the rate of loss can be slowed but the offset may be sufficient to keep bone density and strength above the critical threshold for osteoporotic fracture even in old age. Mild exercise has been found effective in increasing bone density in institutionalised women aged over 75 years.

420/1   (1983)
Osteoporosis and activity (Editorial)
Lancet **i**, 1365-1366
Osteoporosis, Review

420/2   **Adams, R., Andrews, M. & Sussman, M.**   (1983)
Physical activity for patients wearing spinal orthoses
Phys Sports Med **11**, 75
Children, Handicap, Leisure activity, Vertebrae

420/3   **Aisenbrey, J.A.**   (1987)
Exercise in the prevention and management of osteoporosis
Phys Ther **67**, 1100-1104
Review

420/4   **Alexander, M.J.L.**   (1985)
Biochemical aspects of lumbar spine injuries in athletes: A review
Can J Appl Sport Sci **10**, 1-20
Hazards, JOINTS, Review

420/5   **Aloia, J.F.**   (1981),
Exercise and skeletal health
J Am Geriatr Soc **29**, 104-107
Osteoporosis, Review

420/6   **Aloia, J.F.**   (1982)
Estrogen and exercise in prevention and treatment of osteoporosis
Geriatrics **37**, 81-85
Osteoporosis, Review

420/7   **Aloia, J.F., Cohn, S.H., Ostuni, J.A., Cane, R. & Ellis, K.J.**   (1978)
Prevention of involutional bone loss by exercise
Ann Intern Med **89**, 356-358
Adult, Exercise programme, Female, Intervention, Menopause, Radius

420/8   **Aloia, J.F., Vaswani, A.N., Yeh, J.K. & Cohn, S.H.**   (1988)
Premenopausal bone mass is related to physical activity
Arch Intern Med **30**, 121-123
Adult, Comparative, Female, Leisure activity, Radius, Vertebrae

420/9   **Åström, J., Ahnqvist, S., Beertems, J. & Jónsson, B.**   (1987)
Physical activity in women sustaining fracture of the neck of the femur
J Bone Joint Surg (Br) **69**, 381-383
Adult, Case-control, Customary activity, Female, Femur, Leisure activity

420/10   **Avioli, L. V. (Ed.)**   (1984)
Functional adaption in bone tissue
Calcif Tissue Int (Suppl) **36**
Review

420/11   **Ayalon, J., Simkin, A., Leichter, I. & Raifmann, S.**   (1987)
Dynamic bone loading exercises for postmenopausal women: Effect on the density of the distal radius
Arch Phys Med Rehabil **68**, 280-283
Adult, Exercise programme, Female, Intervention, Menopause, Osteoporosis, Radius

420/12   **Bates, P.**   (1985)
Shin splints-a literature review
Br J Sports Med **19**, 132-137
Hazards, Review

420/13   **Beverley, M., Prinsley, P., Dziewulski, P., Burdett-Smith, P. & Evans, M.**   (1988)
Bone density response to limited isometric exercise
J Bone Joint Surg (Br) **70**, 153
Adult, Elderly, Exercise programme, Female, Intervention, Menopause, MUSCLE STRENGTH

420/14 **Blessing, D.L.** (1987)
The physiologic effects of eight weeks of
aerobic dance with and without hand
held weights
Am J Sports Med **15**, 508-510
Adult, Exercise programme, Intervention,
MUSCLE STRENGTH

420/15 **Block, J.E., Genant, H.K. & Black,
D.** (1986)
Greater vertebral bone mass in exercising
young men
West J Med **145**, 39-42
Adult, Comparative, Leisure activity,
Male, Vertebrae

420/16 **Block, J.E., Smith, R., Black, D. &
Genant, H.K.** (1987)
Does exercise prevent osteoporosis?
J Am Med Ass **257**, 3115-3117
Review

420/17 **Bonn, D.** (1987)
Hormones for healthy bones
New Scientist **19 Feb**, 32-35
Review

420/18 **Brewer, V., Meyer, B.M., Keele,
M.S., Upton, S.J. & Hagan,
R.D.** (1983)
Role of exercise in prevention of
involutional bone loss
Med Sci Sports Exerc **15**, 445-449
Adult, Body composition, Comparative,
Female, Leisure activity, Marathon,
Radius, Running, Vigorous

420/19 **Burr, D.B., Martin, R.B. & Martin,
P.A.** (1983)
Lower extremity loads stimulated bone
formation in vertebral column:
implications for osteoporosis
Spine **8**, 681-685
Adult, Exercise programme, Intervention,
Osteoporosis, Vertebrae

420/20 **Cann, C.E., Martin, M.C., Genant,
H.K. & Jaffe, R.B.** (1984)
Decreased spinal mineral content in
amenorrheic women
J Am Med Ass **251**, 626-629
Adult, Amenorrhea, Athlete,
Comparative, Female, Hazards,
MENSTRUAL FUNCTION,
REPRODUCTIVE HORMONES,
Vertebrae, Vigorous

420/21 **Chalmers, J. & Ho, K.C.** (1970)
Geographical variations in senile
osteoporosis: the association with
physical activity
J Bone Joint Surg (Br) **52**, 667-675
Adult, Comparative, Customary activity,
Female, Male, Osteoporosis

420/22 **Chow, R.K., Harrison, J.E. &
Notarius, C.** (1987)
Effect of two randomised exercise
programmes on bone mass of healthy
postmenopausal women
Br Med J **295**, 1441-1444
Adult, AEROBIC CAPACITY, Exercise
programme, Female, Intervention,
Menopause

420/23 **Chow, R.K. & Harrison,
J.E.** (1987)
Relationship of kyphosis to physical
fitness and bone mass on post-
menopausal women
Am J Phys Med **66**, 219-227
Adult, Female, Menopause, Vertebrae

420/24 **Chow, R.K., Harrison, J.E., Brown,
C.F. & Hajek, V.** (1986)
Physical fitness effect on bone mass in
postmenopausal women
Arch Phys Med Rehabil **67**, 231-4
Adult, AEROBIC CAPACITY, Female,
Femur, Menopause, MUSCLE
STRENGTH

420/25   Chow, R.K., Harrison, J.E.,
Sturtridge, W., Josse, R., Murray, T.M.,
Bayley, A., Dorman, J. & Hammond,
T.   (1987)
The effect of exercise on bone mass of
osteoporotic patients on fluoride
treatment
Clin Invest Med **10**, 59-63
*Adult, AEROBIC CAPACITY, Elderly,
Exercise programme, Intervention,
Osteoporosis*

420/26   Claus-Walker, J., Carter, R.E.,
Campos, R.J. & Spencer, W.A.   (1979)
Sitting, muscular exercises, and collagen
metabolism in tetraplegia
Am J Phys Med **58**, 285-293
*Adult, Handicap, Male, MUSCLE
STRENGTH, Osteoporosis*

420/27   Cohn, S.H., Abesamis, C.,
Yasumura, S., Aloia, J.F., Zanzi, I. &
Ellis, K.J.   (1977)
Comparative skeletal mass and radial
bone mineral content in black and white
women
Metabolism **26**, 171-178
*Adult, Comparative, Elderly, Female,
MUSCLE STRENGTH, Radius*

420/28   Cooper, C., Barker, D.J.P., Morris,
J. & Briggs, R.S.J.   (1987)
Osteoporosis, falls, and age in fracture of
the proximal femur
Br Med J **295**, 13-15
*Adult, Case-control, Elderly, Female,
Femur, Osteoporosis,*

420/29   Cummings, S.R., Kelsey, J.L.,
Nevitt, M.C. & O'Dowd, K.J.   (1985)
Epidemiology of osteoporosis and
osteoporotic fractures
Epidemiol Rev **7**, 178-208
Osteoporosis, Review

420/30   Daffner, R.H. & Gehweiler, J.
A.   (1982)
Stress fractures in runners
J Am Med Ass **247**, 1039-1041
Adult, Hazards, Male, Running

420/31   Dalen, N., Laftman, P., Ohlsen, H.
& Stromberg, L.   (1985)
The effect of athletic activity on the bone
mass in human diaphyseal bone
Orthopedics **8**, 1139-1141
*Adult, Comparative, Leisure activity,
Male*

420/32   Dalsky, G.P.   (1987)
Exercise: its effect on bone mineral
content
Clin Obstet Gynecol **30**, 820-832
Review

420/33   Dequeker, J. & Van Tendeloo,
G.   (1982)
Metacarpal bone mass and upper-
extremity strength in 18-year-old boys
Invest Radiol **17**, 427-429
*Adult, Male, MUSCLE STRENGTH,
Weight*

420/34   Doyle, F., Brown, J. & Lachance,
C.   (1970)
Relation between bone mass and muscle
weight
Lancet **i**, 391-393
*Adult, Female, Male, MUSCLE
STRENGTH, Vertebrae*

420/35   Drinkwater, B.L., Nilson, K.,
Chesnut, C.H., Bremner, W.J.,
Shainholtz, S. & Southworth,
M.B.   (1984)
Bone mineral content of amenorrheic and
eumenorrheic athletes
N Engl J Med **311**, 277-281
*Adult, Amenorrhea, Athlete,
Comparative, Female, Hazards,
MENSTRUAL FUNCTION,
REPRODUCTIVE HORMONES,
Radius, Running, Vertebrae, Vigorous,
Weight*

420/36   Drinkwater, B.L., Nilson, K., Olt, S. & Chesnut, C.H.   (1986)
Bone mineral density after resumption of menses in amenorrheic athletes
J Am Med Ass **256,** 380-382
Adult, Amenorrhea, Athlete, Female, MENSTRUAL FUNCTION, REPRODUCTIVE HORMONES, Vertebrae

420/37   Falch, J.A.   (1982)
The effect of physical activity on the skeleton
Scand J Soc Med (Suppl) **29,** 55-58
Review

420/38   Fisher, E.C., Nelson, M.E., Frontera, W.R., Turksoy, R.N. & Evans, W.J.   (1986)
Bone mineral content and levels of gonadotropins and estrogens in amenorrheic running women
J Clin Endocrinol Metab **62,** 1232-1236
Adult, Amenorrhea, AEROBIC CAPACITY, Athlete, Body composition, Comparative, Female, Hazards, MENSTRUAL FUNCTION, Radius, REPRODUCTIVE HORMONES, Running, Vertebrae, Vigorous, Weight

420/39   Goodman, C.E.   (1985)
Osteoporosis: protective measures of nutrition and exercise
Geriatrics **40,** 59-70
Exercise programme, Osteoporosis, Review

420/40   Goodman, C.E.   (1987)
Osteoporosis and physical activity
AAOHN J **35,** 539-542
Review

420/41   Harrison, J.E.   (1984)
Neutron activation studies and the effect of exercise on osteoporosis
J Med Clin Exp Theor **15,** 285-294
Adult, Female, Radius, Vertebrae

420/42   Heath, H. 3rd.   (1985)
Athletic women, amenorrhea, and skeletal integrity
Ann Intern Med **102,** 258-60
Athlete, Hazards, MENSTRUAL FUNCTION, Review

420/43   Huddleston, A.L., Rockwell, D., Kulund, D.N. & Harrison, R.B.   (1980)
Bone mass in lifetime tennis athletes
J Am Med Ass **244,** 1107-1109
Comparative, Elderly, Leisure activity, Male, Radius, Vigorous

420/44   Jacobson, P.C., Beaver, W., Grubb, S.A., Taft, T.N. & Talmage, R.V.   (1984)
Bone density in women: college athletes and older athletic women
J Orthop Res **2,** 328-332
Adult, Comparative, Elderly, Female, Menopause, Leisure activity, Radius, Swimming, Vertebrae

420/45   Jones, H.H., Priest, J.D., Hayes, W.C., Tichenor, C.C. & Nagel, D.A.   (1977)
Humeral hypertrophy in response to exercise
J Bone Joint Surg **59,** 204-208
Adult, Athlete, Comparative, Female, Leisure activity, Male, Vigorous

420/46   Jones, K.P., Ravnikar, V.A., Tulchinsky, D. & Schiff, I.   (1985)
Comparison of bone density in amenorrheic women due to athletics, weight loss, and premature menopause
Obstet Gynecol **66,** 5-8
Adult, Amenorrhea, Athlete, Body composition, Comparative, Endocrine, Female, Hazards, MENSTRUAL FUNCTION, Radius, REPRODUCTIVE HORMONES, Vigorous

420/47   Korcok, M.   (1982)
Add exercise to calcium in osteoporosis prevention
J Am Med Ass **247,** 1106, 1112
Osteoporosis, Review

420/48   **Kriska, A.M., Sandler, R.B., Cauley, J.A., LaPorte, R.E., Hom, D.L. & Pambianco, G.**   (1988)
The assessment of historical physical activity and its relation to adult bone parameters
Am J Epidemiol **127**, 1053-1063
Adult, Female, Leisure activity, Menopause, Radius

420/49   **Krølner, B. & Toft, B.**   (1983)
Vertebral bone loss: an unheeded side effect of therapeutic bed rest
Clin Sci **64**, 537-540
Adult, Inactivity, Intervention, Osteoporosis, Vertebrae

420/50   **Krølner, B., Toft, B., Nielsen, S.P. & Tøndevold, E.**   (1983),
Physical exercise as prophylaxis against involutional vertebral bone loss: a controlled trial
Clin Sci **64**, 541-546
Adult, AEROBIC CAPACITY, Elderly, Exercise programme, Female, Intervention, Menopause, Osteoporosis, Radius, Vertebrae

420/51   **Krølner, B., Tøndevold, E., Toft, B., Berthelsen, B. & Nielsen, S.P.**   (1982)
Bone mass of the axial and the appendicular skeleton in women with Colles' fracture ; its relation to physical activity
Clin Physiol **2**, 147-157
Adult, AEROBIC CAPACITY, Customary activity, Female, Menopause, Radius, Vertebrae

420/52   **Lane, N.E., Bloch, D.A., Jones, H.H., Marshall, W.H. Jr, Wood, P.D. & Fries, J.F.**   (1986)
Long-distance running, bone density, and osteoarthritis
J Am Med Ass **255**, 1147-1151
Adult, Comparative, Elderly, Female, JOINTS, Leisure activity, Male, Running.

420/53   **Lanyon, L.E.**   (1984)
Functional strain as a determinant for bone remodelling
Calcif Tissue Int **36**, S56-61
Animal, Intervention

420/54   **Lindberg, J.S., Fears, W.B., Hunt, M.M., Powell, M.R., Boll, D. & Wade, C.E.**   (1984)
Exercise-induced amenorrhea and bone density
Ann Intern Med **101**, 647-648
Adult, Amenorrhea, Body composition, Comparative, Female, Hazards, Menopause, MENSTRUAL FUNCTION, Radius, REPRODUCTIVE HORMONES, Running, Vertebrae, Vigorous

420/55   **Linnell, S.L., Stager, J.M., Blue, P.W., Oyster, N. & Robertshaw, D.**   (1984)
Bone mineral content and menstrual regularity in female runners
Med Sci Sports Exerc **16**, 343-348
Adult, Amenorrhea, Athlete, Body composition, Comparative, Female, Hazards, MENSTRUAL FUNCTION, Radius, Running, Vigorous, Weight

420/56   **Luchini, M.A., Sarokhan, A.J. & Michell, L.J.**   (1983)
Acute displaced femoral-shaft fractures in long-distance runners
J Bone Joint Surg (Am) **65**, 689-691
Adult, Hazards, Marathon, Running, Vigorous

420/57   **Lukert, B.P.**   (1982)
Osteoporosis – A Review and Update
Arch Phys Med Rehabil **63**, 480-487
Review

420/58   Marcus, R., Cann, C.E., Madvig, P., Minkoff, J., Goddard, M., Bayer, M., Martin, M.C., Gaudiani, L., Haskell, W. & Genant, H.K.   (1985)
Menstrual function and bone mass in elite women distance runners. Endocrine and metabolic features
Ann Intern Med **102**, 158-63,
Adult, AEROBIC CAPACITY, Amenorrhea, Athlete, Body composition, Comparative, Endocrine, Female, Hazards, Marathon, MENSTRUAL FUNCTION, Radius, REPRODUCTIVE HORMONES, Running, Vertebrae, Vigorous, Wei

420/59   Margulies, J.Y., Simkin, A., Leichter, I., Bivas, A., Steinberg, R., Giladi, M., Stein, M., Kashtan, H. & Milgrom, C.   (1986)
Effect of intense physical activity on the bone-mineral content in the lower limbs of young adults
J Bone Joint Surg (Am) **68**, 1090-1093
Adult, Hazards, Intervention, Male, Occupational activity

420/60   Martin, A.D. & Houston, C.S.   (1987)
Osteoporosis, calcium and physical activity
Can Med Ass J **136**, 587-593
Review

420/61   Martin, R.B. & Gutman, W.   (1978)
The effect of electric fields on osteoporosis of disuse
Calcif Tissue Res **25**, 23-27
Animal, Femur, Inactivity, Osteoporosis

420/62   Matheson, G.O., Clement, D.B. & McKenzie, D.C.   (1987)
Stress fractures in athletes: A study of 320 cases
Am J Sports Med **15**, 46-58
Adult, Athlete, Hazards, Leisure activity, Vigorous

420/63   Matsuda, J.J., Zernicke, R.F., Vailas, A.C., Pedrini, V.A., Pedrini-Mille, A. & Maynard, J.A.   (1986)
Structural and mechanical adaption of immature bone to strenuous exercise
J Appl Physiol **60**, 2028-2034
Animal, Exercise programme, GROWTH, Hazards, Intervention, Vigorous

420/64   McArthur, J.   (1984)
Amenorrhoeic athletes: at risk of developing osteoporosis?
Br J Sports Med **18**, 253-255
Hazards, Review

420/65   McDonald, R., Hegenauer, J. & Saltman, P.   (1986)
Age-related differences in the bone mineralization pattern of rats following exercise
J Gerontol **41**, 445-452
Animal, Comparative, Elderly, Exercise programme, Femur, Intervention

420/66   Meleski, B.W., Malina, R.M. & Bouchard, C.   (1981)
Cortical bone, body size, and skeletal maturity in ice hockey players 10 to 12 years of age
Can J Appl Sport Sci **6**, 212-217
Children, GROWTH, Leisure activity, Male

420/67   Milgrom, C., Giladi, M., Stein, M., Kashtan, H., Margulies, J.Y., Chisin, R., Steinberg, R. & Aharonson, Z.   (1985)
Stress fractures in military recruits
J Bone Joint Surg (Br) **67-B**, 732-735
Adult, Cohort, Hazards, Male, Occupational activity

420/68   Montoye, H., Smith, E.L. Jr. & Farder, D.   (1980)
Bone mineral in senior tennis players
Scand J Sports Sci **2**, 26-32
Elderly, Leisure activity, Male

420/69   Nelson, M.E., Fisher, E.C., Catsos, P.D., Meredith, C.N., Turksoy, R.N. & Evans, W.J.   (1986)
Diet and bone status in amenorrheic runners
Am J Clin Nutr **43**, 910-916
Adult, Amenorrhea, AEROBIC CAPACITY, Athlete, Body composition, Comparative, ENERGY BALANCE, Female, Hazards, MENSTRUAL FUNCTION, Radius, REPRODUCTIVE HORMONES, Running, Vertebrae, Vigorous, Weight

420/70   Nilsson, B.E., Andersson, S.M., Havdrup, T. & Westlin, N.E.   (1978)
Ballet-dancing and weight-lifting – effects on BMC
Am J Roent **131**, 541-542
Adult, Comparative, Female, GROWTH, Leisure activity, Male, Radius, Vigorous

420/71   Notelovitz, M.   (1986)
Post-menopausal osteoporosis: A practical approach to its prevention
Acta Obstet Gynecol Scand (Suppl 134) **134**, 67-80
Osteoporosis, Review

420/72   Orava, A., Puranen, J. & Ala-Ketola, L.   (1978)
Stress fractures caused by physical exercise
Acta Orthop Scand **49**, 19-27
Adult, Athlete, Hazards, Leisure activity

420/73   Oyster, N., Morton, M. & Linnell, S.L.   (1984)
Physical activity and osteoporosis in post-menopausal women
Med Sci Sports Exerc **16**, 44-50
Comparative, Elderly, Female, Leisure activity, Menopause, Osteoporosis, REPRODUCTIVE HORMONES, Weight

420/74   Petrofsky, J.S., Heaton, H. 3rd & Phillips, C.A.   (1983)
Outdoor bicycle for exercise in paraplegics and quadriplegics
J Biomed Eng **5**, 292-296
Adult, Exercise programme, Handicap, MUSCLE STRENGTH

420/75   Plato, C.C. & Norris, A.H.   (1980)
Bone measurements of the second metacarpal and grip strength
Hum Biol **52**, 131-149
Adult, Male, Elderly, MUSCLE STRENGTH

420/76   Pocock, N.A., Eisman, J. A., Yeates, M.G., Sambrook, P.N. & Eberl, S.   (1986)
Physical fitness is a major determinant of femoral neck and lumbar spine bone mineral density
J Clin Invest **78**, 618-621
AEROBIC CAPACITY, Elderly, Femur, Vertebrae

420/77   Reid, I. R., Mackie, M. & Ibbertson, H.K.   (1986)
Bone mineral content in Polynesian and white New Zealand women
Br Med J **292**, 1547-1548
Adult, Comparative, Customary activity, Endocrine, Female, Radius

420/78   Riggs, B.L. & Melton, L.J. 3rd   (1986)
Involutional Osteoporosis
N Engl J Med **314**, 1676-1686
Osteoporosis, Review

420/79   Rubin, C.T. & Lanyon, L.E.   (1984)
Regulation of bone formation by applied dynamic loads
J Bone Joint Surg (Am) **66**, 397-402
Animal, Intervention

420/80 **Rubin, C.T., Pratt, G.W., Porter, A.L., Lanyon, L.E. & Poss, R.** (1987)
The use of ultrasound in vivo to determine acute change in the mechanical properties of bone following intense physical activity
J Biomech **20**, 723-727
Acute exercise, Adult

420/81 **Rundgren, A., Aniansson, A., Ljungberg, P. & Wetterqvist, H.** (1984)
Effects of a training programme for elderly people on mineral content of the heel bone
Arch Gerontol Geriatr **3**, 243-248
Elderly, Exercise programme, Female, Intervention

420/82 **Sandler, R.B., Cauley, J.A., Hom, D.L., Sashin, D. & Kriska, A.M.** (1987)
The effects of walking on the cross-sectional dimensions of the radius in postmenopausal women
Calcif Tissue Int **41**, 65-69
Adult, Female, Leisure activity, Longitudinal, Menopause, MUSCLE STRENGTH, Radius

420/83 **Schneider, V.S. & McDonald, J.** (1984)
Skeletal calcium homeostasis and countermeasures to prevent disuse osteoporosis
Calcif Tissue Int **36**, S151-154
Adult, Inactivity, Intervention, Male, Osteoporosis

420/84 **Sherin, K.** (1983)
Aerobic exercise. Can you answer the questions your patients ask?
Postgraduate Med **73**, 157-164
AEROBIC CAPACITY, Review

420/85 **Silbermann, M., von der Mark, K., van Menxel, M. & Reznick, A.Z.** (1987)
Effect of short-term physical stress on DNA and collagen synthesis in the femur of young and old mice
Gerontology **33**, 49-56
Animal, Comparative, Elderly, Exercise programme, Femur, Intervention

420/86 **Simkin, A., Ayalon, J. & Leichter, I.** (1987)
Increased trabecular bone density due to bone-loading exercises in postmenopausal osteoporotic women
Calcif Tissue Int **40**, 59-63
Adult, Exercise programme, Female, Intervention, Menopause, Osteoporosis, Radius

420/87 **Sinaki, M., McPhee, M.C., Hodgson, S.F., Merritt, J.M. & Offord, K.P.** (1986)
Relationship between bone-mineral density of spine and strength of back extensors in healthy post-menopausal women
Mayo Clin Proc **61**, 116-122
Adult, Female, Menopause, MUSCLE STRENGTH, Vertebrae

420/88 **Sinaki, M. & Mikkelsen, B.A.** (1984)
Postmenopausal spinal osteoporosis: flexion versus extension exercises
Arch Phys Med Rehabil **65**, 593-596
Adult, Comparative, Exercise programme, Female, Hazards, Intervention, Menopause, Osteoporosis, Vertebrae

420/89 **Smith, D.M., Khairi, M.R.A., Norton, J. & Johnston, C.C.** (1976)
Age and activity effects on rate of bone mineral loss
J Clin Invest **58**, 716-721.
Adult, Comparative, Customary activity, Elderly, Female, Leisure activity, Longitudinal, Menopause, Radius

420/90 **Smith, E.L. Jr, Reddan, W. & Smith, P.E.** (1981)
Physical activity and calcium modalities for bone mineral increase in aged women
Med Sci Sports Exerc **13**, 60-64
Elderly, Exercise programme, Female, Longitudinal, Radius

420/91   Smith, E.L. Jr., Smith, P.E.,
Ensign, C.J. & Shea, M.M.   (1984)
Bone involution decrease in exercising
middle-aged women
Calcif Tissue Int **36**, S129-138
*Adult, Exercise programme, Female,
Longitudinal, Radius*

420/92   Smith, E.L. Jr. & Raab,
D.M.   (1986)
Osteoporosis and physical activity
Acta Med Scand (Suppl) **711**, 149-156
Review

420/93   Smith, R.   (1985)
Exercise and osteoporosis
Br Med J **290**, 1163-1164
Osteoporosis, Review

420/94   Smith, R.   (1987)
Osteoporosis: cause and management
Br Med J **294**, 329-332
Osteoporosis, Review

420/95   Snyder, A.C., Wenderoth, M.P. &
Johnston, C.C. Jr.   (1986)
Bone mineral content of elite lightweight
amenorrheic oarswomen
Hum Biol **58**, 863-869
*Adult, Amenorrhea, Athlete, Body
composition, Comparative, Female,
Hazards, Leisure activity, MENSTRUAL
FUNCTION, Radius, Vertebrae*

420/96   Sowers, M., Wallace, R.B. &
Lemke, J.H.   (1985)
Correlates of forearm bone mass among
women during maximal bone
mineralization
Prev Med **14**, 585-596
*Adult, Body composition, Female, Leisure
activity, Radius, Occupational activity*

420/97   Stillman, R.J., Lohman, T.G.,
Slaughter, M.H. & Massey, B.H.   (1986)
Physical activity and bone mineral
content in women aged 30 to 85 years
Med Sci Sports Exerc **5**, 576-580
*Adult, Body composition, Comparative,
Customary activity, Elderly, Female,
Radius*

420/98   Suominen, H., Heikkinen, E.,
Vainio, P. & Lahtinen, T.   (1984)
Mineral density of calcaneus in men at
different ages: a population study with
special reference to life-style factors
Age Ageing **13**, 273-281
*Adult, AEROBIC CAPACITY,
Comparative*

420/99   Warren, M.P., Brooks-Gunn, J.,
Hamilton, L.H., Warren, L.F. &
Hamilton, W.G.   (1986),
Scoliosis and fractures in young ballet
dancers. Relation to delayed menarche
and secondary amenorrhea.
N Engl J Med **314**, 1348-1353
*Amenorrhea, Children, Cohort, Female,
Hazards, MENSTRUAL FUNCTION,
REPRODUCTIVE HORMONES*

420/100   Whedon, G.D.   (1984)
Disuse osteoporosis; physiological
aspects
Calcif Tissue Int (Suppl) **36**, 146-150
Inactivity, Review

420/101   White, M.K., Martin, R.B.,
Yeater, R.A., Butcher, R.L. & Radin,
E.L.   (1984)
The effects of exercise on the bones of
postmenopausal women
Int Orthop **7**, 209-214
*Adult, Exercise programme, Female,
Intervention, Menopause, Osteoporosis*

420/102   Wilby, J., Linge, K., Reilly, T. &
Troup, J.D.G.   (1987)
Spinal shrinkage in females: circadian
variation and the effects of circuit weight
training
Ergonomics **30**, 47-54
*Adult, Female, MUSCLE STRENGTH,
PERCEIVED EXERTION, Vertebrae*

420/103   Williams, J.A., Wagner, J.,
Wasnich, R. & Heilbrun, L.   (1984)
The effect of long-distance running upon
appendicular bone mineral content
Med Sci Sports Exerc **16**, 223-227
*Adult, Intervention, Leisure activity,
Male, Marathon, Running*

420/104   **Woo, S.L., Kuei, S.C., Amiel, D.,
Gomez, M.A., Hayes, W.C., White, F.C.
& Akeson, W.H.**   (1981)
The effect of prolonged physical training
on the properties of long bone: A study of
Wolff's Law
J Bone Joint Surg (Am) **63**, 780-786
*Animal, Exercise programme, Femur,
Intervention*

420/105   **Wyshak, G., Frisch, R.E.,
Albright, T.E., Albright, N.L. & Schiff,
I.**   (1987)
Bone fractures among former college
athletes compared with nonathletes in
menopausal and postmenopausal years
Obstet Gynecol **69**, 121-125
*Adult, Athlete, Cohort, Female, Leisure
activity, Menopause, Vigorous*

420/106   **Yeater, R.A. & Martin,
R.B.**   (1984)
Senile osteoporosis. The effects of
exercise
Postgraduate Med **75**, 147-163
Review

420/107   **Yeh, C-K & Rodan, G.A.**   (1984)
Tensile forces enhance prostaglandin E
synthesis in osteoblastic cells grown on
collagen ribbons
Calcif Tissue Int (Suppl) **36**, S67-S71
Animal

KEYWORDS are listed in the appendix in addition the following specific keywords have been used in this section:

Amenorrhea
Cortisol
Height
Growth hormone

Summary of evidence: exercise is a hazard if over-use in severe athletic training occurs.

THE PROBLEM

Can exercise stimulate growth of the skeletal system or the cardio-respiratory system so as to increase the dimensions of those systems in later life? Some have advocated vigorous activity programmes in schools in the hope that this would be so.

SCOPE

This section contains references on the effects of exercise on growth in children particularly relating to height, cardiac size and ventilatory capacity. There are also references to overuse injuries and to hormone levels.

METHODOLOGICAL DIFFICULTIES

A fundamental difficulty is the variable growth curve in children and the impossibility of knowing what dimensions the individual would have reached without the extra exercise. Longitudinal studies in which exercise is eventually discontinued and in which measured values are related to mean growth curves provide some insight. There are also problems in quantifying and controlling for relevant customary exercise on a long term basis.

EVIDENCE

There is no evidence that exercise promotes additional growth in children. Studies of athletic youngsters, who are an elite group already self-selected because of large dimensions for age, show that once training is discontinued their cardiac dimensions and functional capacity drop back to within the 95% confidence limit of the mean curve. Hormone studies show that growth hormone is released during exercise but it is also released during sleep and provides no firm basis for assuming that vigorous exercise would produce extra growth. Over-use can be a hazard in children if competitive training schedules are severe. Prolonged exposure to repetitive vigorous movements can cause damage, for instance to epiphyseal joints leaving permanent impairment. Positive informed attitudes to exercise should nevertheless be encouraged from an early age for the good reasons set out in other sections.

430/1   **Bailey, D.A., Malina, R.M. & Rasmussen, R.L.**   (1978)
The influence of exercise, physical activity and athletic performance on the dynamics of human growth. In: Human Growth (Eds.) Falkner, F. and Tanner, J.M.
Balliere Tindall, London 475-505
Review

430/2   Bernick, M.J.E., Brich, W.B.M., Peltenberg, A.L., Zonderland, M.L. & Huisveld, I.A.   (1983)
Height, body composition, biological maturation and training in relation to socio-economic status in girl gymnasts, swimmers and controls
Growth **47**, 1-12
Athlete, Body composition, Children, Comparative, Height, Leisure activity, Swimming, Vigorous

430/3   Beunen, G., Malina, R.M., Ostyn, M., Renson, R., Simons, J. & Van Gerven, D.   (1983)
Fatness, growth and motor fitness of Belgian boys 12 through 20 years of age
Hum Biol **55**, 599-614
Body composition, Children, Height, JOINTS, Male, MUSCLE STRENGTH, Weight

430/4   Beunen, G., Ostyn, M., Renson, R., Simons, J. Swalus, P. & Van Gerven, D.   (1974)
Skeletal maturation and physical fitness of 12-15 year old boys
Acta Paed Belg **28**, 221-232
BONES, Children, Comparative, Leisure activity, Male

430/5   Beunen, G., Ostyn, M., Simons, J., Renson, R. & Van Gerven, D.   (1981)
Chronological and biological age related to physical fitness in boys 12 to 19 years
Ann Hum Biol **8**, 321-332
Children, Leisure activity, Male

430/6   Buckler, J.M.H. & Brodie, D.A.   (1977)
Growth and maturity characteristics of schoolboy gymnasts
Ann Hum Biol **4**, 455-464
Athlete, Children, Leisure activity, Male

430/7   Bunt, J.C., Boileau, R.A., Bahr, J.M. & Nelson, R.A.   (1986)
Sex and training differences in human growth hormone levels during prolonged exercise
J Appl Physiol **61**, 1796-1801
Acute exercise, Adult, Comparative, Female, Growth hormone, Leisure activity, Male, REPRODUCTIVE HORMONES

430/8   Caine, D.J. & Linder, K.J.   (1984)
Growth plate injury: A threat to long distance runners
Phys Sports Med **12**, 118-124
Children, Hazards, Review

430/9   Caldarone, G., Leglise, M. & Giampietro, M.   (1986)
Anthropometric measurements, body composition, biological maturation and growth predictions in young male gymnasts of high agonistic level
J Sports Med Phys Fitness **26**, 406-415
Body composition, Children, Height, Leisure activity, Male, Vigorous

430/10   Greene, S.A., Torresani, T. & Prader, A.   (1987)
Growth hormone response to a standardised exercise test in relation to puberty and stature
Arch Dis Child **62**, 53-56
Acute exercise, Children, Growth hormone, Height

430/11   Kobayashi, K., Kitamura, K., Miura, M., Sodeyama, H., Murase, Y., Miyashita, M. & Matsui, H.   (1978)
Aerobic power as related to body growth and training in Japanese boys
J Appl Physiol **44**, 666-672
AEROBIC CAPACITY, Athlete, Children, Cohort, Comparative, Height, Male

**430/12   Meleski, B.W., Shoup, R.F. &
Malina, R.M.**   (1982)
Size, physique and body composition of
competitive swimmers 11 through 20
years of age
Hum Biol **54**, 609-625
*Athlete, Body compostion, Children,
Female, Swimming, Vigorous*

430/13   Micheli, L.J.   (1983)
Overuse injuries in children's sports: the
growth factor
Orthop Clin North America **14**, 337-360
Review

430/14   Orave, S. & Puranen, J.   (1978)
Exertion injuries in adolescent athletes
Br J Sports Med **12**, 4-10
*Athlete, Children, Hazards, JOINTS,
Leisure activity, Vigorous*

430/15   Parizkova, J.   (1974)
Particularities of lean body mass and fat
development in growing boys as related
to their motor activity
Acta Paed Belg (Suppl) **28**, 233-243
*AEROBIC CAPACITY, Body
composition, Children, Height, Leisure
activity, Longitudinal, Male, Weight*

430/16   Parizkova, J.   (1968)
Longitudinal study of the development of
body composition and body build in boys
of various physical activity
Hum Biol **40**, 212-225
*Body compostion, Children, Height,
Leisure activity, Longitudinal, Male,
Weight*

**430/17   Peltenburg, A.L., Erich, W.B.,
Bernink, M.J.E., Zonderland, M.L. &
Huisveld, I.A.**   (1984)
Biological maturation, body
composition, and growth of female
gymnasts and control groups of
schoolgirls and girl swimmers, aged 8 to
14 years: a cross-sectional survey of 1064
girls
Int J Sports Med **5**, 36-42
*Body composition, Children,
Comparative, Female, Height, Leisure
activity, MENSTRUAL FUNCTION,
Swimming, Weight*

430/18   Rarick, G.L. (Ed)   (1973)
Physical activity, Human growth and
development
Academic Press, NY
Review

430/19   Rowley, S.   (1986)
The effect of intensive training on young
athletes. A review of the research
literature
The Sports Council
*Children, Hazards, MUSCLE
STRENGTH, Review*

**430/20   Sakamoto, K. & Grunewald,
K.K.**   (1987)
Beneficial effects of exercise on growth of
rats during intermittent fasting
J Nutr **117**, 390-395
*Animal, Exercise programme,
Intervention*

430/21   Salmela, J.H.   (1979)
Growth patterns of elite French-
Canadian female gymnasts
Can J Appl Sport Sci **4**, 219-222
*Athlete, Body compostion, Children,
Female, Height, Intervention, Leisure
activity, Weight*

430/22   Shephard, R.J.   (1982)
Physical activity and growth
Chicago: Year Book Publishers.
Review

430/23   **Sprynarová, S.**   (1987)
The influence of training on physical and
functional growth before, during and
after puberty
Eur J Appl Physiol **56,** 719-724
*AEROBIC CAPACITY, Athlete,
Children, Comparative, Leisure activity,
Male, Vigorous*

430/24   **Thorland, W.G., Johnson, G.O.,
Housh, T.J. & Refsell, M.J.**   (1983)
Anthropometric characteristics of elite
adolescent competitive swimmers
Hum Biol **55,** 735-748
*Athlete, Body composition, Children,
Swimming, Vigorous*

430/25   **VanHelder, W.P., Casey, K. &
Radomski, M.W.**   (1987)
Regulation of growth hormone during
exercise by oxygen demand and
availability
Eur J Appl Physiol **56,** 628-632
*Acute exercise, Adult, Growth hormone,
Male*

430/26   **Walsh, B.T., Puig-Antich, J.,
Goetz, R., Gladis, M., Novacenko, H.,
Glassman, A.H.**   (1984)
Sleep and growth hormone secretion in
women athletes
Electroencephalogr Clin Neurophysiol **57,**
528-533
*Adult, Amenorrhea, Athlete, Female,
Growth hormone, MENSTRUAL
FUNCTION, SLEEP*

430/27   **Winter, J.S.D.**   (1974)
The metabolic response to exercise and
exhaustion in normal and growth-
hormone-deficient children
Can J Physiol Pharmacol **52,** 575-582
*Acute exercise, Children, Comparative,
Cortisol, Endocrine*

KEYWORDS are listed in the appendix in addition the following specific keywords have been used in this section:

Calorie intake
Metabolic rate
Obesity

Summary of evidence: exercise ameliorates diseases associated with obesity, cures obesity and prevents weight gain

THE PROBLEM

The prevalence of obesity is high in the so-called developed countries; 7% of the adult population of the United Kingdom are severely obese, that is more than 30% above that regarded by life insurance underwriters as desirable weight for height. Obesity is associated with many chronic diseases of middle age such as hypertension, late-onset diabetes and CHD, arthritis, and bronchitis; it also increases the risk of complications during surgery. Over-weight people are twice as likely as their normal weight peers to die before the age of 65. Since body fat is stored when there is an excess of calorie intake over calorie expenditure, could increasing expenditure through regular moderate exercise cure obesity? It has also been a long-standing hope that exercise would cause long-term increases in resting metabolic rate or enhance dietary-induced thermogenesis. This would explain why some active people remain thin despite an apparently high calorie intake.

SCOPE

This section contains references dealing primarily with the effects of various kinds of exercise in both normal and obese subjects on body fat, lean body mass, hormone status, adipose cells, metabolic rate and dietary intake. It contains studies of men and women, studies in all ages including children, a few background studies and a few animal studies.

METHODOLOGICAL DIFFICULTIES

Studies of the effects of exercise on obesity are partially confounded if there is a change in dietary intake. This is difficult to measure and control. Exercise can induce changes in both muscle and fat, the net effect being no change in body mass. It is therefore necessary to assess body fat. The techniques for this have a low reliability and/or are tedious and expensive.

EVIDENCE

Exercise has a part to play in the prevention of weight gain as well as in the management of the overweight and obese states when they have developed. Weight loss in normal individuals can be achieved by increasing customary levels of exercise. An increase in energy expenditure does not necessarily lead to a corresponding increase in appetite or energy intake even in the absence of dietary restriction. Thus, over a period of many months there is a calorie deficit and weight is lost. There is no good evidence that exercise promotes an increase in metabolic rate above that directly associated with the exercise. Exercise appears to attenuate the risks associated with obesity of developing other chronic diseases even before weight has been lost. The risk of heart attack in obese people even if they remain over-weight can be reduced by vigorous exercise. Obese exercisers have been found to have a risk of suffering a heart attack no greater than normal exercisers, whereas those obese people who were sedentary had five times this risk (see 231.1). Although the very obese are limited by a reduced exercise tolerance this does not preclude a suitably graded walking programme. Dietary restriction must, therefore, be the major part of any treatment of gross obesity, but even in these cases moderate exercise can have a small but significant contribution in the long term. Any given activity has a higher calorie cost for the overweight individual than for their thin counterparts; this increases the effect of the exercise on physical capabilities (see section 110) as well as contributing more to the calorie deficit achieved.

510/1   **Allen, D.W. & Quigley, B.M.**   (1977)
The role of physical activity in the control of obesity
Med J Aust **2**, 434-438
Obesity, Review

510/2   **Baecke, J.A.H., van Staveren, W.A. & Burema, J.**   (1983)
Food consumption, habitual physical activity and body fatness in young Dutch adults
Am J Clin Nutr **37**, 278-86
Adult, Body composition, Calorie intake, Female, Leisure activity, Male, Occupational activity

510/3   **Ballor, D.L., Katch, V.L., Becque, M.D. & Marks, C.**   (1988)
Resistance weight training during caloric restriction enhances lean body weight maintenance
Am J Clin Nutr **47**, 19-25
Adult, Body composition, Comparative, Exercise programme, Female, Intervention, MUSCLE STRENGTH

510/4   **Belko, A.Z., Van Laon, M., Barbieri, T.F. & Mayclin, P.**   (1987)
Diet, exercise, weight loss, and energy expenditure in moderately overweight women
Int J Obes **11**, 93-104
Adult, AEROBIC CAPACITY, Body composition, Calorie intake, Exercise programme, Female, Intervention, Metabolic rate, Weight

510/5   **Berkowitz, R.I., Agras, W. S., Korner, A.F., Kraemer, H.C. & Zeanah, C.H.**   (1985)
Physical activity and adiposity: A longitudinal study from birth to childhood
J Pediatr **106**, 734-738
Body composition, Children, Cohort, Customary activity

510/6   **Binkhorst, R.A., Heevel, J. & Noordeloos, A.M.**   (1984)
Energy expenditure of (severe) obese subjects during submaximal and maximal exercise
Int J Sports Med **5**, 71-73
Acute exercise, Adult, Metabolic rate, Obesity

510/7   **Björntorp, P.**   (1978)
Physical training in the treatment of obesity
Int J Obes **2**, 149-156
Obesity, Review

510/8   **Björntorp, P.**   (1983)
Physiological and clinical aspects of exercise in obese persons
Exerc Sport Sci Rev **11**, 159-180
Review

510/9   Björntorp, P., De Jounge, K.,
Krotkiewski, M., Sullivan, L., Sjöström,
L. & Sternberg, J.   (1973)
Physical training in human obesity. iii.
Effects of long-term physical training on
body composition
Metabolism **22**, 1467-1475
*Adult, AEROBIC CAPACITY, Body
composition, CARBOHYDRATE
TOLERANCE, Exercise programme,
Intervention, Obesity, Weight*

510/10   Björntorp, P., De Jounge, K.,
Sjöström, L. & Sullivan, L.   (1970)
The effect of physical training on insulin
production in obesity
Metabolism **19**, 631-640
*Adult, AEROBIC CAPACITY, Body
composition, CARBOHYDRATE
TOLERANCE, Exercise programme,
Intervention, MUSCLE STRENGTH,
Weight*

510/11   Blair, D. & Buskirk, E.R.   (1987)
Habitual daily energy expenditure and
activity levels of lean and adult-onset and
child-onset obese women
Am J Clin Nutr **45**, 540-550
*Adult, Comparative, Customary activity,
Female, Obesity*

510/12   Blair, S.N., Blair, A., Pate, R.R.,
Howe, H.G., Rosenberg, M. & Parker,
G.M.   (1981)
Interactions among dietary patterns,
physical activity and skinfold thickness
Res Quart **52**, 505-511
*Adult, Body composition, Calorie intake,
Comparative, Leisure activity*

510/13   Blaza, S. & Garrow, J.S.   (1983)
Thermogenic response to temperature,
exercise and food stimuli in lean and
obese women, studied by 24 h direct
calorimetry
Br J Nutr **49**, 171-180
*Acute exercise, Adult, Body composition,
Calorie intake, Female, Metabolic rate,
Obesity, Weight*

510/14   Blomquist, B., Borjeson, M.,
Larsson, Y., Persson, B. & Sterky,
G.   (1965)
Effect of activity on the body
measurements and work capacity of
overweight boys
Acta Paediatr Scand **54**, 566-572
*Body composition, CARDIAC
PERFORMANCE, Children, Exercise
programme, Male, Intervention, Obesity*

510/15   Bloom, W.L. & Eidex,
M.F.   (1967)
Inactivity as a major factor in adult
obesity
Metabolism **16**, 679-684
*Adult, Comparative, Metabolic rate,
Obesity*

510/16   Bloom, W.L. & Eidex,
M.F.   (1967)
The comparison of energy expenditure in
the obese and lean
Metabolism **16**, 685-692
*Adult, Comparative, Metabolic rate,
Obesity*

510/17   Boileau, R.A., Buskirk, E.R.,
Horstman, D.H., Mendez, J. & Nicholas,
W.C.   (1971)
Body composition changes in obese and
lean men during physical conditioning
Med Sci Sports **3**, 183-189
*Adult, AEROBIC CAPACITY, Body
composition, Exercise programme,
Intervention, Male, Obesity*

510/18   Boileau, R.A., Lohman, T.G. &
Slaughter, M.H.   (1985)
Exercise and body composition of
children and youth
Scand J Sports Sci **7**, 17-27
Children, Review

510/19   Bradfield, R.B., Paulos, J. & Grossman, L.   (1971)
Energy expenditure and heart rate of obese high school girls
Am J Clin Nutr **24**, 1482-1484
Body composition, Children, Comparative, Customary activity, Female, Obesity

510/20   Bray, G.A., Whipp, B.J., Koyal, S.N. & Wasserman, K.   (1977)
Some respiratory and metabolic defects of exercise in moderately obese men
Metabolism **26**, 403-412
Acute exercise, Adult, Body composition, BLOOD PRESSURE, CARBOHYDRATE TOLERANCE, Comparative, GROWTH, Male, Obesity, RESPIRATORY FUNCTION, Weight

510/21   Brown, W.J. & Jones, P.R.M.   (1977)
The distribution of body fat in relation to habitual activity
Ann Hum Biol **4**, 537-550
Adult, Body composition, Leisure activity

510/22   Brownell, K.D. & Kaye, F.S.   (1982)
The distribution of body fat in relation to habitual activity
Am J Clin Nutr **35**, 277-283
Children, Intervention, Leisure activity, Obesity, Weight

510/23   Buskirk, E.R.   (1986)
Introduction to the symposium: exercise in the treatment of obesity
Med Sci Sports Exerc **18**, 1-2
Review

510/24   Buskirk, E.R. & Taylor, H.L.   (1957)
Maximal oxygen uptake and its relation to body composition, with special reference to physical activity and obesity
J Appl Physiol **11**, 72-78
Adult, AEROBIC CAPACITY, Body composition, Comparative, Leisure activity, Male

510/25   Dale, D.V., Saris, W.H.M., Schoffelen, P.F.M. & Hoor F.T.   (1987)
Does exercise give an additional effect in weight reduction regimes?
Int J Obes **11**, 367-375
Adult, AEROBIC CAPACITY, Body Composition, Calorie intake, Exercise programme, Female, Intervention, Metabolic rate, Obesity, Weight

510/26   Davies, C.T.M., Godfrey, S., Light, M., Sargeant, A.J. & Zeidifard, E.   (1975)
Cardiopulmonary responses to exercise in obese girls and young women
J Appl Physiol **38**, 373-376
Adult, AEROBIC CAPACITY, Body composition, Children, Female, Obesity, RESPIRATORY FUNCTION

510/27   Despres, J.P., Bouchard, C., Savard, R., Tremblay, A., Marcotte, M. & Theriault, G.   (1984)
Level of physical fitness and adipocyte lipolysis in humans
J Appl Physiol **56**, 1157-61
Adult, AEROBIC CAPACITY, Body composition, Exercise programme, Intervention, Male, Vigorous

510/28   Despres, J.P., Bouchard, C., Savard, R., Tremblay, A., Marcotte, M. & Theriault, G.   (1984)
The effect of a 20 week endurance training program on adipose tissue morphology and lipolysis in men and women
Metabolism **33**, 235-238
Adult, Body composition, Exercise programme, Female, Intervention, Male, Vigorous, Weight

510/29   Donahoe, C.P. Jr., Lin, D.H., Kirschenbaum, D.S. & Keesey, R.E.   (1984)
Metabolic consequences of dieting and exercise in the treatment of obesity
J Consult Clin Psychol **52**, 827-836
Adult, Body composition, Exercise programme, Female, Intervention, Metabolic rate, Obesity

510/30   Dudleston, A.K. & Bennion, M.   (1970)
Effect of diet and/or exercise on obese college women
J Am Dietetics Assoc **56,** 126-129
Adult, Exercise programme, Female, Intervention, Obesity

510/31   Dumitrescu, C., Mihalache, N., Mirodon, Z. & Perianu, S.   (1981)
The behaviour of some biologic parameters in obese patients after short-term exercise under restrictive diets
Med Interne **19,** 199-204
Acute exercise, Adult, CARBOHYDRATE TOLERANCE, Female, Obesity

510/32   Durrant, M.L., Royston, J.P. & Wloch, R.T.   (1982)
Effect of exercise on energy intake patterns in lean and obese humans
Physiol Behav **38,** 703-710
Acute exercise, Adult, Calorie intake, Comparative, Obesity

510/33   Epstein, L.H., Koeske, R., Zidansek, J. & Wing, R.R.   (1983)
Effects of weight loss on fitness in obese children
Am J Dis Child **137,** 654-657
AEROBIC CAPACITY, Calorie intake, Children, Female, Intervention, Leisure activity, Male, Obesity, Weight

510/34   Epstein, L.H. & Wing, R.R.   (1980)
Aerobic exercise and weight
Addictive Behaviours **5,** 371-388
Hazards, Review

510/35   Epstein, L.H., Wing, R.R., Koeske, R. & Valoski, A.   (1984)
Effects of diet plus exercise on weight change in parents and children
J Consult Clin Psychol **52,** 827-836
Children, Exercise programme, Intervention, Obesity, Weight

510/36   Epstein, L.H., Wing, R.R., Penner, B.C & Kress, M.J.   (1985)
Effect of diet and controlled exercise on weight loss in obese children
J Pediatr **107,** 358-361
Children, Exercise programme, Female, Intervention, Obesity, Weight

510/37   Epstein, L.H., Wing, R.R. & Valoski, A.   (1985)
Childhood obesity
Pediatr Clin North Am **32,** 363-379
Children, Obesity, Review

510/38   Farebrother, M.J.B.   (1979)
Respiratory function and cardiorespiratory response to exercise on obesity
Br J Dis Chest **73,** 211-229
Obesity, RESPIRATORY FUNCTION, Review

510/39   Flatt, J.P.   (1987)
Dietary fat, carbohydrate balance, and weight maintanance: effects of exercise
Am J Clin Nutr **45,** 296-306
Review

510/40   Forbes, G.B.   (1985)
Body composition as affected by physical activity and nutrition
Fed Proc **44,** 343-347
Review

510/41   Foss, M.L., Lampman, R.M. & Schteingart, D.E.   (1980)
Extremely obese patients: improvements in exercise tolerance with physical training and weight loss
Arch Phys Med Rehabil **61,** 119-124
Adult, Calorie intake, Exercise programme, Intervention, Obesity, Weight

510/42   Franklin, B.A. & Rubenfire, M.   (1980)
Losing weight through exercise
J Am Med Ass **244,** 377-379
Obesity, Review

510/43   Franklin, B.A., Buskirk, E.R.,
Hodgson, J.L., Gahagen, H., Kollias, J. &
Mendez, J.   (1979)
Effects of physical conditioning on
cardiorespiratory function, body
composition and serum lipids in relatively
normal-weight and obese middle-aged
women
Int J Obes **3**, 97-109
*Adult, AEROBIC CAPACITY, Body
composition, Female, Intervention,
LIPIDS, Obesity, RESPIRATORY
FUNCTION*

510/44   Freedman-Akabas, S., Colt, E.,
Kissileff, H.R. & Pi-Sunyer, F.X.   (1985)
Lack of sustained increase in VO2
following exercise in fit and unfit subjects
Am J Clin Nutr **41**, 545-549
*Acute exercise, Adult, Comparative,
Female, Leisure activity, Male, Metabolic
rate*

510/45   Fripp, R.R., Hodgson, J.L.,
Kwiterovich, P.O., Werner, J.C., Schuler,
H.G. & Whitman, V.   (1985)
Aerobic capacity, obesity, and
atherosclerotic risk factors in male
adolescents
Pediatrics **75**, 813-818
*AEROBIC CAPACITY, BLOOD
PRESSURE, Body composition,
Children, LIPIDS, Male, Obesity,
PRIMARY PREVENTION, Weight*

510/46   Gardner, A.W.   (1988)
Longitudinal study of energy expenditure
in males during steady-state exercise
J Gerontol **43**, B22-25
*Acute exercise, Adult, Comparative,
Leisure activity, Longitudinal, Metabolic
rate*

510/47   Gardner, A.W., Poehlman, E.T.,
Sedlock, D.A., Corrigan, D.L. &
Siconolfi, S.   (1988)
A longitudinal study of energy
expenditure in males during steady-state
exercise
J Gerontol **43**, B22-25
*Acute exercise, Adult, AEROBIC
CAPACITY, Leisure activity,
Longitudinal, Male, Metabolic rate,
Weight*

510/48   Garrow, J.S.   (1981)
Treat obesity seriously. A clinical manual
Churchill Livingstone
Obesity, Review

510/49   Garrow, J.S.   (1986)
Effect of exercise on obesity
Acta Med Scand (Suppl 711) **220**, 67-73
Obesity, Review

510/50   Garrow, J.S., Halliday, B., Hesp,
R., Stallet, S.F. & Warwick,
P.M.   (1977)
Weight loss, resting metabolic rate,
physical activity and body composition in
obese women on a reducing diet
Proc Nutr Soc **36**, 112A
*Adult, Body composition, Calorie intake,
Exercise programme, Female,
Intervention, Metabolic rate, Obesity,
Weight*

510/51   Garthwaite, S.M., Cheng, H. &
Bryan, J.E.   (1986)
Ageing, exercise and food restriction:
effects on body composition
Mech Ageing Dev **36**, 187-196
*Adult, Body composition, Calorie intake,
Comparative, Elderly, Leisure activity*

510/52   Glick, Z. & Kaufmann,
N.A.   (1976)
Weight and skinfold thickness changes
during a physical training course
Med Sci Sports **8**, 109-112
*Adult, Body composition, Intervention,
Occupational activity*

510/53   Glick, Z. & Shvartz, E.   (1983)
Physiologic responses to exercise in
normal and obese women
Int J Obes **7**, 37-44
Acute exercise, Adult, Comparative,
Female, Obesity

510/54   Gossain, V.V., Srivastava, L.,
Rovner, D.R. & Turek, D.   (1983)
Plasma glucagon in simple obesity: effect
of exercise
Am J Med Sci **286**, 4-10
Acute exercise, Adult, Comparative,
Female, GROWTH

510/55   Gwinup, G.   (1975)
Effect of exercise alone on the weight of
obese women
Arch Intern Med **135**, 676-680
Adult, Body composition, Female,
Intervention, Leisure activity, Obesity

510/56   Hadjiolova, I., Mintcheva, L.,
Dunev, S., Daleva, M., Handjiev, S. &
Balabanski, L.   (1982)
Physical working capacity in obese
women after an exercise programme for
body weight reduction
Int J Obes **6**, 405-410
Adult, AEROBIC CAPACITY, Exercise
programme, Female, Intervention,
Obesity, RESPIRATORY FUNCTION,
Weight

510/57   Hagan, R.D., Upton, S.J., Wong, L.
& Whittam, J.   (1986)
The effects of aerobic conditioning and/
or caloric restriction in overweight men
and women
Med Sci Sports Exerc **18**, 87-94
Adult, AEROBIC CAPACITY, Body
composition, Calorie intake, Exercise
programme, Female, Intervention,
LIPIDS, Male, Obesity, Running, Weight

510/58   Henson, L.C., Poole, D.C.,
Donahue, C.P. & Heber, D.   (1987)
Effects of exercise training on resting
energy expenditure during caloric
restriction
Am J Clin Nutr **46**, 893-899
Adult, AEROBIC CAPACITY, Body
composition, Calorie intake, Exercise
programme, Female, Intervention,
Metabolic rate

510/59   Hickson, J.F. Jr., Hartung, G.H.,
Pate, T.D., Kendall, S.C., McMahon,
J.C. & Moore, C.M.   (1986)
Effect of short-term energy intake level
and exercise on oxygen consumption in
men
Eur J Appl Physiol **55**, 198-201
Acute exercise, Adult, Calorie intake,
Male, Metabolic rate

510/60   Hill, J.O   (1987)
Effects of exercise and food restriction on
body composition and metabolic rate in
obese women
Am J Clin Nutr **46**, 622-630
Adult, Body composition, Calorie intake,
Exercise programme, Female,
Intervention, Metabolic rate, Obesity

510/61   Ho, S.S.   (1987)
Assessment of overweight and physical
activity among adolescents and youths in
Hong Kong
Public Health **101**, 457-464
Adult, Children, Customary activity,
Female, Leisure activity, Male, Weight

510/62   Holm, G., Jacobsson, B., Holm, J.,
Björntorp, P., & Smith, U.   (1977)
Effects of submaximal exercise on
adipose tissue metabolism in man
Int J Obes **1**, 249-257
Acute exercise, Adult, Body composition,
Calorie intake, CARBOHYDRATE
TOLERANCE, Endocrine, LIPIDS,
Obesity, Weight

510/63   **Horton, E.S.** (1986)
Metabolic aspects of exercise and weight reduction
Med Sci Sports Exerc **18**, 10-18
Review

510/64   **Huttunen, N., Knip, M. & Paavilainen, T.** (1986)
Physical activity and fitness in obese children
Int J Obes **10**, 519-525
AEROBIC CAPACITY, Body composition, Children, Comparative, Intervention, Leisure activity, Weight

510/65   **Jones, N.L., Heigenhauser, J.F., Kuksis, A., Matsos, C.G., Sutton, J.R. & Toews, C.J.** (1980)
Fat metabolism in heavy exercise
Clin Sci **59**, 469-478
Acute exercise, Adult, Male, RESPIRATORY FUNCTION, Vigorous

510/66   **Kahle, E.B., Walker, R.B., Eisenman, P.A., Behall, K.M., Hallfrisch, J. & Reiser, S.** (1982)
Moderate diet control in children: the effects on metabolic indicators that predict obesity-related degenerative diseases
Am J Clin Nutr **35**, 950-957
Calorie intake, CARBOHYDRATE TOLERANCE, Children, Exercise programme, Intervention, LIPIDS, Male, Obesity, PRIMARY PREVENTION, Weight

510/67   **Katch, V., Becque, M.D., Marks, C., Moorehead, C. & Rocchini, A.** (1988)
Oxygen uptake and energy output during walking of obese male and female adolescents
Am J Clin Nutr **47**, 26-32
Acute exercise, AEROBIC CAPACITY, Children, Comparative, Female, Male, Metabolic rate

510/68   **Klinzing, J.E. & Hazelton, I.** (1982)
The effects of exercise and weight change on cardiorespiratory endurance
J Sports Med Phys Fitness **22**, 469-476
Adult, BLOOD PRESSURE, Body composition, Calorie intake, Exercise programme, Intervention, Weight

510/69   **Komorowski, J.M., Owczarczyk, I. & Janiszewski, M.** (1984)
Effect of chronic exercise on certain aspects of hormonal function in obesity
Endokrynol Pol **35**, 157-163
Adult, Exercise programme, Female, Intervention, Obesity, REPRODUCTIVE HORMONES

510/70   **Krotkiewski, M.** (1983)
Physical training in the prophylaxis and treatment of obesity, hypertension and diabetes
Scand J Rehabil Med (Suppl) **9**, 55-70
Adult, BLOOD PRESSURE, Body composition, CARBOHYDRATE TOLERANCE, Female, Intervention, Male, MUSCLE METABOLISM, Obesity, Weight

510/71   **Krotkiewski, M. & Björntorp, P.** (1986)
Muscle tissue in obesity with different distribution of adipose tissue. Effects of physical training
Int J Obes **10**, 331-341
Adult, AEROBIC CAPACITY, BLOOD PRESSURE, Body composition, CARBOHYDRATE TOLERANCE, Exercise programme, Female, Intervention, LIPIDS, Male, MUSCLE STRENGTH, Obesity, Weight

510/72   **Krotkiewski, M., Mandroukas, K., Sjöström, L., Sullivan, L., Wetterqvist, H. & Björntorp, P.** (1979)
Effects of long-term physical training on body fat, metabolism, and blood pressure in obesity
Metabolism **28**, 650-658
Adult, BLOOD PRESSURE, Body composition, CARBOHYDRATE TOLERANCE, Exercise programme, Female, Intervention, LIPIDS, Obesity, Weight

510/73   **Krotkiewski, M., Sjöstrom, L., Sullivan, L., Lundberg, P.A., Lindstedt, G., Wetterqvis, H. & Björntorp, P.** (1984)
The effect of acute and chronic exercise on thyroid hormones in obesity
Acta Med Scand **216**, 269-275
Acute exercise, Adult, AEROBIC CAPACITY, BLOOD PRESSURE, Body composition, CARBOHYDRATE TOLERANCE, Exercise programme, Female, Intervention, Obesity

510/74   **Krotkiewski, M., Toss, L., Björntorp, P. & Holm, G.** (1981)
The effect of a very-low-calorie diet with and without chronic exercise on thyroid and sex hormones, plasma proteins, oxygen uptake, insulin and c peptide concentrations in obese women
Int J Obes **5**, 287-293
Adult, AEROBIC CAPACITY, Body composition, Female, Intervention, LIPIDS, Obesity, REPRODUCTIVE HORMONES,

510/75   **Kukkonen, K., Rauramaa, R., Siitonen, O. & Hanninen, O.** (1982)
Physical training of obese middle-aged persons
Ann Clin Res (Suppl 34) **14**, 80-85
Adult, AEROBIC CAPACITY, Female, Intervention, Leisure activity, Male, Obesity, Weight

510/76   **Lampman, R.M., Schteingart, D.E. & Foss, M.L.** (1986)
Exercise as a partial therapy for the extremely obese
Med Sci Sports Exerc **18**, 19-24
Obesity, Review

510/77   **Lennon, D., Nagle, F., Stratman, F., Shrago, E. & Dennis, S.** (1985)
Diet and exercise training effects on resting metabolic rate
Int J Obes **9**, 39-47
Adult, AEROBIC CAPACITY, Body composition, Calorie intake, Exercise programme, Female, Intervention, Leisure activity, Male, Metabolic rate, Weight

510/78   **Leon, A.S., Conrad, J., Hunninghake, D.B. & Serfass, R.** (1979)
Effect of a vigorous walking program on body composition, and carbohydrate and lipid metabolism of obese young men
Am J Clin Nutr **33**, 1776-1787
Adult, Body composition, BLOOD PRESSURE, CARBOHYDRATE TOLERANCE, Exercise programme, Intervention, LIPIDS, Male, Obesity, Weight

510/79   **Lewis, S., Haskell, W.L., Klein, H., Halpern, J. & Wood, P.D.** (1975)
Prediction of body composition in habitually active middle-aged men
J Appl Physiol **39**, 221-225
Adult, Body composition, Leisure activity, Male

510/80   **Lewis, S., Haskell, W.L., Wood, P.D., Manoogian, N., Bailey, J.E. & Pereira, M.** (1976)
Effects of physical activity on weight reduction in obese middle-aged women
Am J Clin Nutr **29**, 151-156
Adult, BLOOD PRESSURE, Body composition, Exercise programme, Female, Intervention, LIPIDS, Obesity, Vigorous

510/81   Lincoln, J.E.   (1972)
Calorie intake, obesity and physical
activity
Am J Clin Nutr **25**, 390-394
Adult, Calorie intake, Comparative,
Leisure activity, Male, Obesity,
Occupational activity, Weight

510/82   McKenzie, T.L., Buono, M. &
Nelson, J.   (1984)
Modification of coronary heart disease
(CHD) risk factors in obese boys through
diet and exercise
Am Corr Ther J **38**, 37-35
Children, Intervention, Leisure activity,
Male, PRIMARY PREVENTION

510/83   McMurray, R.G., Ben-Ezra, V.,
Forsythe, W.A. & Smith, A.T.   (1985)
Response of endurance-trained subjects
to caloric deficits induced by diet or
exercise
Med Sci Sports Exerc **17**, 574-579
Adult, Acute exercise, AEROBIC
CAPACITY, Calorie intake, Leisure
activity

510/84   Moody, D.L., Kollias, J. & Buskirk,
E.R.   (1969)
The effect of a moderate exercise
program on body weight and skinfold
thickness in overweight college women
Med Sci Sports **1**, 75-80
Adult, Body composition, Exercise
programme, Female, Intervention, Weight

510/85   Oscai, L.B. & Williams,
B.T.   (1968)
Effect of exercise on overweight middle-
aged males
J Am Geriatr Soc **16**, 794-797
Adult, Body composition, Exercise
programme, Intervention, Male, Running,
Weight

510/86   Pacy, P.J., Barton, N., Webster,
J.D. & Garrow, J.S.   (1985)
The energy cost of aerobic exercise in fed
and fasted normal subjects
Am J Clin Nutr **42**, 764-768
Acute exercise, Adult, Metabolic rate

510/87   Pacy, P.J., Webster, J.D. &
Garrow, J.S.   (1986)
Exercise and obesity
Sports Med **3**, 89-113
Obesity, Review.

510/88   Parizkova, J.   (1974)
Proportions of lean body mass and fat
development in growing boys as related
to their motor activity
Acta Paed Belg (Suppl) **28**, 233-243
Body composition, Children, Customary
activity, Male

510/89   Parizkova, J. & Eiselt, E.   (1968)
Longitudinal study of changes in
anthropometric indicators and body
composition in old men of various
physical activity
Hum Biol **40**, 331-344
Body composition, Comparative, Elderly,
Leisure activity, Male, RESPIRATORY
FUNCTION

510/90   Pavlou K.N., Steffee, W.P., Lerman
R.H. & Burrows, B.   (1985)
Effects of dieting and exercise on lean
body mass, oxygen uptake and strength
Med Sci Sports Exerc **17**, 466-471
Adult, AEROBIC CAPACITY, Body
composition, Exercise programme,
Intervention, Male, MUSCLE
STRENGTH, Vigorous

510/91   Pena, M., Barta, L., Regoly-Merei,
A. & Tichy, M.   (1980)
The influence of physical exercise upon
the body composition of obese children
Act Paed Acad Scientific Hungaricae **21**,
9-14
Body composition, Children, Intervention,
Obesity

510/92   **Petroiu, A., Schneider, F., Lungu, G., Mihalas, G., Varadeanu, A. & Man, I.**   (1984)
Lipidogram structure and the exercise capacity in obesity
Physiologie **21**, 117-120
Acute exercise, Adult, BLOOD PRESSURE, Female, LIPIDS, Obesity, PERCEIVED EXERTION

510/93   **Poehlman, E.T., Tremblay, A., Marcotte, M., Perusse, L., Theriault, G. & Bouchard, C.**   (1987)
Heredity and changes in body composition and adipose tissue metabolism after short term exercise training
Eur J Appl Physiol **56**, 398-402
Adult, AEROBIC CAPACITY, Body composition, Exercise programme, Intervention, Male, Weight

510/94   **Pollock, M.L. & Jackson, A.**   (1977)
Body composition: measurement and changes resulting from physical training. In: Toward an understanding of human performance (Ed.) Burke, E.J.
Movement Publications, NY
Adult, Body composition, Exercise programme, Intervention

510/95   **Porikos, K.P. & Pi-Sunyer, F.X.**   (1984)
Regulation of food intake in human obesity: Studies with caloric dilution and exercise
Clin Endocrinol Metab **13**, 547-561
Review

510/96   **Prentice, A.M., Black, A.E., Coward, W.A., Davies, H.L., Goldberg, G.R., Murgatroyd, P.R., Ashford, J., Sawyer M. & Whitehead, R.G.**   (1986)
High levels of energy expenditure in obese women
Br Med J **292**, 983-987
Adult, Calorie intake, Comparative, Customary activity, Female, Metabolic rate, Obesity

510/97   **Sasaki, J., Shindo, M., Tanaka, H., Ando, M. & Arakawa, K.**   (1987)
A long-term aerobic exercise program decreases the obesity index and increases the high density lipoprotein cholesterol concentration in obese children
Int J Obes **11**, 339-345
Body composition, Children, Exercise programme, Intervention, LIPIDS, Obesity, Weight

510/98   **Schaeffer, O.**   (1974)
The relative roles of diet and physical activity on blood lipids and obesity
Am Heart J **88**, 673-674
Adult, Body composition, LIPIDS, Obesity, Occupational activity

510/99   **Scheen, A.J., Pirnay, F., Luyckx, A.S. & Lefebvre, P.J.**   (1983)
Metabolic adaptation to prolonged exercise in severely obese subjects
Int J Obes **7**, 221-229
Acute exercise, Adult, CARBOHYDRATE TOLERANCE, Male, Obesity, RESPIRATORY FUNCTION

510/100   **Schneider, D.A., Knowlton, R.G. & Blatchford, F.W.**   (1985)
The free fatty acid responses to prolonged walking of moderately obese middle aged persons
Hum Biol **57**, 365-373
Acute exercise, Adult, Body composition, Comparative, LIPIDS, Obesity

510/101   **Segal, K.R. & Gutin, B.**   (1983)
Thermic effects of food and exercise in lean and obese women
Metabolism **32**, 581-589
Acute exercise, Adult, Calorie intake, Comparative, Female, Obesity,

510/102   **Segal, K.R., Gutin, B., Nyman, A.M. & Pi-Sunyer, F.X.**   (1985)
Thermic effect of food at rest, during exercise, and after exercise in lean and obese men of similar body weight
J Clin Invest **76**, 1107-1112
Acute exercise, Adult, Body composition, Calorie intake, Comparative, Male, Metabolic rate, Obesity

510/103   **Segal, K.R., Presta, E. & Gutin, B.**   (1984)
Thermic effect of food during graded exercise in normal weight and obese men
Am J Clin Nutr **40**, 995-1000
Acute exercise, Adult, AEROBIC CAPACITY, Comparative, Male, Metabolic rate, Obesity

510/104   **Segal, K.R., Gutin, B., Albu, J. & Pi-Sunyer, F.X.**   (1987)
Thermic effects of food and exercise in lean and obese men of similar lean body mass
Am J Physiol **252**, E110-117
Acute exercise, Adult, AEROBIC CAPACITY, ANAEROBIC CAPACITY, Body composition, CARBOHYDRATE TOLERANCE, Comparative, Male, Metabolic rate, Obesity,

510/105   **Sheldahl, L.M.**   (1986)
Special ergometric techniques and weight reduction
Med Sci Sports Exerc **18**, 25-30
Exercise programme, Obesity, Review

510/106   **Sidney, K.H., Shephard, R.J. & Harrison, J.**   (1977)
Endurance training and body composition of the elderly
Am J Clin Nutr **30**, 326-33
Body composition, BONES, Elderly, Exercise programme, Female, Intervention, Male, Weight

510/107   **Sopko, G., Leon, A.S., Jacobs, D.R. Jr., Foster, N., Moy, J., Kuba, K., Anderson, J.T., Casal, D., McNally, C. & Frantz, I.**   (1985)
The effects of exercise and weight loss on plasma lipids in young obese men
Metabolism **34**, 227-236
Adult, AEROBIC CAPACITY, Body composition, Exercise programme, Intervention, LIPIDS, Male, Weight

510/108   **South-Paul, J.E. & Tenholder, M.F.**   (1985)
The assessment of improved physiologic function with a short term exercise program in mildly to moderately obese people
Milit Med **150**, 35-37
Adult, Calorie intake, Female, Male, Obesity

510/109   **Stern, J.S.**   (1984)
Is obesity a disease of inactivity?
Res Publ Assoc Res Nerv Ment Dis **62**, 131-139
Obesity, Review

510/110   **Sunnegårdh, J., Bratteby, L.E., Hagman, U., Samuelson, G. & Sjolin, S.**   (1986)
Physical activity in relation to energy intake and body fat in 8- and 13-year-old children in Sweden
Acta Paediat Scand **75**, 955-963
Body composition, Calorie intake, Children, Customary activity, Female, Leisure activity, Male

510/111   **Tagliaferro, A.R., Kertzer, R. & Davis, J.R.**   (1986)
Effects of exercise-training on the thermic effect of food and body fatness of adult women
Physiol Behav **38**, 703-710
Adult, Body composition, Exercise programme, Female, Intervention, Metabolic rate

510/112   Thompson, K., Jarvie, G., Lahey, B. & Cureton, K.   (1982)
Exercise and obesity: etiology, physiology, and intervention
Psychol Bull **91**, 55-79
Obesity, Review

510/113   Thomson, M. & Cruickshank, F.   (1979)
Survey into the eating and exercise habits of New Zealand pre-adolescents in relation to overweight and obesity
NZ Med J **89**, 7-9
Body composition, Children, Female, GROWTH, Leisure activity, Male

510/114   Tremblay, A., Despres, J.P. & Bouchard, C.   (1984)
Adipose tissue characteristics of ex-obese long-distance runners
Int J Obes **8**, 641-648
Adult, Comparative, Leisure activity, LIPIDS, Male, Obesity, Running

510/115   Tremblay, A., Fontaine, E., Poehlman, E.T., Mitchell, D., Perron, L. & Bouchard, C.   (1986)
The effect of exercise-training on resting metabolic rate in lean and moderately obese individuals
Int J Obes **10**, 511-517
Adult, Body composition, Comparative, Exercise programme, Female, Intervention, Male, Metabolic rate, Obesity, Weight

510/116   Vroman, N.B., Buskirk, E.R. & Hodgson, J.L.   (1983)
Cardiac output and skin blood flow in lean and obese individuals during exercise in the heat
J Appl Physiol **55**, 69-74
Acute exercise, Adult, Body composition, CARDIAC PERFORMANCE, Comparative, Male, Obesity.

510/117   Ward, D.S. & Bar-Or, O.   (1986)
Role of the physician and physical education teacher in the treatment of obesity at school
Pediatrician **13**, 44-51
Review

510/118   Warwick, P.M. & Garrow, J.S.   (1981)
The effect of addition of exercise to a regime of dietary restriction on weight loss, nitrogen balance , resting metabolic rate and spontaneous physical activity in three obese women in a metabolic ward
Int J Obes **5**, 25-32
Adult, Body composition, Female, Intervention, METABOLIC FUNCTION, Obesity

510/119   Waxman, M.S. & Stunkard, A.J.   (1980)
Caloric intake and expenditure of obese boys
J Pediatr **96**, 187-193
Calorie intake, Children, Comparative, Customary activity, Male, Obesity

510/120   Welle, S.   (1984)
Metabolic responses to a meal during rest and low-intensity exercise
Am J Clin Nutr **40**, 990-994
Acute exercise, Adult, CARBOHYDRATE TOLERANCE, LIPIDS, Metabolic rate

510/121   Whipp, B.J. & Davis, J.A.   (1984)
The ventilatory stress of exercise in obesity
Am Rev Respir Dis (Suppl) **129**, S90-92
RESPIRATORY FUNCTION, Review

510/122   Widhalm, K., Maxa, E. & Zyman, H.   (1978)
Effect of diet and exercise upon the cholesterol triglyceride content of plasma lipoproteins in overweight children
Eur J Paediatr **127**, 121-126
Children, Exercise programme, Intervention, LIPIDS, Weight

510/123   **Wilkinson, P.W., Parkin, J.M., Pearlson, G., Strong, H. & Sykes, P.**   (1977)
Energy intake and physical activity in obese children
Br Med J **1**, 756
Calorie intake, Children, Comparative, Customary activity, Female, Leisure activity, Male, Obesity

510/124   **Williams, C.L.**   (1984)
Prevention and treatment of childhood obesity in a public school setting
Pediatr Ann **13**, 482-490
Review

510/125   **Wirth, A.**   (1987)
Metabolic effects and body fat mass changes in obese subjects on a very-low-calorie diet with and without intensive physical training
Ann Nutr Metab **31**, 378-386
Adult, Body composition, Calorie intake, Exercise programme, Intervention, Obesity

510/126   **Woo, R.**   (1985)
The effect of increasing physical activity on voluntary food intake and energy balance
Int J Obes (Suppl 2) **9**, 155-160
Adult, Body composition, Calorie intake, Exercise programme, Female, Intervention, Metabolic rate, Obesity, Weight

510/127   **Woo, R., Garrow, J.S. & Pi-Sunyer, F.X.**   (1982)
Effect of exercise on spontaneous calorie intake in obesity
Am J Clin Nutr **36**, 470-477
Adult, Body composition, Calorie intake, Exercise programme, Female, Intervention, Metabolic rate, Obesity, Weight

510/128   **Woo, R., Garrow, J.S. & Pi-Sunyer, F.X.**   (1982)
Voluntary food intake during prolonged exercise in obese women
Am J Clin Nutr **36**, 478-484
Adult, BLOOD PRESSURE, Body composition, Calorie intake, Exercise programme, Female, Intervention, Metabolic rate, Obesity, Weight

510/129   **Worsley, A., Coonan, W., Leitch, D. & Crawford, D.**   (1984)
Slim and obese children's perceptions of physical activities
Int J Obes **8**, 201-211
Body composition, Children, Leisure activity, Obesity

510/130   **Young, J.C., Treadway, J.L., Balon, T.W., Gavras, H.P. & Ruderman, N.B.**   (1986)
Prior exercise potentiates the thermic effect of carbohydrate load
Metabolism **35**, 1048-1053
Acute exercise, Adult, AEROBIC CAPACITY, Body composition, CARBOHYDRATE TOLERANCE, Metabolic rate

510/131   **Zahorska-Markiewicz, B.**   (1980)
Thermic effect of food and exercise in obesity
Eur J Appl Physiol **44**, 231-235
Acute exercise, Adult, Calorie intake, Comparative, Female, Metabolic rate, Obesity

520 CARBOHYDRATE TOLERANCE

KEYWORDS are listed in the appendix in addition the following specific keywords have been used in this section:

Glucose tolerance (Glucose tolerance tests)
Insulin sensitivity (Glucose clamp)
Type 1 (Diabetes – severe, juvenile onset)
Type 2 (Diabetes – mild, late onset)

Summary of evidence: exercise ameliorates diabetes mellitus, cures mild late-onset diabetes mellitus and prevents impaired glucose tolerance

THE PROBLEM

Glucose tolerance deteriorates with increasing age and is associated with the development of late-onset diabetes mellitus (Type 2). Can exercise improve glucose tolerance and reduce the incidence of diabetes? Is exercise hazardous in those with severe diabetes (Type 1)?

SCOPE

This section contains references dealing primarily with changes produced by exercise in glucose tolerance and insulin sensitivity in those suffering from diabetes mellitus and normal subjects. It contains studies of men and women, studies of all age groups, studies of sedentary and athletic groups, and some background studies.

METHODOLOGICAL DIFFICULTIES

Exercise can reduce obesity as well as changing glucose tolerance. Obesity is also associated with the development of diabetes so the possible effects of the exercise may be confounded.

EVIDENCE

The sensitivity of body tissues to insulin increases with vigorous rhythmic exercise. This is manifest as a more rapid return of blood glucose to normal levels after a glucose 'meal' (glucose tolerance test) and a decreased insulin requirement for a given intake of carbohydrate. Glucose tolerance deteriorates with increasing age and is exacerbated by obesity. This age effect can be reversed with exercise. Thus, moderate rhythmic exercise appears to reduce the risk in both normal and obese middle-aged people that they will develop diabetes. Those who already have diabetes of mature-onset (Type 2) are relatively insensitive to the insulin they produce; exercise increases the insulin sensitivity of their skeletal muscle cells which ameliorates their disease. The combination of these two effects means that some patients who are prepared to include vigorous exercise as a permanent part of their lifestyle find that insulin injections or other drug treatment become unnecessary. Individuals with severe early-onset diabetes also stand to gain from the general health benefits of exercise in particular the reduction in risk of developing coronary heart disease. Exercise is not hazardous for them provided they are able to balance their calorie intake and their insulin to provide for the extra energy output.

520/1   (1982)
Diabetes and exercise-Proceedings of the symposium, Olympia, Greece, September 21-22, (1980)
Curr Probl Clin Biochem **11**, 1-199
Review

520/2   Baevre, H., Sovik, O., Wisnes, A. & Heiervang, E.   (1985)
Metabolic responses to physical training in young insulin-dependent diabetics
Scand J clin Lab Invest **45**, 109-114
AEROBIC CAPACITY, Children, Endocrine, Exercise programme, GROWTH, Insulin sensitivity, Intervention, LIPIDS,

520/3   Bakth, S., Arena, J., Lee, W., Torres, R., Haider, B., Patel, B.C., Lyons, M.M. & Regan, T.J.   (1986)
Arrhythmia susceptibility and myocardial composition in diabetes. The influence of physical conditioning
J Clin Invest **77**, 382-395
Animal, CARDIAC PERFORMANCE, Endocrine, Exercise programme, HAZARDS-CVS, Intervention, LIPIDS, Type 1

520/4   Barnard, R.J., Massey, M.R., Cherny, S., O'Brien, L.T. &Pritikin, N.   (1983),
Long-term use of a high-complex-carbohydrate, high-fiber, low-fat diet and exercise in the treatment of NIDDM patients
Diabetes Care **6**, 268-273
Adult, Leisure activity, LIPIDS, Longitudinal, Type 2

520/5   Berger, M., Berchtold, P., Cüppers, H.J., Drost, H., Kley, H.K., Muller, W.A., Weigelmann, W., Zimmerman-Telschow, H., Gries, F.A., Kruskemper, H.L. & Zimmerman, H.   (1977)
Metabolic and hormonal effects of muscular exercise in juvenile type diabetes
Diabetologia **13**, 355-365
Acute exercise, Adult, Endocrine, GROWTH, Male, Type 1

520/6   Berger, M., Kemmer, F.W., Becker, K., Herberg, L., Schwenen, M., Gjinavivci, A. & Berchtold, P.   (1979)
Effect of physical training on glucose tolerance and on glucose metabolism of skeletal muscle in anaesthetized rats
Diabetologia **16**, 179-184
Animal, Exercise programme, Glucose tolerance, Insulin sensitivity, Intervention, MUSCLE METABOLISM

520/7   Berger, M. & Lefebvre, P.   (1982)
Is exercise beneficial to patients with type I diabetes mellitus? Transcript of a controversy debate
Curr Probl Clin Biochem **11**, 101-114
Review

520/8   Björntorp, K. & Lindgarde, F.   (1985)
Impaired physical fitness and insulin secretion in normoglycaemic subjects with familial aggregation of type 2 diabetes mellitus
Diabetes Res **2**, 151-156
Acute exercise, Adult, Glucose tolerance, Insulin sensitivity, Male, Type 2

520/9   Björntorp, P., De Jounge, K., Sjöström, L. & Sullivan, L.   (1973)
Physical training in human obesity. ii. Effects on plasma insulin in glucose-intolerant subjects without marked hyperinsulinemia
Scand J clin Lab Invest **32**, 41-45
Adult, AEROBIC CAPACITY, Body composition, ENERGY BALANCE, Exercise programme, Glucose tolerance, Intervention, Weight

520/10   Björntorp, P., DeJounge, K., Sjöström, L. & Sullivan, L.   (1970)
The effect of physical training on insulin production in obesity
Metabolism **19**, 631-37
Adult, AEROBIC CAPACITY, Body composition, Exercise programme, ENERGY BALANCE, GLUCOSE TOLERANCE, INSULIN SENSITIVITY, Intervention, MUSCLE STRENGTH, Weight

520/11   Björntorp, P., Fahen, M., Grimby, G., Gustafson, A., Holm, J., Renström, P. & Schersten, T.   (1972)
Carbohydrate and lipid metabolism in middle age and physically well-trained men
Metabolism **21**, 1037-1044
Adult, AEROBIC CAPACITY, Body composition, Comparative, Glucose tolerance, Leisure activity, LIPIDS, Male, MUSCLE METABOLISM

520/12   Björntorp, P. & Krotkiewski, M.   (1985)
Exercise treatment in diabetes mellitus
Acta Med Scand **217**, 3-7
Review

520/13   Bloom, S.R., Johnson, R.H., Park, D.M., Rennie, M.J. &Sulaiman, W.R.   (1976)
Differences in the metabolic and hormonal response to exercise between racing cyclists and untrained individuals
J Physiol **258**, 1-18
Acute exercise, Adult, Comparative, Cycling, GROWTH, Male, Vigorous

520/14   Bogardus, C., Ravussin, E., Robbins, D.C., Wolfe, R.R.,Horton, E.S. & Sims E.A.   (1984)
Effects of physical training and diet therapy on carbohydrate metabolism in patients with glucose intolerance and non-insulin-dependent diabetes mellitus
Diabetes **33**, 311-318
Adult, AEROBIC CAPACITY, Body composition, Exercise programme, Insulin sensitivity, Intervention, Type 2, Vigorous

520/15   Campaigne, B.N., Gilliam, T.B., Spencer, M.L., Lampman, R.M. & Schork, M.A.   (1984)
Effects of a physical activity program on metabolic control and cardiovascular fitness in children with insulin-dependent diabetes mellitus
Diabetes Care **7**, 57-62
AEROBIC CAPACITY, Children, Exercise programme, Intervention, Type 1, Weight

520/16   Caron, D., Poussier, P., Marliss, E.B. & Zinman, B.   (1982)
The effect of postprandial exercise on meal related glucose intolerance in insulin-dependent diabetes mellitus
Diabetes Care **5**, 364-369
Acute exercise, Adult, RESPIRATORY FUNCTION, Type 1

520/17   Cederholm, J. & Wibell, L.   (1985)
Glucose tolerance and physical activity in a Health Survey of middle-aged subjects
Acta Med Scand **217**, 373-378
Adult, Glucose tolerance, Female, Leisure activity, Male, Occupational activity, Weight

520/18   Cederholm, J. & Wibell, L.   (1986)
The relationship of blood pressure to blood glucose and physical leisure time activity
Acta Med Scand **219**, 37-46
Adult, BLOOD PRESSURE, Comparative, Glucose tolerance, Female, Leisure activity, Male. Occupational activity, PRIMARY PREVENTION, Weight,

520/19   Clark, M.G., Rattigan, S. & Clark, D.G.   (1983)
Obesity with insulin resistance: Experimental insights
Lancet **ii**, 1236-1240
ENERGY BALANCE, Review

520/20   Costill, D.L., Cleary, P., Fink, W.J., Foster, C., Ivy, J.L. & Witzmann, F.   (1979)
Training adaptions in skeletal muscle of juvenile diabetics
Diabetes **28**, 818-822
Adult, AEROBIC CAPACITY, Exercise programme, Intervention, LIPIDS, Male, MUSCLE METABOLISM, Running, Type 1

520/21   Craig, B.W., Hammons, G.T., Gartwaite, S.M., Jarett, J. & Holloszy, J.O.   (1981)
Adaptations of fat cells to exercise: response to glucose uptake and oxidation to insulin
J Appl Physiol **51**, 1500-1506
Animal, Exercise programme, Insulin sensitivity, Intervention

520/22   Davis, T.A. & Karl, I.E.   (1986)
Response of muscle protein turnover to insulin after acute exercise and training
Biochem J **240**, 651-657
Acute exercise, Animal, Exercise programme, Insulin sensitivity, Intervention, MUSCLE METABOLISM

520/23   DeFronzo, R.A., Sherwin, R.S. & Kraemer, N.   (1987)
Effect of physical training on insulin action in obesity
Diabetes **36**, 1379-1385
Adult, ENERGY BALANCE, Female, Glucose tolerance, INSULIN SENSITIVITY, Intervention

520/24   Donahue, R.P., Orchard, T.J., Becker, D.J., Kuller, L.H. & Drash, A.L.   (1988)
Physical activity, insulin sensitivity, and the lipoprotein profile in young adults: the Beaver County Study
Am J Epidemiol **127**, 95-103
Adult, Female, Insulin sensitivity, Leisure activity, LIPIDS, Male

520/25   Galbo, H., Hedeskoy, C.J., Capito, K. & Vinten, J.   (1981)
The effect of physical training on insulin secretion of the rat pancreatic islets
Acta Physiol Scand **111**, 75-79
Animal, Body composition, Glucose tolerance, Intervention, Swimming

520/26   Gavin, J.R. 3rd, Heath, G.W., Ponser, J.M., Hagberg, J.M., Bloomfield, S.A. & Holloszy, J.O.   (1982)
Improvement in insulin sensitivity with acute exercise
Diabetes (Suppl 2) **31**, 32A
Acute exercise, Adult, AEROBIC CAPACITY, Glucose tolerance, Inactivity, Insulin sensitivity

520/27   Gunnarsson, R., Wallberg-Henriksson, H., Rossner, S. & Wahren, J.   (1987)
Serum lipid and lipoprotein levels in female type I diabetics: relationship to aerobic capacity and glycaemic control
Diabete Metab **13**, 417-421
Adult, AEROBIC CAPACITY, Female, Glucose tolerance, LIPIDS, Type 1

520/28   Heath, G.W., Gavin, J.R. 3rd, Hinderliter, J.M., Hagberg, J.M., Bloomfield, S.A. & Holloszy, J.O.   (1983)
Effects of exercise and lack of exercise on glucose tolerance and insulin sensitivity
J Appl Physiol **55**, 512-517
Acute exercise, Adult, AEROBIC CAPACITY, Body composition, Exercise programme, Glucose sensitivity, Inactivity, Intervention

520/29   Hollenbeck, C.B., Haskell, W.L, Rosenthal, M. & Reaven, G.M.   (1984)
Effect of habitual physical activity on regulation of insulin-stimulated glucose disposal in older males
J Am Geriatr Soc **33**, 273-277
AEROBIC CAPACITY, Body composition, Comparative, Elderly, Insulin sensitivity, Leisure activity, Male, Weight

520/30 Holloszy, J.O., Schultz, J., Kusnierkiewicz, J., Hagberg, J.M. & Ehsani, A.A. (1986)
Effects of exercise on glucose tolerance and insulin resistance
Acta Med Scand (Suppl 711) **220**, 55-65
Adult, AEROBIC CAPACITY, Body composition, Exercise programme, Glucose tolerance, Intervention, Male, Type 2

520/31 Holm, G. & Björntorp, P. (1980)
Metabolic effects of physical training
Acta Paediatr Scand (Suppl 283) **9**, 9-14
Review

520/32 Holm, G. & Stromblad, G. (1983)
Type I diabetes and physical exercise
Acta Med Scand **671**, 95-8
Review, Type 1

520/33 Hubinger, A., Ridderskamp, I., Lehmann, E. & Gries, F.A. (1985)
Metabolic response to different forms of physical exercise in type I diabetics and the duration of the glucose lowering effect
Eur J Clin Invest **5**, 197-203
Acute exercise, Adult, AEROBIC CAPACITY, Endocrine, GROWTH, Type 1

520/34 Hultman, E.H. (1986)
Carbohydrate metabolism during hard exercise and in the recovery period after exercise
Acta Physiol Scand (Suppl 556) **128**, 75-82
Review

520/35 Huttunen, N.P., Kaar, M.L., Knip, M., Mustonen, A., Puukka, R. & Akerblom, H.K. (1984)
Physical fitness of children and adolescents with insulin-dependent diabetes mellitus
Ann Clin Res **16**, 1-5
Children, Type 1

520/36 Ivy, J.L., Frishberg, B.A., Farrell, S.W., Miller, W.J. & Sherman, W.M. (1985)
Effects of elevated and exercise-reduced muscle glycogen levels on insulin sensitivity
J Appl Physiol **59**, 154-159
Acute exercise, Adult, Glucose tolerance, Male, MUSCLE METABOLISM

520/37 Iwasaki, M., Kobayashi, M., Ohgaku, S., Maegawa, H. &Shigeta, Y. (1982)
Effect of acute exercise on insulin binding to erythrocytes in type II diabetes
Endocrinol Jpn **29**, 561-566
Acute exercise, Adult, Insulin sensitivity, Type 2

520/38 Jakober, B., Schmulling, R.M. & Eggstein, M. (1983)
Carbohydrate and lipid metabolism in type I diabetics during exhaustive exercise
Int J Sports Med **4**, 104-108
Acute exercise, Adult, Endocrine, LIPIDS, Male, Type 1, Vigorous

520/39 Jarrett, R.J., Shipley, M.J. & Hunt, R. (1986)
Physical activity, glucose tolerance, and diabetes mellitus: The Whitehall study
Diabetic Med **3**, 549-551
Adult, Glucose tolerance, Leisure activity, Male, Type 2, Weight

520/40 Jung, K. (1982)
Physical exercise therapy in juvenile diabetes mellitus
J Sports Med **22**, 23
Endocrine, Glucose tolerance, GROWTH, Intervention, MUSCLE STRENGTH, PERCEIVED EXERTION

520/41   Kahle, E.B., O'Dorisio, T.M., Walker, R.B., Eisenman, P.A., Reiser, S., Cataland, S. & Zipf, W.B.   (1986)
Exercise adaptation responses for gastric inhibitory polypeptide (GIP) and insulin in obese children. Possible extra-pancreatic effects
Diabetes **35**, 579-582
Children, ENERGY BALANCE, Exercise programme, Glucose tolerance, Intervention, Weight

520/42   Kemmer, F.W. & Berger, M.   (1984)
Exercise in therapy and the life of diabetic patients
Clin Sci **67**, 279-283
Review, Type 1, Type 2

520/43   King, D.S., Dalsky, G.P., Staten, M.A., Clutter, W.E., Van Houte, D.R. & Holloszy, J.O.   (1987)
Insulin action and secretion in endurance-trained and untrained humans
J Appl Physiol **63**, 2247-2252
Adult, AEROBIC CAPACITY, Body composition, Comparative, Insulin sensitivity

520/44   Kjær, M. & Galbo, H.   (1988)
Effrect of physical training on the capacity to secrete epinephrine
J Appl Physiol **64**, 11-16
Acute exercise, Adult, Athlete, Endocrine, Male

520/45   Koivisto, V.A. & Groop, L.   (1982)
Physical training in juvenile diabetes
Ann Clin Res **14**, 74-79
Review, Type 1

520/46   Koivisto, V.A., Somam, V.R. & Felig, P.   (1980)
Effects of acute exercise on insulin binding to monocytes in obesity
Metabolism **29**, 168
Acute exercise, Adult, ENERGY BALANCE

520/47   Koivisto,V.A., Soman, V.R., Conrad, P., Hendler, R., Nadel, E. & Felig, P.   (1979)
Insulin binding to monocytes in trained athletes
J Clin Invest **64**, 1011-1015
Acute exercise, Adult, AEROBIC CAPACITY, Athlete, Comparative, Insulin sensitivity

520/48   Koivisto, V.A. & Yki-Järvinen, H.   (1987)
Effect of exercise on insulin binding and glucose transport in adipocytes of normal humans
J Appl Physiol **63**, 1319-1323
Acute exercise, Adult, Insulin sensitivity, Male

520/49   Krotkiewski, M., Bjorntorp, P., Holm, G., Marks, V., Morgan, L., Smith, U. & Feurle, G.E.   (1984)
Effects of physical training on insulin, connecting peptide (C-peptide), gastric inhibitory polypeptide (GIP) and pancreatic polypeptide (PP) levels in obese subjects
Int J Obes **8**, 193-199
Adult, BLOOD PRESSURE, Body composition, Exercise programme, ENERGY BALANCE, Female, Glucose tolerance, Intervention, LIPIDS

520/50   Krotkiewski, M. & Górski, J.   (1986)
Effects of muscular exercise on plasma C-peptide and insulin in obese non-diabetics and diabetics, type II
Clin Physiol **6**, 499-506
Acute exercise, Adult, Body composition, ENERGY BALANCE, Female, Type 2

520/51   Krotkiewski, M., Lonnroth, P., Mandroukas, K., Wroblewski, Z., Rebuffe-Scrive, M., Holm, G., Smith, U. & Björntorp, P.   (1985)
The effects of physical training on insulin secretion and effectiveness and on glucose metabolism in obesity and type 2 (non-insulin-dependent) diabetes mellitus
Diabetologia **28**, 881-890
Adult, AEROBIC CAPACITY, BLOOD PRESSURE, Body composition, ENERGY BALANCE, Exercise programme, Female, Glucose tolerance, Insulin sensitivity, Intervention, LIPIDS, Type 2, Vigorous, Weight

520/52   Lampman, R.M., Schteingart, D.E., Santinga, J.T., Savage, P.J., Hydrick, C.R., Bassett, D.R. & Block, W.D.   (1987)
The influence of physical training on glucose tolerance, insulin sensitivity, and lipid and lipoprotein concentrations in middle-aged hypertriglyceridaemic, carbohydrate intolerant men
Diabetologia **30**, 380-385
Adult, AEROBIC CAPACITY, BLOOD PRESSURE, Exercise programme, Glucose tolerance, Insulin sensitivity, LIPIDS, Intervention, Male, Type 2

520/53   Landt, K.W., Campaigne, B.N., James, F.W. & Sperling, M.A.   (1985)
Effects of exercise training on insulin sensitivity in adolescents with type I diabetes
Diabetes Care **8**, 461-465
AEROBIC CAPACITY, Body composition, Children, Exercise programme, Insulin sensitivity, Intervention, Type 1.

520/54   LaPorte, R.E., Dorman, J.S., Tajima, N. Cruikshank, K.J., Orchard, T.J., Cavender, D.E., Becker, D.J. & Drash, A.L.   (1986)
Pittsburgh insulin-dependent diabetes mellitus morbidity and mortality study: physical activity and diabetic complications
Pediatrics **78**, 1027-1033
Adult, Cohort, Female, Leisure activity, Male, PRIMARY PREVENTION, Type 1

520/55   Larsson, Y.   (1980)
Physical exercise and juvenile diabetes – Summary and Conclusions
Acta Paediatr Scand (Suppl) **283**, 120-122
Review, Type 1

520/56   Larsson, Y., Persson, B., Sterky, G. & Thoren, C.   (1964)
Functional adaptation to vigorous training and exercise in diabetic and non-diabetic adolescents
J Appl Physiol **19**, 629-635
Acute exercise, AEROBIC CAPACITY, CARDIAC PERFORMANCE, Children, Exercise programme, Intervention, Male, Type 1, Vigorous,

520/57   Larsson, Y., Sterky, G., Ekengren, K. & Moller, T.   (1962)
Physical fitness and the influence of training in diabetic adolescent girls
Diabetes **11**, 109-117
Children, Exercise programme, Female, Intervention, LIPIDS, Type 1

520/58   LeBlanc, J., Nadeua, A.I., Richard, D. & Tremblay, A.   (1981)
Studies on the sparing effect of exercise on insulin requirements in human subjects
Metabolism **30**, 1119-1124
Acute exercise, Adult, AEROBIC CAPACITY, Athlete, Body composition, Comparative, Female, Glucose tolerance, Inactivity, Leisure activity, Male,

520/59   **Lindgarde, F., Malmquist, J. & Balke, B.** (1983)
Physical fitness, insulin secretion, and glucose tolerance in healthy males and mild type-2 diabetes
Acta Diabetol Lat **20**, 33-40
Adult, AEROBIC CAPACITY, Comparative, Exercise programme, Glucose tolerance, Intervention, Male, Type 2

520/60   **Lindgärde, F. & Saltin, B.** (1981)
Daily physical activity, work capacity, and glucose tolerance in lean and obese normoglycaemic middle-age men
Diabetologia **20**, 134-138
Adult, AEROBIC CAPACITY, Body composition, Comparative, ENERGY BALANCE, Glucose tolerance, Leisure activity, LIPIDS, Male, Occupational activity

520/61   **Lipman, R.L., Raskin, P., Love, T., Triebwasser, J., LeCocq, F.R. & Schnure, J.J.** (1972)
Glucose intolerance during decreased physical activity in man
Diabetes **21**, 101-107
Adult, Animal, Glucose tolerance, Inactivity, Intervention, Male

520/62   **Ludvigsson, J.** (1980)
Physical exercise in relation to degree of metabolic control in juvenile diabetes
Acta Paediatr Scand (Suppl) **283**, 45-49
Children, Leisure activity, Longitudinal, Type 1

520/63   **Maehlum, S., Dahl-Jorgensen, K. & Meen, H.D.** (1982)
Diabetes mellitus and physical activity
Scand J Soc Med (Suppl) **29**, 209-216
Review

520/64   **Mikines, K.J., Kjaer, M., Hagen, C., Sonne, B., Richter, E.A. & Galbo, H.** (1985)
The effect of training on responses of beta-endorphin and other pituitary hormones to insulin-induced hypoglycemia
Eur J Appl Physiol **54**, 476-479
Adult, AEROBIC CAPACITY, Athlete, Endocrine, GROWTH, Male, MOOD

520/65   **Minuk, H. L, Vranic, M., Marless, E.B., Hanna, A.K., Albisser, A.M. & Zinman, B.** (1981)
Glucoregulatory and metabolic responses to exercise in obese non-insulin-dependent diabetics
Am J Physiol **240**, E458-464
Acute exercise, Adult, Comparative, ENERGY BALANCE, Type 2

520/66   **Misbin, R.I., Moffa, A.M. & Kappy, M.S.** (1983)
Insulin binding to monocytes in obese patients treated with carbohydrate restriction and changes in physical activity
J Clin Endocrinol Metab **56**, 273-278
Adult, ENERGY BALANCE, Glucose tolerance, Insulin sensitivity

520/67   **Mondon, C.E., Dolkas, C.B. & Reaven, G.V.** (1980)
Site of enhanced insulin sensitivity in exercise trained rats at rest
Am J Physiol **239**, E169-177
Animal, Exercise programme, Glucose tolerance, Insulin sensitivity, Intervention

520/68   **Naveri, H., Kuoppasalmi, K. & Harkonen, M.** (1985)
Metabolic and hormonal changes in moderate and intense long-term running exercises
Int J Sports Med **6**, 276-281
Acute exercise, Adult, ENERGY BALANCE, GROWTH, LIPIDS, Male, MUSCLE METABOLISM

520/69   Nelson, J.D., Poussier, P., Marliss, E.B., Albisser, A.M. & Zinman, B. (1982)
Metabolic response of normal man and insulin-infused diabetics to postprandial exercise
Am J Physiol **242**, E309-16
Acute exercise, Adult, Comparative, Endocrine, Type 1

520/70   Olefsky, J.M. & Kolterman, O.G. (1981)
Mechanisms of insulin resistance in obesity and noninsulin-dependent (Type II) Diabetes
Am J Med **70**, 151-168
ENERGY BALANCE, Review, Type 2

520/71   Perron, L., Mitchell, D. & Tremblay, A. (1986)
The role of body fat in insulin sensitivity of endurance athletes
Diabete Metab **12**, 233-238
Adult, AEROBIC CAPACITY, Athlete, Body composition, Comparative, Insulin sensitivity, Leisure activity

520/72   Rauramaa, R. (1984)
Relationship of physical activity, glucose tolerance, and weight management
Prev Med **13**, 37-46
ENERGY BALANCE, Glucose tolerance, Insulin sensitivity, PRIMARY PREVENTION, Review

520/73   Reitman, J.S., Vasquez, B., Klimes, I. & Nagulesparan, M. (1984)
Improvement of glucose homeostasis after exercise training in non-insulin-dependent diabetes
Diabetes Care **7**, 434-441
Adult, Exercise programme, Glucose tolerance, Intervention, Type 2, Vigorous

520/74   Richter, E.A., Ruderman, N.B. & Schneider, S.H. (1981)
Diabetes and exercise
Am J Med **70**, 201-209
Review

520/75   Rönnemaa, T., Mattilla. K., Lehtonen, A. & Kallio, V. (1986)
A controlled randomised study on the effect of long-term physical exercise on the metabolic control in type 2 diabetic patients
Acta Med Scand. **220**, 219-224
Adult, AEROBIC CAPACITY, Exercise programme, Glucose tolerance, Intervention, Type 2, Weight

520/76   Rosenthal, M., Haskell, W.L., Solomon, R., Widstrom, A. & Reaven, G.M. (1983)
Demonstration of a relationship between level of physical training and insulin-stimulated glucose utilization in normal humans
Diabetes **32**, 408-411
Adult, AEROBIC CAPACITY, Glucose tolerance

520/77   Rowland, T.W., Swadba, L.A., Biggs, D.E., Burke, E.J. & Reiter, E.O. (1985)
Glycemic control with physical training in insulin-dependent diabetes mellitus
Am J Dis Child **139**, 307-310
AEROBIC CAPACITY, Children, Exercise programme, Intervention, Type 1, Weight

520/78   Ruderman, N.B., Ganda, O.P. & Johansen, K. (1979)
The effect of physical training on glucose tolerance and plasma lipids in maturity-onset diabetes
Diabetes (Suppl 1) **28**, 89-92
Adult, AEROBIC CAPACITY, Exercise programme, Glucose tolerance, Intervention, LIPIDS, Male, Type 2

520/79 Saltin, B., Lindgarde, F., Houston, M., Horlin, R., Nygaard, E. & Gad, P. (1979)
Physical training and glucose tolerance in middle-aged men with chemical diabetes
Diabetes (Suppl 1) **28**, 30-32
Adult, Body composition, Comparative, Exercise programme, Glucose tolerance, Intervention, Male, MUSCLE METABOLISM, MUSCLE STRENGTH, Type 2

520/80 Satao, Y., Hayamizu, S. & Yamamoto, C. (1986)
Improved insulin sensitivity in carbohydrate and lipid metabolism after physical training
Int J Sports Med **7**, 307-310
Adult, Exercise programme, Insulin sensitivity, Intervention, LIPIDS

520/81 Schernthaner, G., Muhlhauser, I., Seebacher, C., Templ, H., Sinzinger, H. & Silberbauer, K. (1982)
Activation of platelet in vivo function and plasma levels of catecholamines and growth hormone during bicycle exercise in juvenile diabetes and healthy individuals
Curr Probl Clin Biochem **11**, 69-83
Acute exercise, Children, COAGULATION, GROWTH, Type 1

520/82 Schneider, S.H., Amorosa, L.F., Khachadurian, A.K. & Ruderman, N.B. (1984)
Studies on the mechanism of improved glucose control during regular exercise in type 2 (non-insulin-dependent) diabetes
Diabetologia **26**, 355-360
Adult, AEROBIC CAPACITY, Exercise programme, Glucose tolerance, Intervention, Male, Type 2

520/83 Schneider, S.H. & Ruderman, N.B. (1986)
Exercise and physical training in the treatment of diabetes mellitus
Compr Ther **12**, 49-56
Review

520/84 Seals, D.R., Hagberg, J.M., Allen, W.K., Hurley, B.F., Dalsky, G.P., Ehsani, A.A. & Holloszy, J.O. (1984)
Glucose tolerance in young and older athletes and sedentary men
J Appl Physiol **56**, 1521-1525
Adult, AEROBIC CAPACITY, Body composition, Comparative, Glucose tolerance, Insulin sensitivity, Male, Weight

520/85 Sherwin, R.S. & Koivisto, V.A. (1981)
Keeping in step: Does exercise benefit the diabetic?
Diabetologia **20**, 84-86
Review

520/86 Sills, I.N. & Cerny, F.J. (1983)
Responses to continuous and intermittent exercise in healthy and insulin-dependent diabetic children
Med Sci Sports Exerc **15**, 450-454
Acute exercise, AEROBIC CAPACITY, Children, Comparative, Endocrine, GROWTH, Male, Type 1

520/87 Soman, V.R., Koivisto, V.A., Deibert, D., Felig, P. & DeFronzo, R.A. (1979)
Increased insulin sensitivity and insulin binding to monocytes after physical training
N Engl J Med **301**, 1200-1204
Adult, AEROBIC CAPACITY, Exercise programme, Insulin sensitivity, Intervention, Male, Weight

520/88 Stein, R., Goldberg, N., Kalman, F. & Chesler, R. (1984)
Exercise and the patient with Type I diabetes mellitus
Pediatr Clin North Am **31**, 665-673
Review, Type 1

520/89   Taylor, R., Zimmet, P., Raper, L.R. & Ringrose, H.   (1984)
Physical activity and prevalence of diabetes in Melanesian and Indian men in Fiji
Diabetologia **27**, 578-582
Adult, Body composition, Glucose tolerance, Occupational activity, Type 2, Weight

520/90   Trovati, M., Carta, Q., Cavalot, F., Vitali, S., Banaudi, C., Lucchina, P.G., Fiocchi, F., Emanuelli, G. & Lenti, G.   (1984)
Influence of physical training on blood glucose control, glucose tolerance, insulin secretion, and insulin action in non-insulin-dependent diabetic patients
Diabetes Care **7**, 416-420
Adult, AEROBIC CAPACITY, Exercise programme, Glucose tolerance, Intervention, Male, Type 2

520/91   Trovati, M., Tamponi, G., Marra, S., Lorenzati, R., Schinco, P., Bazzan, M., Vitali, S., Cavalot, F., Pagano, G. & Lenti, G.   (1983)
Exercise-induced changes of Factor VIII complex in healthy subjects and in type-I diabetics: relation between growth hormone and Von Willebrand Factor increments
Horm Metab Res **15**, 316-320
Acute exercise, Adult, AEROBIC CAPACITY, COAGULATION, GROWTH, Male, Type 1

520/92   Vicari, A.M., Margonato, A., Petrelli, P., Vicedomini, G.G. & Pozza, G.   (1984)
Plasma beta-thromboglobulin concentration at rest and after physical exercise in complicated and uncomplicated diabetes mellitus
Diabete Metab **10**, 235-238
Acute exercise, Adult, COAGULATION, Comparative, Type 1

520/93   Vranic, M. & Berger, M.   (1979)
Exercise and diabetes mellitus
Diabetes **28**, 147-160
Review

520/94   Vranic, M., Horvath, S. & Wahren, J.   (1979)
Exercise and diabetes: an Overview. Summary of the conference on diabetes and exercise
Diabetes (Suppl 1) **28**, 107-110
Review

520/95   Wallberg, H., Gunnarsson, R., Henriksson, J., DeFronzo, R.A., Ostman, J., Felig, P. & Wahren, J.   (1981)
Physical training in diabetes: Dissociation between changes in insulin sensitivity and blood glucose regulation
Clin Res **29**, 426A
Adult, AEROBIC CAPACITY, Exercise programme, Insulin sensitivity, Intervention, LIPIDS, MUSCLE METABOLISM, Type 1

520/96   Wallberg-Henriksson, H.   (1986)
Repeated exercise regulates glucose transport capacity in skeletal muscle
Acta Physiol Scand **127**, 39-43
Animal, Customary activity, Intervention, Swimming

520/97   Wallberg-Henriksson, H., Gunnarsson, R., Henriksson, J., DeFronzo, R.A., Felig, P., Östman, J. & Wahren, J.   (1982)
Increased peripheral insulin sensitivity and muscle mitochondrial enzymes but unchanged blood glucose control in type I diabetics after physical training
Diabetes **31**, 1044-1050
Adult, AEROBIC CAPACITY, Exercise programme, Glucose tolerance, Insulin sensitivity,Intervention, LIPIDS, Male, MUSCLE METABOLISM, Type 1

520/98   **Wallberg-Henriksson, H., Gunnarsson, R., Rössner, S. & Wahren, J.**   (1986)
Long-term physical training in female type 1 (insulin-dependent) diabetic patients: Absence of significant effect on glycaemic control and lipoprotein levels
Diabetologia **29**, 53-57
Adult, AEROBIC CAPACITY, Exercise programme, Female, Intervention, LIPIDS, Type 1, Weight

520/99   **Wirth, A., Holm, G. & Björntorp, P.**   (1982)
Effect of physical training on insulin uptake by the perfused rat liver
Metabolism **31**, 457-462
Animal, Exercise programme, Intervention

520/100   **Wirth, A., Holm, G., Nilsson, B., Smith, U. & Björntorp, P.**   (1980)
Insulin kinetics and insulin binding to adipocytes in physically trained and food restricted rats
Am J Physiol **238**, E108-115
Animal, Comparative

520/101   **Wolfe, P.I. & DiCarlo, S.**   (1983)
Fatigue rate during anaerobic and aerobic exercise in insulin-dependent diabetics and nondiabetics
Phys Ther **63**, 500-504
Acute exercise, Adult, MUSCLE STRENGTH, Type 1

520/102   **Zander, E., Schulz, B., Chlup, R., Woltansky, P. & Lubs, D.**   (1985)
Muscular exercise in type I-diabetics. II. Hormonal and metabolic responses to moderate exercise
Exp Clin Endocrinol **85**, 95-104
Acute exercise, Adult, AEROBIC CAPACITY, Type 1

520/103   **Zinman, B., Murray, F.T., Vranic, M., Albisser, A.M., Leibel, B.S., McClean, P.A. & Marliss, E.B.**   (1977)
Glucoregulation during moderate exercise in insulin treated diabetics
J Clin Endocrinol Metab **45**, 641-652
Acute exercise, Adult, AEROBIC CAPACITY, Comparative, Type 1

520/104   **Zinman, B. & Vranic, M.**   (1985)
Diabetes and exercise
Med Clin North Am **69**, 145-157
Review, Type 1, Type 2

520/105   **Zinman, B., Vranic, M., Albisser, M., Leibel, B.S. & Marliss, E.B.**   (1979)
The role of insulin in the metabolic response to exercise in diabetic man
Diabetes (Suppl 1) **28**, 76-81
Acute exercise, Adult, AEROBIC CAPACITY, Comparative, Type 1

520/106   **Zinman, B., Zuniga-Guajardo, S. & Kelly, D.**   (1984)
Comparison of the acute and long-term effects of exercise on glucose control in type I diabetes
Diabetes Care **7**, 515-519
Acute exercise, Adult, AEROBIC CAPACITY, Exercise programme, Intervention, Type 1

520/107   **Zorzano, A., Balon, T.W., Goodman, M.N. & Ruderman, N.B.**   (1986)
Glycogen depletion and increased insulin sensitivity and responsiveness in muscle after exercise
Am J Physiol **251**, E664-669
Acute exercise, Animal, Insulin sensitivity, MUSCLE METABOLISM

520/108   **Zorzano, A., Balon, T.W., Jakubowski J.A., Goodman, M.N., Deykin, M. D. & Ruderman, N.B.** (1986)
Effects of insulin and prior exercise on prostaglandin release from perfused rat muscle. Evidence that prostaglandins do not mediate changes in glucose uptake
Biochem J **240,** 437-443
Acute exercise, Animal, Endocrine

KEYWORDS are listed in the appendix in addition the following specific keywords have been used in this section:

Amenorrhea
Androgens
Contraception
Dysmenorrhea
Endometriosis
Endorphins
Fertility (excluding amenorrhea)
FSH (Follicle stimulation hormone)
LH (Luteinising hormone)
Menarche
Menstrual cycle (any changes in cycle, oligomenorrhea)
Menopause
Oestrogens
Premenstrual symptoms
PRL (Prolactin)
Progesterone

Summary of evidence: strenuous exercise reduces reproductive function which may reduce bone density

THE PROBLEM

Can exercise cure or ameliorate dysmenorrhea or pre-menstrual syndrome? Is strenuous exercise hazardous during menstrual periods? Does the amenorrhea and late menarche associated with repeated intense exercise carry any long term health risks or threat to future fertility?

SCOPE

This section contains references dealing primarily with changes produced by exercise on menstrual status, the pattern of menstrual cycling, menstrual abnormalities and hormone profiles.

METHODOLOGICAL DIFFICULTIES

The reproductive hormones are numerous and of low plasma concentration. Their function is interrelated and depends crucially on their monthly pattern of rise and fall and in some cases on surges which last only for a few hours. It is therefore difficult without continuous monitoring of blood levels to obtain an adequately complete picture. Many factors such as gynaecological age, parity, menstrual phase, body fat, diet and psychological pressure can confound studies of the effects of exercise.

EVIDENCE

There is no evidence that exercise can relieve menstrual abnormalities, there is also no reason why menstruating women should not take exercise; female athletes have won Olympic medals during their menstrual periods. However, intense athletic activity, the stress of a competitive situation and low body fat stores combine in some, especially young nulliparous individuals, to reduce or stop menstrual flow or to delay menarche. This has been observed in marathon runners and in ballet dancers. The effect appears to be reversible and there is as yet no evidence of permanent impairment of fertility. The changes in hormone profiles associated with amenorrhea may lead to loss of bone density, although the bone-loading influence of the exercise may offset this hormonal effect to some extent (see section 420). Long term studies remain to be completed. (See also 630)

610/1   **(1982)**   Running jumping and . . . amenorrhoea (editorial)
Lancet *ii,* **638-640**
Amenorrhea, Female, REPRODUCTIVE HORMONES Review

610/2   **Abraham, S.F., Beaumont, P.J., Fraser, I.S. & Llewellyn-Jones, D.**   (1982)
Body weight, exercise and menstrual status among ballet dancers in training
Br J Obstet Gynaecol **89,** 507-510
Amenorrhea, Children, Exercise programme, Female, Hazards, Intervention, Menarche, Menstrual cycle, Vigorous, Weight

610/3   **Baker, E.R.**   (1981)
Menstrual dysfunction and hormonal status in athletic women: A review
Fertil Steril **36,** 691-696
Amenorrhea, Athlete, Hazards, REPRODUCTIVE HORMONES, Review

610/4   **Baker, E.R., Mathur, R.S., Kirk, R.F., Landgrebe, S.C., Moody, L.O. & Williamson, H.O.**   (1982)
Plasma gonadotropins, prolactin, and steroid hormone concentrations in female runners immediately after a long-distance run
Fertil Steril **38,** 38-41
Acute exercise, Adult, Androgens, Endocrine, Female, FSH, LH, Menstrual cycle, PRL, REPRODUCTIVE HORMONES, Running, Vigorous

610/5   **Baker, E.R., Mathur, R.S., Kirk, R.F. & Williamson, H.O.**   (1981)
Female runners and secondary amenorrhea: correlation with age, parity, mileage, and plasma hormonal and sex-hormone-binding globulin concentrations
Fertil Steril **36,** 183-187
Adult, Amenorrhea, Androgens, Body composition, Comparative, Endocrine, Female, Fertility, Leisure activity, LH, Menarche, Menstrual cycle, Oestrogens, Running

610/6   **Bale, P. & Davies, J.**   (1983)
Effects of menstruation and contraceptive pill on the performance of physical education students
Br J Sports Med **17,** 46-50
Adult, Amenorrhea, Contraception, Dysmenorrhea, Female, Menstrual cycle, Menstrual function, Occupational activity

610/7   **Bernstein, L., Ross, R.K., Lobo, R., Hanisch, R., Krailo, M.D. & Henderson, B.E.**   (1987)
The effects of moderate physical activity on menstrual cycle patterns in adolescence: implications for breast cancer prevention
Br J Cancer **55,** 681-685
Amenorrhea, Body composition, Cancer, Children, Female, Leisure activity, Menarche, Menstrual cycle,

610/8   **Bonen, A., Belcastro, A.N., Ling, W.Y. & Simpson, A.A.**   (1981)
Profiles of selected hormones during menstrual cycles of teenage athletes
J Appl Physiol **50,** 545-551
Adult, Athlete, Children, Comparative, Female, FSH, LH, Menstrual cycle, Oestrogens, PRL, Progesterone, REPRODUCTIVE HORMONES, Swimming, Vigorous

610/9   **Bonen, A., Haynes, F.J., Watson-Wright, W., Sopper, M.M., Pierce, G.N., Low, M.P. & Graham, T.E.**   (1983)
Effects of menstrual cycle on metabolic responses to exercise
J Appl Physiol **55,** 1506-1513
Acute exercise, Adult, AEROBIC CAPACITY, CARBOHYDRATE TOLERANCE, Comparative, Endocrine, Female, FSH, GROWTH, LH, Menstrual Cycle, REPRODUCTIVE HORMONES

610/10   **Bonen, A., Ling, W.Y., MacIntyre, K.P., Neil, R., McGrail, J.C. & Belcastro, A.N.**   (1979)
Effects of exercise on the serum concentrations of FSH, LH, progesterone,and estradiol
Eur J Appl Physiol **42,** 15-23
Acute exercise, Adult, Endocrine, Exercise programme, Female, FSH, Intervention, LH, Menstrual cycle, Oestrogens, Progesterone, REPRODUCTIVE HORMONES

610/11   **Boyden, T.W., Pamenter, R.W., Grosso, D., Stanforth, P.R., Rotkis, T.C. & Wilmore, J.H.**   (1982)
Prolactin responses, menstrual cycles, and body composition of women runners
J Clin Endocrinol Metab **54,** 711-714
Adult, Body composition, Endocrine, Exercise programme, Female, Intervention, Menstrual cycle, PRL, REPRODUCTIVE HORMONES, Running, Vigorous

610/12   **Boyden, T.W., Pamenter, R.W., Stanforth, P.R., Rotkis, T.C. & Wilmore, J.H.**   (1984)
Impaired gonadotropin responses to gonadotropin-releasing hormone stimulation in endurance-trained women
Fertil Steril **41,** 359-363
Adult, Body composition, Exercise programme, Female, Hazards, Intervention, Menstrual cycle, REPRODUCTIVE HORMONES, Running

610/13   **Boyden, T.W., Pamenter, R.W., Stanforth, P.R., Rotkis, T.C. & Wilmore, J.H.**   (1983)
Sex steroids and endurance running in women
Fertil Steril **39,** 629-632
Androgens, Body composition, Endocrine, Exercise programme, Female, Menstrual function, Metabolic function, Oestrogens, REPRODUCTIVE HORMONES, Weight

610/14   **Brisson, G.R., Dulac, S., Peronnet, F. & Ledoux, M.**   (1982)
The onset of menarche: a late event in pubertal progression to be affected by physical training
Can J Appl Sport Sci **7,** 61-67
Female, Menarche, Review

610/15   **Brisson, G.R., Volle, M.A., DeCarufel, D., Desharnais, M. & Tanaka, M.**   (1980)
Exercise-induced dissociation of the blood prolactin response in young women according to their sports habits
Horm Metab Res **12,** 201-205
Acute exercise, Adult, AEROBIC CAPACITY, Comparative, Endocrine, Female, Leisure activity, PRL, REPRODUCTIVE HORMONES

610/16   **Bullen, B.A., Skrinar, G.S., Beitins, I.Z., Carr, D.B., Reppert, S.M., Dotson, C.O., Fencl, M., Gervino, E.V. & McArthur, J.W.**   (1984)
Endurance training effects on plasma hormonal responsiveness and sex hormone excretion
J Appl Physiol **56,** 1453-1463
Acute exercise, Adult, AEROBIC CAPACITY, Body composition, Endocrine, Endorphins, Exercise programme, GROWTH, Female, FSH, Intervention, Leisure activity, LH, Menstrual cycle, Oestrogens, PRL, Prog

610/17   Bullen, B.A., Skrinar, G.S., Beitins, I.Z., von Mering, G., Turnbull, B.A. & McArthur, J.W.   (1985)
Induction of menstrual disorders by strenuous exercise in untrained women
N Engl J Med **312**, 1349-1353
Adult, AEROBIC CAPACITY, Body composition, Endocrine, Exercise programme, Female, FSH, Hazards, Intervention, LH, Menstrual cycle, Menstrual function, Oestrogens, REPRODUCTIVE HORMONES, Running, Vigor

610/18   Calabrese, L.H., Kirkendall, D., Floyd, M., Rapoport, S., Williams, G.W., Weuiker, G.G. & Bergfeldt, J.A.   (1983)
Menstrual abnormalities, nutritional patterns and body composition in female classical ballet dancers
Phys Sports Med **11**,
Adult, Amenorrhea, Body composition, ENERGY BALANCE, Female, Leisure activity, Menarche, Menstrual cycle, Vigorous

610/19   Canty, A.P.   (1984)
Can aerobic exercise relieve the symptoms of premenstrual syndrome (PMS)?
J School Health **54**, 410-411
Female, Premenstrual symptoms, Review

610/20   Carr, D.B., Bullen, B.A., Skrinar, G.S., Arnold, M.A., Rosenblatt, M., Beitins, I.Z., Martin, J.B. & McArthur, J.W.   (1981)
Physical conditioning facilitates the exercise induced secretion of beta-endorphin and beta-lipotropin in women
N Engl J Med **305**, 560-563
Adult, Endorphins, Endocrine, Exercise programme, Female, Intervention, MOOD

610/21   Casper, R.F., Wilkinson, D. & Cotterell, M.A.   (1984)
The effect of increased cardiac output on luteal phase gonadal steroids: a hypothesis for runners amenorrhea
Fertil Steril **41**, 364-368
Adult, Amenorrhea, CARDIAC PERFORMANCE, Female, Hazards, LH, Oestrogens, Progesterone, REPRODUCTIVE HORMONES

610/22   Chang, F.E., Dodds, W.G., Sullivan, M., Kim, M.H. & Malarkey, W.B.   (1986)
The acute effects of exercise on prolactin and growth hormone secretion: comparison between sedentary women and women runners with normal and abnormal menstrual cycles
J Clin Endocrinol Metab **62**, 551-556
Acute exercise, Amenorrhea, Body composition, Comparative, Endocrine, Female, GROWTH, Hazards, Leisure activity, LH, Oestrogens, PRL, REPRODUCTIVE HORMONES, Running, Vigorous

610/23   Chang, F.E., Richards, S.R., Kim, M.H. & Malarkey, W.B.   (1984)
Twenty four-hour prolactin profiles and prolactin responses to dopamine in long distance running women
J Clin Endocrinol Metab **59**, 631-635
Adult, Amenorrhea, Androgens, Comparative, Endocrine, Female, FSH, Hazards, Leisure activity, LH, Menarche, Menstrual cycle, Oestrogens, PRL, REPRODUCTIVE HORMONES, Running, Vigorous

610/24   Chin, N.W., Chang, F.E., Dodds, W.G., Kim, M.H. & Malarkey, W.B.   (1987)
Acute effects of exercise on plasma catecholamines in sedentary and athletic women with normal and abnormal menses
Am J Obstet Gynecol **157**, 938-944
Acute exercise, Adult, Amenorrhea, Comparative, Endocrine, Female, LH

610/25   Cramer, D.W., Wilson, E., Stillman, R.J., Berger, M.J., Belisle, S., Schiff, I., Albrecht, B., Gibson, M., Stadel, B.V. & Schoenbaum, S.C.   (1986)
The relation of endometriosis to menstrual characteristics, smoking, and exercise
J Am Med Ass **255**, 1904-1908
Adult, Comparative, Endometriosis, Female, Leisure activity, Menstrual cycle, URO-GENITAL TRACT

610/26   Cumming, D.C., Vickovic, M.M., Wall, S.R. & Fluker, M.R.   (1985)
Defects in pulsatile LH release in normally menstruating runners
J Clin Endocrinol Metab **60**, 810-812
Adult, Comparative, Endocrine, Female, Hazards, Leisure activity, LH, Menstrual cycle, REPRODUCTIVE HORMONES, Running

610/27   Cumming, D.C., Vickovic, M.M., Wall, S.R., Fluker, M.R. & Belcastro, A.N.   (1985)
The effect of acute exercise on pulsatile release of luteinizing hormone in women runners
Am J Obstet Gynecol **153**, 482-485
Acute exercise, Adult, Endocrine, Female, Hazards, Leisure activity, LH, Running

610/28   Dale, E., Gerlach, D. & Wilhite, A.   (1979)
Menstrual dysfunction in distance runners
Obstet Gynecol **54**, 47-53
Adult, Amenorrhea, Androgens, Body composition, Dysmenorrhea, Endocrine, Female, FSH, Hazards, Leisure activity, LH, Menstrual cycle, Oestrogens, Progesterone, REPRODUCTIVE HORMONES, Running, Vigorous

610/29   Dale, E. & Goldberg, D.L.   (1982)
Implications of nutrition in athletes' menstrual cycle irregularities
Can J Appl Sport Sci **7**, 74-78
Adult, Body composition, Endocrine, ENERGY BALANCE, Female, LIPIDS, Menstrual cycle, Running

610/30   De Bruyn-Prevost, P., Masset, C. & Sturbois, X.   (1984)
Physiological response from 18-25 years women to aerobic and anaerobic physical fitness tests at different periods during the menstrual cycle
J Sports Med Phys Fitness **24**, 144-148
Adult, AEROBIC CAPACITY, ANAEROBIC CAPACITY, Female, Menstrual cycle

610/31   Dixon, G., Eurman, P., Stern, B.E., Schwartz, B. & Rebar, R.W.   (1984)
Hypothalamic function in amenorrheic runners
Fertil Steril **42**, 377-383
Adult, Amenorrhea, Body composition, Comparative, Endocrine, Endorphins, Female, FSH, LH, Metabolic function, MOOD, Oestrogens, REPRODUCTIVE HORMONES

610/32   Ellison, P.T. & Lager, C.   (1986)
Moderate recreational running is associated with lowered salivary progesterone profiles in women
Am J Obstet Gynecol **154**, 1000-1003
Adult, Comparative, Female, Hazards, Leisure activity, Menstrual cycle, Progesterone, REPRODUCTIVE HORMONES, Running

610/33   Fears, W.B., Glass, A.R. & Vigersky, R.A.   (1983)
Role of exercise in the pathogenesis of the amenorrhea associated with anorexia nervosa
J Adolesc Health Care **4**, 22-24
Amenorrhea, Children, FSH, LH, Leisure activity

610/34   Frisch, R.E.   (1985)
Fatness, menarche, and female fertility
Perspect Biol Med **28**, 611-633
Body composition, REPRODUCTIVE HORMONES, Review

610/35   Frisch, R.E.   (1987)
Body fat, menarche, fitness and fertility
Hum Reprod **2**, 521-533
Review

610/36   Frisch, R.E., Gotz-Welbergen,
A.V., McArthur, J.W., Albright, T.,
Witschi, J., Bullen, B.A., Birnholz, J.,
Reed, R.B. & Hermann, H.   (1981)
Delayed menarche and amenorrhea of
college athletes in relation to age of onset
of training
J Am Med Ass **246**, 1559-1563
*Adult, Amenorrhea, Athlete, Body
composition, Comparative, Female,
Hazards, Leisure activity, Menarche,
Menstrual cycle, Running, Swimming,
Vigorous, Weight*

610/37   Frisch, R.E., Wyshak, G. &
Vincent, L.   (1980)
Delayed menarche and amenorrhea in
ballet dancers
N Engl J Med **303**, 17-19
*Amenorrhea, Body composition, Children,
Female, Hazards, Leisure activity,
Menarche, Menstrual cycle, Vigorous*

610/38   Galle, P.C., Freeman, E.W., Galle,
M.G., Huggins, G.R. & Sondheimer,
S.J.   (1983)
Physiologic and psychologic profiles in a
survey of women runners
Fertil Steril **39**, 633-639
*Adult, Athlete, Comparative, Female,
Leisure activity, Menstrual cycle,
MOOD, Running*

610/39   Golub, L.J., Menduke, H. & Lang,
W.R.   (1960)
Further evaluation of a therapeutic
exercise for teenage dysmenorrhoea
Obstet Gynec (N.Y.) **16**, 469-471
*Children, Dysmenorrhea, Exercise
programme, Female, Intervention,*

610/40   Goulding, A.   (1986)
Athletic amenorrhoea: a risk factor for
osteoporosis in later life?
NZ Med J **99**, 765-767
Amenorrhea, BONES, Review

610/41   Green, B.B., Daling, J.R., Weiss,
N.S., Liff, J.M. & Koepsall, T.   (1986)
Exercise as a risk factor for infertility with
ovulatory dysfunction
Am J Public Health **76**, 1432-1436
*Adult, Comparative, Female, Fertility,
Hazards, Leisure activity, Vigorous*

610/42   Hale, R.W., Kosasa, T., Krieger, J.
& Pepper, S.   (1983)
A marathon: the immediate effect on
female runners' luteinizing hormone,
follicle-stimulating hormone, prolactin,
testosterone, and cortisol levels
Am J Obstet Gynecol **146**, 550-556
*Acute exercise, Adult, Androgens,
Comparative, Endocrine, Female, FSH,
Leisure activity, LH, Marathon,
Menopause, PRL, REPRODUCTIVE
HORMONES, Running, Swimming,
Vigorous*

610/43   Haywood, K.M.   (1980)
Strength and flexibility in gymnasts
before and after menarche
Br J Sports Med **14**, 189-192
*Children, Female, JOINTS, Menarche,
MUSCLE STRENGTH*

610/44   Hirata, K., Nagasaka, T., Hirai, A.,
Hirashita, M., Takahata, T. & Nunomura,
T.   (1986)
Effects of human menstrual cycle on
thermoregulatory vasodilation during
exercise
Eur J Appl Physiol **54**, 559-565
*Acute exercise, Adult, Female, Menstrual
cycle*

610/45   Howlett, T.A., Tomlin, S.,
Ngahfoong, L., Rees, L.H., Bullen, B.A.,
Skrinar, G.S. & McArthur, J.W.   (1984)
Release of beta-endorphin and met-
enkephalin during exercise in normal
women: response to training
Br Med J **288**, 1950-1952
*Acute exercise, Adult, Endocrine,
Endorphins, Exercise programme,
Female, Intervention, MOOD,
REPRODUCTIVE HORMONES*

610/46   **Hutton, J.D.**   (1986)
Effect of exercise on puberty, periods and
pregnancy
NZ Med J **99**, 6-8
*Adult, Amenorrhea, Body composition,
Endocrine, Female, Leisure activity,
Menstrual cycle, Oestrogens,
Progesterone, PREGNANCY*

610/47   **Israel, R.G., Sutton, M. & O'Brien,
K.F.**   (1985)
Effects of aerobic training on primary
dysmenorrhea symptomatology in
college females
J Am Coll Health **33**, 241-244
*Adult, Dysmenorrhea, Exercise
programme, Female, Intervention,
Menstrual cycle*

610/48   **Jacobs, H.S.**   (1982)
Amenorrhoea in athletes
Br J Obstets Gynae **89**, 498-500
Amenorrhea, Athlete, Hazards, Review

610/49   **Jurkowski, J.E., Jones, N.L.,
Toews, C.J. & Sutton, J.R.**   (1981)
Effects of menstrual cycle on blood
lactate, O2 delivery, and performance
during exercise
J Appl Physiol **51**, 1493-1499
*Acute exercise, Adult, CARDIAC
PERFORMANCE, Endocrine, Female,
Menstrual cycle, Oestrogens,
Progesterone, REPRODUCTIVE
HORMONES, Vigorous,*

610/50   **Jurkowski, J.E., Jones, N.L.,
Walker, W.C., Younglaie, E.V. & Sutton,
J.R.**   (1978)
Ovarian hormonal responses to exercise
J Appl Physiol **44**, 109-114
*Acute exercise, Adult, Endocrine, Female,
FSH, LH, Menstrual function,
Oestrogens, Progesterone,
REPRODUCTIVE HORMONES*

610/51   **Katch, F.I. & Spiak, D.L.**   (1984)
Validity of the Mellits and Cheek method
for body-fat estimation in relation to
menstrual cycle status in athletes and
non-athletes below 22 per cent fat
Ann Hum Biol **11**, 389-396
*Adult, Amenorrhea, Athlete, Body
composition, Comparative, Female,
Leisure activity, Menstrual cycle*

610/52   **Laatikainen, T., Virtanen, T. &
Apter, D.**   (1986)
Plasma immunoreactive beta-endorphin
in exercise-associated amenorrhea
Am J Obstet Gynecol **154**, 94-97
*Amenorrhea, Children, Endocrine,
ENDORPHINS, Female, FSH, Hazards,
Leisure Activity, LH, MOOD,
Oestrogens, PRL, REPRODUCTIVE
HORMONES, Running,*

610/53   **LLoyd, T., Buchanan, J.R., Bitzer,
S., Waldman, C.J., Myers, C. & Ford,
B.G.**   (1987)
Interrelationships of diet, athletic
activity, menstrual status, and bone
density in collegiate women
Am J Clin Nutr **46**, 681-684
*Adult, Athlete, BONES, Comparative,
Female, Leisure activity, Menarche,
Menstrual cycle*

610/54   **Loucks, A.B.**   (1986)
Does exercise training affect reproductive
hormones in women?
Clin Sports Med **5**, 535-557
*Amenorrhea, Female, Hazards,
REPRODUCTIVE HORMONES,
Review*

610/55   **Loucks, A.B. & Horvath, S.M.**   (1984)
Exercise-induced stress responses of amenorrheic and eumenorrheic runners
J Clin Endocrinol Metab **59**, 1109-1120
Acute exercise, Adult, AEROBIC CAPACITY, Amenorrhea, Androgens, Body composition, Comparative, Endocrine, Female, FSH, Hazards, LH, MOOD, Oestrogens, PRL, REPRODUCTIVE HORMONES, Vigorous

610/56   **Loucks, A.B. & Horvath, S.M.**   (1985)
Atheletic amneorrhea: a review
Med Sci Sports Exerc **17**, 56-72
Amenorrhea, Athlete, Hazards, REPRODUCTIVE HORMONES, Review

610/57   **Loucks, A.B., Horvath, S.M. & Freedson, P.S.**   (1984)
Menstrual status and validation of body fat prediction in athletes
Hum Biol **56**, 383-392
Adult, Amenorrhea, Athlete, Body composition, Comparative, Female, Hazards, Leisure activity, MUSCLE STRENGTH, Running

610/58   **Malina, R.M.**   (1983)
Menarche in athletes: A synthesis and hypothesis
Ann Hum Biol **10**, 1-24
Athlete, Menarche, Review

610/59   **Malina, R.M., Spirduso, W., Tate, C. & Baylor, A.**   (1978)
Age at menarche and selected menstrual characteristics in athletes at differenct competitive levels in different sports
Med Sci Sports **10**, 218-222
Adult, Athlete, Children, Dysmenorrhea, Female, Leisure activity, Menarche, Running, Swimming,

610/60   **Mathur, D.N. & Toriola, A.L.**   (1982)
Age at menarche in Nigerian athletes
Br J Sports Med **16**, 250-252
Adult, Athlete, Comparative, Female, Leisure activity

610/61   **McArthur, J.W.**   (1985)
Endorphins and exercise in females: possible connection with reproductive dysfunction
Med Sci Sports Exerc **17**, 82-88
Endocrine, Endorphins, Female, Menstrual cycle, MOOD, REPRODUCTIVE HORMONES, Review

610/62   **McArthur, J.W., Bullen, B.A., Beitins, I.Z., Pagano, M., Badger, T.M. & Klibanski, A.**   (1980)
Hypothalamic amenorrhea in runners of normal body composition
Endocr Res Comm **7**, 13-25
Adult, Amenorrhea, Body composition, Female, FSH, Hazards, Leisure activity, LH, Oestrogens, REPRODUCTIVE HORMONES

610/63   **Nesheim, B-I. & Bergsjø, P.**   (1982)
Physical activity and reproductive function in women
Scand J Soc Med (Suppl) **29**, 77-81
PREGNANCY, REPRODUCTIVE HORMONES, Review

610/64   **Notelovitz, M., Fields, C., Caramelli, K., Dougherty, M. & Schwartz, A.L.**   (1986)
Cardiorespiratory fitness evaluation in climacteric women: comparison of two methods
Am J Obstet Gynecol **154**, 1009-1013
Acute exercise, Adult, AEROBIC CAPACITY, CARDIAC PERFORMANCE, Female, Menopause, Menstrual cycle

610/65   Øian, P., Augestad, L.B., Molne, K., Oseid, S., Aakvaag, A.   (1984)
Menstrual dysfunction in Norwegian top athletes
Acta Obstet Gynecol Scand **63**, 693-697
Adult, Amenorrhea, Androgens, Athlete, Endocrine, Female, FSH, Hazards, Leisure activity, Menarche, Oestrogens, PRL, REPRODUCTIVE HORMONES, Vigorous

610/66   Osler, D.C. & Crawford, J.D.   (1973)
Examination of the hypothesis of a critical weight at menarche in ambulatory and bedridden mentally retarded girls
Pediatrics **51**, 675-679
Body composition, Female, Handicap, Inactivity, Menarche

610/67   Pellerin-Massicotte, J., Brisson, G.R., St-Pierre, C., Rioux, P. & Rajotte, D.   (1987)
Effect of exercise on the onset of puberty, gonadotropins, and ovarian inhibition
J Appl Physiol **63**, 1165-1173
Animal, Exercise programme, FSH, Intervention, LH, Menarche, REPRODUCTIVE HORMONES

610/68   Peltenburg, A.L., Erich, W.B., Thijssen, J.J., Veeman, W., Jansen, M., Bernink, M.J., Zonderland, M.L., van den Brande, J.L. & Huisveld, I.A.   (1984)
Sex hormone profiles of premenarcheal athletes
Eur J Appl Physiol **52**, 385-392
Androgens, Athlete, Body composition, Children, Comparative, Endocrine, Female, FSH, Hazards, Leisure activity, LH, Menarche, Menstrual function, Oestrogens, REPRODUCTIVE HORMONES, Swimming, Vigorous

610/69   Plismane, S.O., Ozolin, P.P. & Merten, A.A.   (1984)
Effect of the ovarian cycle on blood supply to the limbs during exertion
Hum Physiol **10**, 208-211
Acute exercise, Adult, CARDIAC PERFORMANCE, Female, Menstrual cycle,

610/70   Price, W.A., Dimarzio, L.R. & Gardner, P.R.   (1986)
Biopsychosocial approach to premenstrual syndrome
Am Fam Physician **33**, 117-122
Premenstrual symptoms, Review

610/71   Prior, J.C., Cameron, K., Yuen, B.H. & Thomas, J.   (1982)
Menstrual cycle changes with marathon training: anovulation and short luteal phase
Can J Appl Sport Sci **7**, 173-177
Adult, Female, Leisure activity, Marathon, Menstrual cycle, Running

610/72   Prior, J.C., Vigna, Y., Sciarretta, D., Alojada, N. & Schulzer, M.   (1987)
Conditioning exercise decreases premenstrual symptoms: A prospective, controlled 6-month trial
Fertil Steril **47**, 402-408
Adult, Comparative, Exercise programme, Female, Intervention, Menstrual cycle, MOOD, Premenstrual symptoms

610/73   Prior, J.C., Vigna, Y. & Alojada, N.   (1986)
Conditioning exercise decreases pre-menstrual symptoms
Eur J Appl Physiol **55**, 349-355
Adult, Exercise programme, Female, Intervention, Menstrual cycle, Oestrogens, Premenstrual symptoms, Progesterone, Weight

610/74   Puhl, J.L. & Brown, C.H. (Eds.)   (1986)
The menstrual cycle and physical activity
Human Kinetics Publishers Inc., Champaign, Ill.
Review

610/75   **Rebar, R.W. & Cumming, D.C.** (1981)
Reproductive function in women athletes
J Am Med Ass **246**, 1590
Athlete, Female, Review

610/76   **Richards, S.R., Chang, F.E., Bossetti, B., Malarkey, W.B. & Kim, M.H.** (1985)
Serum carotene levels in female long-distance runners
Fertil Steril **43**, 79-81
Adult, Amenorrhea, Androgens, Comparative, Endocrine, Female, FSH, LH, Menstrual cycle, Oestrogens, PRL, REPRODUCTIVE HORMONES

610/77   **Ronkainen, H.** (1985)
Depressed follicle-stimulating hormone, luteinizing hormone, and prolactin responses to the luteinizing hormone-releasing hormone,thyrotropin-releasing hormone, and metoclopramide test in endurance runners in the hard-training season
Fertil Steril **44**, 755-759
Adult, Comparative, Endocrine, Female, FSH, Hazards, Leisure activity, LH, Menstrual cycle, Oestrogens, PRL, Progesterone, REPRODUCTIVE HORMONES, Running, Vigorous

610/78   **Ronkainen, H., Pakarinen, A. & Kauppila, A.** (1984)
Pubertal and menstrual disorders of female runners, skiers and volleyball players
Gynecol Obstet Invest **18**, 183-189
Adult, Athlete, Comparative, Dysmenorrhea, Female, Hazards, Leisure activity, Menarche, Menstrual cycle, Running, Vigorous

610/79   **Ronkainen, H., Pakarinen, A., Kirkinen, P. & Kauppila, A.** (1985)
Physical exercise-induced changes and season-associated differences in the pituitary-ovarian function of runners and joggers
J Clin Endocrinol Metab **60**, 416-422
Adult, Androgens, Comparative, Endocrine, Female, FSH, Leisure activity, LH, Menarche, Menstrual cycle, Oestrogens, PRL, Progesterone, REPRODUCTIVE HORMONES, Running, Vigorous

610/80   **Russell, J.B., Mitchell, D.E., Musey, P.I. & Collins, D.C.** (1984)
The role of beta-endorphins and catechol estrogens on the hypothalamic-pituitary axis in female athletes
Fertil Steril **42**, 690-695
Body composition, Children, Comparative, Endocrine, Endorphins, Female, FSH, Leisure activity, Longitudinal, LH, Menstrual cycle, MOOD, Oestrogens, PRL, REPRODUCTIVE HORMONES, Swimming, Vigorous

610/81   **Russell, J.B., Mitchell, D.E., Musey, P.I. & Collins, D.C.** (1984)
The relationship of exercise to anovulatory cycles in female athletes: hormonal and physical characteristics
Obstet Gynecol **63**, 452-456
Adult, Amenorrhea, Body composition, Comparative, Female, Hazards, Leisure activity, LH, Menstrual cycle, Oestrogens, PRL, REPRODUCTIVE HORMONES, Running, Swimming

610/82   **Sanborn, C.F., Martin, B.J. & Wagner, W.W. Jr.** (1982)
Is athletic amenorrhea specific to runners?
Am J Obstet Gynecol **143**, 859-861
Adult, Amenorrhea, Athlete, Comparative, Cycling, Female, Hazards, Leisure activity, Running, Swimming, Vigorous, Weight

610/83   **Schoene, R.B., Robertson, H.T., Pierson, D.J. & Peterson, A.P.**   (1981)
Respiratory drives and exercise in menstrual cycles of athletic and nonathletic women
J Appl Physiol **50**, 1300-1305
Acute exercise, Adult, AEROBIC CAPACITY, ANAEROBIC CAPACITY, Amenorrhea, Athlete, Comparative, Female, Menstrual cycle, REPRODUCTIVE HORMONES, Respiratory function, Vigorous

610/84   **Schwartz, B., Cumming, D.C., Riordan, E., Selye, M., Yen, S.S. & Rebar, R.W.**   (1981)
Exercise-associated amenorrhea: a distinct entity?
Am J Obstet Gynecol **141**, 662-670
Adult, Amenorrhea, Body composition, Comparative, Endocrine, ENERGY BALANCE, Female, FSH, Hazards, LH, Leisure activity, Menarche, MOOD, Oestrogens, REPRODUCTIVE HORMONES, Running, Weight

610/85   **Shade, A.R.**   (1983)
Gynecologic and obstetric problems of the female dancer
Clin Sports Med **2**, 515-523
Menarche, PREGNANCY, Review, URO-GENITAL TRACT

610/86   **Shangold, M.M., Freeman, R., Thysen B. & Gatz, M.L.**   (1979)
The relationship between long distance running, plasma progesterone and luteal phase length
Fertil Steril **31**, 130
Adult, Endocrine, Female, FSH, Intervention, Leisure activity, LH, Menstrual cycle, PRL, Progesterone, REPRODUCTIVE HORMONES, Running

610/87   **Shangold, M.M.**   (1985)
Athletic amenorrhea
Clin Obstet Gynecol **28**, 664-669
Amenorrhea, Review

610/88   **Shangold, M. M.**   (1986)
Gynecological concerns in young and adolescent physically active girls
Pediatrician **13**, 10-13
Children, Hazards, Review

610/89   **Shangold, M.M., Gatz, M.L. & Thysen, B.**   (1981)
Acute effects of exercise on plasma concentrations of prolactin and testosterone in recreational women runners
Fertil Steril **35**, 699-702
Acute exercise, Adult, Androgens, Endocrine, Female, Leisure activity, PRL, REPRODUCTIVE HORMONES, Running

610/90   **Shangold, M.M. & Levine, H.S.**   (1982)
The effect of marathon training upon menstrual function
Am J Obstet Gynecol **143**, 862-869
Adult, Amenorrhea, Body composition, Dysmenorrhea, Female, Fertility, Hazards, Marathon, Menarche, Running, Vigorous, Weight

610/91   **Sidhu, L.S. & Grewal, R.**   (1980)
Age of menarche in various categories of Indian sportswomen
Br J Sports Med **14**, 199-203
Children, Comparative, Female, Leisure activity, Menarche, Vigorous

610/92   **Stager, J.M.**   (1984)
Reversibility of amenorrhoea in athletes
Sports Med **1**, 337-340
Adult, Amenorrhea, Athlete, Female,

610/93   **Stager, J.M., Robertshaw, D. & Miescher, E.**   (1984)
Delayed menarche in swimmers in relation to age at onset of training and athletic performance
Med Sci Sports Exerc **16**, 550-555
Athlete, Children, Female, Menarche, Menstrual function, Swimming, Vigorous

610/94   Stein T.P., Schluter, M.D. &
Diamond, C.E.   (1983)
Nutrition, protein turnover, and physical
activity in young women
Am J Clin Nutr **38**, 223-228
*Adult, Comparative, ENERGY
BALANCE, Female, Menstrual cycle,
Swimming, Vigorous*

610/95   Stephenson, L.A., Kolka, M.A.,
Wilkerson, J.E.   (1982)
Perceived exertion and anaerobic
threshold during the menstrual cycle
Med Sci Sports Exerc **14**, 218-222
*Acute exercise, Adult, AEROBIC
CAPACITY, ANAEROBIC
CAPACITY, Female, Menstrual cycle,
PERCEIVED EXERTION,
RESPIRATORY FUNCTION*

610/96   Strauss, R.H., Liggett, M.T. &
Lanese, R.R.   (1985)
Anabolic steroid use and perceived effects
in ten weight-trained women athletes
J Am Med Ass **253**, 2871-2873
*Adult, Endocrine, Female, Growth,
Menstrual cycle, MUSCLE STRENGTH*

610/97   Teitz, C.C.   (1982)
Sports medicine concerns in dance and
gymnastics
Pediatr Clin North Am **29**, 1399-1421
JOINTS, Review

610/98   Timonen, S & Procope, B.-
J.   (1971)
Premenstrual syndrome and physical
exercise
Acta Obstet Gynecol Scand **50**, 331-337
*Adult, Dysmenorrhea, Comparative,
Female, Leisure activity, Premenstrual
symptoms*

610/99   Vandenbroucke, J.P., van Laar, A.
& Valkenburg, H.A.   (1982)
Synergy between thinness and intensive
sports activity in delaying menarche
Br Med J **284**, 1907-1908
*Children, Comparative, Female, Hazards,
Leisure activity, Menarche, Vigorous,
Weight*

610/100   Veldhuis, J.D., Evans, W.S.,
Demers, L.M., Thorner, M.O., Wakat,
D.K. & Rogol, A.D.   (1985)
Altered neuroendocrine regulation of
gonadotropin secretion in women
distance runners
J Clin Endocrinol Metab **61**, 557-563
*Adult, Amenorrhea, Androgens, Body
composition, Comparative, Endocrine,
Female, FSH, Hazards, LH, Menarche,
Menstrual cycle, Oestrogens, PRL,
REPRODUCTIVE HORMONES,
Running, Vigorous*

610/101   Villanueva, A.L., Schlosser, C.,
Hopper, B., Liu, J.H., Hoffman, D.I. &
Rebar, R.W.   (1986)
Increased cortisol production in women
runners
J Clin Endocrinol Metab **63**, 133-136
*Amenorrhea, Comparative, Endocrine,
Female, Hazards, Leisure activity,
REPRODUCTIVE HORMONES,
Running*

610/102   Wakat, D.K., Sweeney, K.A. &
Rogol, A.D.   (1982)
Reproductive system function in women
cross-country runners
Med Sci Sports Exerc **14**, 263-269
*Adult, Amenorrhea, Athlete, Body
composition, Comparative, Endocrine,
Female, FSH, Hazards, LH, Leisure
activity, Menarche, Menstrual cycle,
Oestrogens, Progesterone, PRL, Running,
Vigorous.*

610/103   Warren, M.P.   (1980)
The effects of exercise on pubertal
progression and reproductive function in
girls
J Clin Endocrinol Metab **51**, 1150-1157
*Amenorrhea, Body composition, BONES,
Children, Comparative, Endocrine,
Exercise programme, Female, Hazards,
Longitudinal, Menarche,
REPRODUCTIVE HORMONES,
Vigorous, Weight*

610/104   **Webb, J.L., Millan, D.L. & Stoltz,
C.J.**   (1979)
Gynecological survey of American
female athletes competing at the
Montreal Olympic Games
J Sports Med Phys Fitness **19**, 405-412
*Adult, Amenorrhea, Athlete,
Dysmenorrhea, Female, Leisure activity,
Menarche, Menstrual cycle, Vigorous*

610/105   **Webb, J.L. & Proctor,
A.J.**   (1983)
Anthropometric, training and menstrual
differences of three groups of American
collegiate female runners
J Sports Med Phys Fitness **23**, 201-209
*Adult, Amenorrhea, Athlete, Body
composition, Comparative, Female,
Leisure activity, Menarche, Menstrual
cycle, Running, Vigorous*

610/106   **Yahiro, J., Glass, A.R., Fears,
W.B., Ferguson, E.E. & Vigersky,
R.A.**   (1987)
Exaggerated gonadotropin response to
luteinizing hormone-releasing hormone
in amenorrheic runners
Am J Obstet Gynecol **156**, 586-591
*Adult, Amenorrhea, Androgens, Athlete,
Body composition, Endocrine, Female,
FSH, Hazards, Leisure activity, LH,
Oestrogens, Progesterone, PRL*

620 PREGNANCY

KEYWORDS are listed in the appendix in addition the following specific keywords have been used in this section:

Endorphins
Foetal response (to exercise)
Maternal response (to exercise)
Outcome (birth outcome, APGAR score, complications)
Placenta
Uterus

Summary of evidence: hazards are minimal if exercise is sensible

THE PROBLEM

Attitudes to pregnant women are protective with good reason. Is exercise harmful during pregnancy? Conversely, are there adverse effects of a sedentary lifesyle during pregnancy? Is exercise of benefit to pregnant women or the unborn child?

SCOPE

This section contains references dealing primarily with changes produced by customary exercise in pregnant women and on the outcome of their pregnancy. There are also studies of the acute effects of exercise on the mother and the foetus. These include changes with time in plasma levels of hormones and signs of foetal distress using heart rate monitoring. There are a number of animal studies.

METHODOLOGICAL DIFFICULTIES

Rather few human studies have been conducted on small numbers of subjects because of the difficulty of assessing relevant spontaneous customary activity during pregnancy, and controlling for the many factors, other than the mother's exercise habits, which affect the growing foetus. The difficulties in providing the necessary level of monitoring make intervention studies impracticable.

EVIDENCE

The general benefits of physical activity apply as much during pregnancy as at any time. Moderate exercise to which the mother has previously been accustomed does not appear to have an adverse affect on pregnancy. Such exercise during pregnancy may be beneficial to the foetus as well as the mother. It is associated with a lower incidence of abortion and prematurity and does not appear to effect outcome as measured by birth-weight, duration of gestation, and measures of well being of the newborn. However, vigorous exercise continued into the last third of pregnancy may be associated with slightly lower birth weights. The usual guide-lines for safe exercise should be followed rigorously during pregnancy, and those previously unaccustomed to exercise should be content with walking and swimming. Contact sports such as skiing and riding and risk of contact injury should be avoided.

620/1   (1984)
References from Workshop on Physical Activity in Pregnancy (1982)
Am J Perinatol **1,** 272-275
Animal, Female, Review

620/2   **Anderson, T.D.**   (1987)
Exercise and sport in pregnancy
Update **15 Feb.,** 346-352
Review

620/3   **Araki, R.**   (1984)
The investigations on the effect of daily
activity on the uterine contraction during
pregnancy
Nippon Sanka Fujinka Gakkai Zasshi **36**,
589-598
Adult, Customary activity, Female,
Leisure activity, Maternal response,
Uterus

620/4   **Artal, R.**   (1986)
Hormonal responses to exercise in
pregnancy In: Exercise in Pregnancy
(Eds.) Artal, R. & Wiswell, R.
Williams and Wilkins, Baltimore 139-146
Endocrine, Review

620/5   **Artal, R., Paul, R., Romen, Y. &**
Wiswell, R.A.   (1984)
Fetal bradycardia induced by maternal
exercise
Lancet **ii**, 258-60
Acute exercise, Adult, AEROBIC
CAPACITY, Endocrine, Female, Foetal
response, Maternal response, Outcome,
Vigorous

620/6   **Artal, R., Platt, LD., Sperling, M.,**
Kammula, R.K., Jilek, J. & Nakamura,
R.   (1981)
I. Maternal cardiovascular and metabolic
responses in normal pregnancy
Am J Obstet Gynecol **140**, 123-127
Acute exercise, Adult,
CARBOHYDRATE TOLERANCE,
Endocrine, Female, Foetal response,
Maternal response, Outcome

620/7   **Artal, R. & Romen, Y.**   (1986)
Fetal responses to maternal exercise. In:
Exercise in Pregnancy (Eds.) Artal, R. &
Wiswell, R.
Williams and Wilkins, Baltimore 195-204
Foetal response, Review

620/8   **Artal, R. & Wiswell, R.A.**   (1986)
Exercise prescription in pregnancy. In:
Exercise in Pregnancy (Eds.) Artal, R. &
Wiswell, R.
Williams and Wilkins, Baltimore 225-228
Exercise programme, Review

620/9   **Artal, R., Wiswell, R.A.,**
Greenspoon, J. & Romen, Y.   (1986)
Pulmonary responses to exercise in
pregnancy. In: Exercise in Pregnancy
(Eds.) Artal, R. & Wiswell, R.
Williams and Wilkins, Baltimore 147-154
RESPIRATORY FUNCTION, Review

620/10   **Artal, R., Wiswell, R., Romen, Y. &**
Dorey, F.   (1986)
Pulmonary responses to exercise in
pregnancy
Am J Obstet Gynecol **154** , 378-383
Acute exercise, Adult, Comparative,
Female, Foetal response, Maternal
response, RESPIRATORY FUNCTION

620/11   **Bell, A.W., Bassett, J.M.,**
Chandler, J.C. & Boston, R.C.   (1983)
Fetal and maternal endocrine responses
to exercise in the pregnant ewe
J Dev Physiol **5**, 129-141
Acute exercise, Animal, Endocrine, Foetal
response, Maternal response,
REPRODUCTIVE HORMONES

620/12   **Berkowitz, G., Kelsey, J., Holford,**
T. & Berkowitz, R.   (1983)
Physical activity and risk of spontaneous
preterm delivery
J Reprod Med **28**, 581-588
Adult, Case-control, Customary activity,
Exercise programme, Female, Leisure
activity, Occupational activity, Outcome

620/13   **Boehnke, W.W., Chernoff, G.F. &**
Finnell, R.H.   (1987)
Investigation of the teratogenic effects of
exercise on pregnancy outcome in mice
Teratogenesis Carcinog Mutagen **7**, 391-
397
Animal, Exercise programme, Hazards,
Intervention, Outcome

620/14   **Bolton, M.E.**   (1980)
Scuba diving and fetal well-being: a
survey of 208 women
Undersea Biomed Res **7**, 183-189
Adult, Female, Hazards, Outcome

620/15   Bonds, D.R. & Delivoria-
Papadopoulos, M.   (1985)
Exercise during pregnancy–potential
fetal and placental metabolic effects
Ann Clin Lab Sci **15**, 91-99
Review

620/16   Chandler, J.C.D. & Bell,
A.W.   (1983)
Effects of maternal exercise on fetal and
maternal respiration and nutrient
metabolism in the pregnant ewe
J Dev Physiol **31**, 161-176
*Acute exercise, Animal, ENERGY
BALANCE, RESPIRATORY
FUNCTION*

620/17   Cherry, N.   (1987)
Physical demands of work and health
complaints among women working late
in pregnancy
Ergonomics **30**, 689-701
*Adult, Female, Maternal response,
Occupational activity, Outcome*

620/20   Clapp, J.F. 3rd   (1985)
Fetal heart rate response to running in
midpregnancy and late pregnancy
Am J Obstet Gynecol **153**, 251-252
*Acute exercise, Adult, Female, Foetal
response, Leisure activity, Running*

620/18   Clapp, J.F. 3rd & Dickstein,
S.   (1984)
Endurance exercise and pregnancy
outcome
Med Sci Sports Exerc **16**, 556-562
*Adult, Female, Intervention, Leisure
activity, Outcome, Vigorous, Weight*

620/19   Clapp, J.F. 3rd., Wesley, M. &
Sleamaker, R.H.   (1987)
Thermoregulatory and metabolic
responses to jogging prior to and during
pregnancy
Med Sci Sports Exerc **19**, 124-130
*Adult, AEROBIC CAPACITY,
CARBOHYDRATE TOLERANCE,
Female, Intervention, Leisure activity,
MUSCLE METABOLISM,
RESPIRATORY FUNCTION, Running*

620/21   Collings, C.A., Curet, L.B. &
Mullin, J.P.   (1983)
Maternal and fetal responses to a
maternal aerobic exercise program
Am J Obstet Gynecol **145**, 702-707
*Adult, AEROBIC CAPACITY, Exercise
programme, Female, Foetal response,
Intervention, Outcome*

620/22   Collings, C.A. & Curet,
L.B.   (1985)
Fetal heart rate response to maternal
exercise
Am J Obstet Gynecol **151**, 498-501
*Adult, Exercise programme, Female,
Foetal response, Intervention, Maternal
response, Outcome*

620/23   Curet, L.B., Orr, J.H., Rankin,
J.H.G. & Ungerer, T.   (1976)
Effect of exercise on cardiac output and
distribution of uterine blood flow in
pregnant ewes
J Appl Physiol **40**, 725-728
*Animal, CARDIAC PERFORMANCE,
Exercise programme, Intervention,
Placenta*

620/24   Dale, E., Mullinax, K.M. & Bryan,
D.H.   (1982)
Exercise during pregnancy: effects on the
fetus
Can J Appl Sport Sci **7**, 98-103
*Acute exercise, Adult, Comparative,
Female, Foetal response, Leisure activity,
Maternal response, Outcome, Running*

620/25   Dibblee, L. & Graham,
T.E.   (1983)
A longitudinal study of changes in
aerobic fitness, body composition, and
energy intake in primigravid patients
Am J Obstet Gynecol **147**, 908-914
*Adult, AEROBIC CAPACITY, Body
composition, ENERGY BALANCE,
Female, Outcome*

620/26 **Dressendorfer, R.** (1978)
Physical training during pregnancy and
lactation
Phys Sports Med **6**, 2
Review

620/27 **Edwards, M.J., Metcalfe, J.,
Dunham, M.Y. & Paul, M.S.** (1981)
Accelerated respiratory response to
moderate exercise in late pregnancy
Respir Physiol **45**, 229-241
*Acute exercise, Adult, Female,
RESPIRATORY FUNCTION*

620/28 **Erdelyi, G.J.** (1962)
Gynecological survey of female athletes
J Sports Med Phys Fitness **2**, 174-179
*Adult, Female, MENSTRUAL
FUNCTION, Outcome*

620/29 **Erkkola, R.** (1976)
The physical work capacity of the
expectant mother and its effect on
pregnancy, labor and the newborn
Int J Gynaecol Obstet **14**, 153-159
*Adult, Comparative, Leisure activity,
Outcome*

620/30 **Erkkola, R.** (1976)
The influence of physical training during
pregnancy on physical work capacity and
circulatory parameters
Scand J clin Lab Invest **36**, 747-754
*Acute exercise, Adult, BLOOD
PRESSURE, Exercise programme,
Female, Intervention, Maternal response*

620/31 **Erkkola, R. & Rauramo, I.** (1976)
Correlation of maternal physical fitness
during pregnancy with maternal and fetal
pH and lactic acid at delivery
Acta Obstet Gynecol Scand **55**, 441-446
Adult, Comparative, Female, Outcome

620/32 **Fox, M.E., Harris, R.E. & Brekken,
A.L.** (1977)
The active-duty military pregnancy: a
new high-risk category
Am J Obstet Gynecol **129**, 705-707
*Adult, Comparative, Female, Hazards,
Occupational activity, Outcome*

620/33 **Garris, D.R., Kaparek, G.J.,
Overton, S. V. & Alligood, G.R.** (1985)
Effects of exercise on fetal-placental
growth and utero-placental blood flow in
the rat
Biol Neonate **47**, 223-229
*Acute exercise, Animal, Foetal response,
Maternal response, Placenta, Outcome,
Uterus*

620/34 **Gauthier, M.M.** (1986)
Guidelines for exercise during pregnancy:
too little or too much?
Phys Sports Med **14**, 162-169
Review

620/35 **Gilbert, R.D., Cummings, L.A.,
Juchau, M.R. & Longo, L.D.** (1979)
Placental diffusing capacity and fetal
development in exercising or hypoxic
guinea pigs
J Appl Physiol **46**, 828-834
*Animal, Exercise programme, Foetal
response, Intervention, Outcome, Placenta*

620/36 **Gorski, J.** (1985)
Exercise during pregnancy: maternal and
fetal responses. A brief review
Med Sci Sports Exerc **17**, 407-416
Review

620/37 **Hale, R.W.** (1987)
Exercise in pregnancy. How each affects
the other
Postgraduate Med **82**, 61-63
Review

620/38 **Hall, D.C. & Kaufman,
D.A.** (1987)
Effects of aerobic strength conditioning
on pregnancy outcomes
Am J Obstet Gynecol **157**, 1199-1203
*Adult, Female, Intervention, MUSCLE
STRENGTH, Outcome,
PERSONALITY*

620/39   **Hauth, J., Gilstrap, L. & Widmer, K.**   (1982)
Fetal heart rate reactivity before and after maternal jogging during the third trimester
Am J Obstet Gynecol **142,** 545 – 547
Acute exercise, Adult, Female, Foetal response, Leisure activity, Maternal response, Running

620/40   **Hohimer, A.R., Bissonnette, J.M., Metcalfe, J. & McKean, T.A.**   (1984)
Effect of exercise on uterine blood flow in the pregnant pygmy goat
Am J Physiol **246,** H207-212
Animal, Exercise programme, Intervention, Uterus

620/41   **Hollingsworth, D.R. & Moore, T.R.**   (1987)
Postprandial walking exercise in pregnant insulin-dependent (type I) diabetic women: Reduction of plasma lipid levels but absence of a significant effect on glycemic control
Am J Obstet Gynecol **157,** 1359-1363
Adult, CARBOHYDRATE TOLERANCE, Exercise programme, Intervention, LIPIDS, Maternal response, Outcome

620/42   **Hon, E.H. & Wohlgemuth, R.**   (1961)
The electronic evaluation of fetal heart rate
Am J Obstet Gynecol **81,** 361-371
Acute exercise, Adult, Female, Foetal response, Outcome

620/43   **Horvath, S.M.**   (1979)
Review of energetics and blood flow in exercise
Diabetes (Suppl) **28,** 33-38
Review

620/44   **Jarrett, J.C. 2nd & Spellacy, W.N.**   (1983)
Jogging during pregnancy: an improved outcome?
Obstet Gynecol **61,** 705-709
Adult, Female, Outcome, Leisure activity, Running

620/45   **Jenkins, R.R. & Ciconnee, C.**   (1980)
Exercise effect during pregnancy on brain nucleic acids of offspring in rats
Arch Phys Med Rehabil **61,** 124-127
Animal, Exercise programme, Intervention, Outcome, PSYCHOMOTOR PERFORMANCE

620/46   **Jones, R.L., Botti, J.J., Anderson, W.M. & Bennett, N.L.**   (1985)
Thermoregulation during aerobic exercise in pregnancy
Obstet Gynecol **65,** 340-345
Acute exercise, Adult, ENERGY BALANCE, Female, Leisure activity, Maternal response, URO-GENITAL TRACT

620/47   **Jopke, T.**   (1983)
Pregnancy: A time to exercise judgement
Phys Sports Med **11,** 139-148
Review

620/48   **Jovanovic, L., Kessler, A. & Peterson, C.M.**   (1985)
Human maternal and fetal response to graded exercise
J Appl Physiol **58,** 1719-1722
Adult, Acute exercise, CARBOHYDRATE TOLERANCE, Endocrine, Female, Foetal response, Leisure activity, Maternal response

620/49   **Katz, J.**   (1983)
Swimming through your pregnancy, the perfect exercise for pregnant women
Dolphin Books, Doubleday, New York 1-159
Exercise programme, Review, Swimming

620/50   Koos, B.J., Power, G.G. & Longo, L.D.   (1986)
Placental oxygen transfer with considerations for maternal exercise. In: Exercise in Pregnancy (Eds.) Artal, R. & Wiswell, R.
Williams and Wilkins, Baltimore 155-180
Placenta, Review

620/52   Lotgering, F.K., Gilbert, R.D. & Longo, L.D.   (1983)
Exercise responses in pregnant sheep: blood gases, temperatures, and fetal cardiovascular system
J Appl Physiol **55**, 842-850
Acute exercise, Animal, CARDIAC PERFORMANCE, Endocrine, Foetal response, Maternal response, Placenta, Vigorous

620/51   Lotgering, F.K., Gilbert, R.D. & Longo, L.D.   (1983)
Exercise responses in pregnant sheep: Oxygen consumption, uterine blood flow, and blood volume
J Appl Physiol **55**, 834-841
Acute exercise, Animal, CARDIAC PERFORMANCE, Foetal response, Maternal response, Placenta, Uterus, Vigorous

620/53   Lotgering, F.K., Gilbert, R.D. & Longo, L.D.   (1984)
The interactions of exercise and pregnancy: a review
Am J Obstet Gynecol **149**, 560-568
Foetal response, Outcome, Review

620/54   Lotgering, F.K., Gilbert, R.D. & Longo, L.D.   (1985)
Maternal and fetal responses to exercise during pregnancy
Physiol Rev **65**, 1-36
CARDIAC PERFORMANCE, Maternal response, Foetal response, Placenta, Uterus, Review

620/55   Mamelle, N., Laumon, B. & Lazer, P.   (1984)
Prematurity and occupational activity during pregnancy
Am J Epidemiol **119**, 309-322
Adult, Female, Occupational activity, Outcome

620/56   Marsal, K., Logren, O. & Gennser, G.   (1979)
Fetal breathing movements and maternal exercise
Acta Obstet Gynecol Scand **58**, 197-201
Acute exercise, Adult, Female, Foetal response, Maternal response

620/57   Morton, M.J., Paul, M.S., Campos, G.R., Hart, M.V. & Metcalfe, J.   (1985)
Exercise dynamics in late gestation: Effects of physical training
Am J Obstet Gynecol **152**, 91-97
Acute exercise, Adult, CARDIAC PERFORMANCE, Exercise programme, Female, Intervention, Maternal response, Outcome

620/58   Mullinax, K.M. & Dale, E.   (1986)
Some considerations of exercise during pregnancy
Clin Sports Med **5**, 559-570
Review

620/59   Naeye, R.L. & Peters, E.   (1982)
Working during pregnancy: effects on the fetus
Pediatrics **69**, 724-727
Adult, Female, Occupational activity, Outcome, Placenta

620/60   Nagy, L.E. & King, J.C.   (1983)
Energy expenditure of pregnant women at rest or walking self-paced
Am J Clin Nutr **38**, 369-376
Acute exercise, Adult, Comparative, Customary activity, ENERGY BALANCE, Female, Uterus

620/61   Nelson, P.S., Gilbert, R.D. & Longo, L.D.   (1983)
Fetal growth and placental diffusing capacity in guinea pigs following long term maternal exercise
J Dev Physiol **5**, 1-10
Animal, Outcome, Placenta, Vigorous

620/62   Parízková, J.   (1979)
Cardiac microstructure in female and male offspring of exercised rat mothers
Acta Anat **104**, 382-387
Animal, CARDIAC PERFORMANCE, COLLATERALS, Exercise programme, Intervention

620/63   Pernoll, M.L., Metcalfe, J. & Paul, M.   (1978)
Fetal cardiac response to maternal exercise. In: Fetal and Newborn Cardiovascular Physiology (Eds) Longo, L.D. & Reneau, D.D.
Garland Press, New York **2**, 389-398
Foetal response, Review

620/64   Platt, L.D., Artal, R., Semel, J., Sipos, L. & Kammula, R.K.   (1983)
Exercise in pregnancy II. Fetal Responses
Am J Obstet Gynecol **147**, 487 – 490
Acute exercise, Adult, BLOOD PRESSURE, Endocrine, Female, Foetal response, Maternal response

620/65   Pomerance, J.J., Gluck, L. & Lynch, V.A.   (1974)
Physical fitness in pregnancy: its effect on pregnancy outcome
Am J Obstet Gynecol **119**, 153-159
Adult, Comparative, Female, Leisure activity, Outcome, Weight

620/66   Rauramo, I., Andersson, B. & Laatikainen, T.   (1982)
Stress hormones and placental steroids in physical exercise during pregnancy
Br J Obstet Gynaecol **89**, 921-925
Acute exercise, Adult, BLOOD PRESSURE, Endocrine, Female, Foetal response, Maternal response, REPRODUCTIVE HORMONES

620/67   Rauramo, I., Salminen, K. & Laatikainen, T.   (1986)
Release of beta-endorphin in response to exercise in non-pregnant and pregnant women
Acta Obstet Gynecol Scand **65**, 609-612
Acute exercise, Adult, BLOOD PRESSURE, CARBOHYDRATE TOLERANCE, Comparative, Endorphins, Female, Maternal response, MOOD, REPRODUCTIVE HORMONES,

620/68   Smith, A.D., Gilbert, R.D., Lammers, R.J. & Longo, L.D.   (1983)
Placental exchange area in guinea pigs following long term maternal exercise: a sterological analysis
J Dev Physiol **5**, 11-21
Animal, Endocrine, Exercise programme, Intervention, Placenta

620/69   Sørensen, K.E. & Børlum, K.-G.   (1986)
Fetal heart function in response to short-term maternal exercise
Br J Obstet Gynaecol **93**, 310-313
Acute exercise, Adult, CARDIAC PERFORMANCE, Foetal response

620/70   South-Paul, J.E.   (1988)
The effect of participation in a regular exercise program upon aerobic capacity during pregnancy
Ostet Gynecol **71**, 175-179
Adult, AEROBIC CAPACITY, Exercise programme, Intervention, RESPIRATORY FUNCTION

620/71   South-Paul, J.E., Rajagopal, K.R. & Tenholder, M.F.   (1988)
The effects of participation in a regular exercise program upon aerobic capacity during pregnancy
Obstet Gynecol **71**, 175-179
Adult, AEROBIC CAPACITY, Exercise programme, Female, Intervention, RESPIRATORY FUNCTION

620/72   **Speroff, L.**   (1980)
Can exercise cause problems in
pregnancy and menstruation
Contemp Ob/Gyn **16,** 57-63
Review

620/73   **St. John Repovich, W.E., Wiswell,
R.A. & Artal, R.**   (1986)
Sports activities and aerobic exercise
during pregnancy. In: Exercise in
Pregnancy (Eds.) Artal, R. & Wiswell, R.
Williams and Wilkins, Baltimore 205-214
*AEROBIC CAPACITY, Exercise
programme, Review*

620/74   **Taferi, N., Naeye, R.L. & Gobzie,
A.**   (1980)
Effects of maternal under-nutrition and
heavy physical work during pregnancy on
birth weight
Br J Obstet Gynaecol **87,** 222-226
*Adult, ENERGY BALANCE, Female,
Occupational activity, Outcome,
Vigorous, Weight*

620/75   **Treadway, J.L., Dover, E.V.,
Morse, W., Newcome, L. & Craig,
B.W.**   (1986)
Influence of exercise training on maternal
and fetal morphological characteristics in
the rat
J Appl Physiol **60,** 1700-1703
*Animal, Exercise programme, Foetal
response, Intervention, Outcome*

620/76   **Treadway, J.L.**   (1986)
The effects of exercise on milk yield, milk
composition, and offspring growth in rats
Am J Clin Nutr **44,** 481-488
*Animal, Exercise programme,
Intervention, Weight*

620/77   **Ueland, K., Novy, M.J. & Metcalfe,
J.**   (1973)
Cardiorespiratory responses to
pregnancy and exercise in normal women
and patients with heart disease
Am J Obstet Gynecol **115,** 4-10
*Acute exercise, Adult, CARDIAC
PERFORMANCE, Female, Maternal
response, SECONDARY
PREVENTION*

620/78   **Veille, J.C., Hohimer, A.R., Burry,
K. & Speroff, L.**   (1985)
The effect of exercise on uterine activity
in the last eight weeks of pregnancy
Am J Obstet Gynecol **151,** 727-730
*Acute exercise, Adult, Female, Foetal
response, Leisure activity, Maternal
response, Outcome, Uterus*

620/79   **Wallace, J.P., Wiswell, R.A. &
Artal, R.**   (1986)
Maternal cardiovascular response to
exercise during pregnancy. In: Exercise in
Pregnancy (Eds.) Artal, R. & Wiswell, R.
Williams and Wilkins, Baltimore 127-137
CARDIAC PERFORMANCE, Review

620/80   **Wiswell, R.A., Artal, R., Romen, Y.
& Kammula, R.K.**   (1985)
Hormonal and metabolic response to
maximal exercise in pregnancy
Med Sci Sports Exerc **17,** 206
*Adult, AEROBIC CAPACITY,
Comparative, Endocrine, Female*

630 REPRODUCTIVE HORMONES

KEYWORDS are listed in the appendix in addition the following specific keywords have been used in this section:

Androgens
Endorphins
FSH (Follicle stimulating hormone)
LH (Luteinising hormone)
Menarche
Menopause
Oestrogens
PRL (Prolactin)

Summary of evidence: prevention of reproductive cancers may occur, improvement in strength in men may be partly explained and reduced reproductive function in women may be partly explained

THE PROBLEM

Does exercise change circulating levels of reproductive hormones in ways which might affect physical performance, fertility, reproductive function or disease ?

SCOPE

This section contains references dealing with changes produced by exercise in a number of different hormones, mainly those concerned with reproductive function. They include catecholamines, cortisol, gonadotropins, prostaglandins and prolactin. The studies are mainly but not exclusively in women; there are also studies of the effects of exercise in cancer of the reproductive system.

METHODOLOGICAL DIFFICULTIES

The levels of many of these hormones are low and their effectiveness sometimes depends on patterned or pulsatile release. Moreover their effects are modified by many other factors.

EVIDENCE

A history of athletic activity is associated with a reduced risk of cancer of the breast or reproductive system in women. This suggests but does not prove that the association is causal. Changes occur in hormone levels during acute exercise in both men and women. The rise in testosterone which is most marked in males may be associated causally with the increase in muscle substance and strength observed following training (see section 130). The changes in women in F.S.H. and L.H. may in part explain the amenorrhea and oligomenorrhea of young athletes (see section 610).

630/1 **Bachman, G.A., Leiblum, S.R. & Sandler, B.** (1985)
Correlates of sexual desire in post-menopausal women
Maturitas **7**, 211-216
Adult, Exercise programme, Female, Intervention, Menopause, URO-GENITAL TRACT

630/2 **Brisson, G.R., Peronnet, F., Ledoux, M., Pellerin-Massicotte, J., Matton, P., Garceau, F. & Boisvert, P. Jr** (1986)
Temperature-induced hyperprolactinemia during exercise
Horm Metab Res **18**, 283-284,
Acute exercise, Adult, ANAEROBIC CAPACITY, Hazards, PRL

630/3   Carli, G., Martelli, G., Viti, A.,
Baldi, L., Bonifazi, M., Lupo, D. & Prisco,
C.   (1983)
The effect of swimming training on
hormone levels in girls
J Sports Med Phys Fitness **23**, 45-51
Androgens, Children, Endocrine, Female,
Intervention, Menarche, Oestrogens,
PRL, Swimming

630/4   Cook, N.J., Read, G.F., Walker,
R.F., Harris, B. & Riad-Fahmy,
D.   (1986)
Changes in adrenal and testicular activity
monitored by salivary sampling in males
throughout marathon runs
Eur J Appl Physiol **55**, 634-638
Acute exercise, Adult, Androgens,
Endocrine, Leisure activity, Male,
Marathon, Running, Vigorous

630/5   DeMeileir, K., Baeyens, L.,
L'Hermite-Baleriaux, M., L'Hermite, M.
& Hollman, W.   (1985)
Exercise-induced prolactin release is
related to anaerobiosis
J Clin Endocrinol Metab **60**, 1250-1260
Acute exercise, Adult, AEROBIC
CAPACITY, ANAEROBIC
CAPACITY, Male, PRL

630/6   Demers, L.M., Harrison, T.S.,
Halbert, D.R. & Santen, R.J.   (1981)
Effect of prolonged exercise on plasma
prostaglandin levels
Prostaglandins Med **6**, 413-418,
Acute exercise, Adult, Androgens,
Endocrine, FSH, Leisure activity, LH,
Marathon, Running, Vigorous

630/7   Frey, H.   (1982)
The endocrine response to physical
activity
Scand J Soc Med (Suppl) **29**, 71-75
Endocrine, Review

630/8   Frisch, R.E., Wyshak, G., Albright,
N.L., Albright, T.E., Schiff, I., Jones,
K.P., Witschi, J., Shiang, E., Koff, E. &
Marguglio, M.   (1985)
Lower prevalence of breast cancer and
cancers of the reproductive system
among former college athletes compared
to non-athletes
Br J Cancer **52**, 885-891
Adult, Athlete, Cancer, Comparative,
Elderly, Female, Leisure activity,
Menarche

630/9   Galbo, H.   (1985)
The hormonal response to exercise
Proc Nutr Soc **44**, 257-66,
Endocrine, ENERGY BALANCE,
Review

630/10   Keizer, H.A., Poortman, J. &
Bunnik, G.S.   (1980)
Influence of physical exercise on sex-
hormone metabolism
J Appl Physiol **48**, 765-679
Acute exercise, Adult, AEROBIC
CAPACITY, Comparative, Endocrine,
Female, MENSTRUAL FUNCTION,
Oestrogens

630/11   Kuusi, T., Kostiainen, E.,
Vartiainen, E., Pitkänen, L., Ehnholm, C.,
Korhonen, H.J., Nissinen, A. & Puska,
P.   (1984)
Acute effects of marathon running on
levels of serum lipoproteins and
androgenic hormones in healthy males
Metabolism **33**, 527-531
Acute exercise, Adult, Androgens, Leisure
activity, LIPIDS, Male, Marathon,
Running, Vigorous

630/12   Mathur, D.N., Toriola, A.L. &
Dada, O.A.   (1986)
Serum cortisol and testosterone levels in
conditioned male distance runners and
nonathletes after maximal exercise
J Sports Med Phys Fitness **26**, 245-250
Acute exercise, Adult, Androgens,
Comparative, Endocrine, Leisure activity,
Male

630/13   **Remes, K., Kuoppasalmi, K. &**
Adlercreutz, H.   (1985)
Effect of physical exercise and sleep
deprivation on plasma androgen levels:
modifying effect of physical fitness
Int J Sports Med **6,** 131-135
Acute exercise, Adult, Androgens,
Comparative, Intervention, LH, Male,
Occupational activity

630/14   **Rogol, A.D., Veldhuis, J.D. &**
Williams, F.T.   (1984)
Pulsatile secretion of gonadotropins and
prolactin in endurance-trained men:
relation to the endogenous opiate system
J Androl **5,** 21
Adult, Endorphins, Leisure activity, Male

630/15   **Semmens, J.B., Rouse, I.L., Beilin,**
L.J. & Masarei, J.R.   (1983)
Relationships between age, body weight,
physical fitness and sex-hormone-
binding globulin capacity
Clin Chim Acta **133,** 295-300
Adult, Androgens, Comparative,
Endocrine, Female, Leisure activity,
LIPIDS, Male, Oestrogens, Weight

630/16   **Webb, M.L., Wallace, J.P., Hamill,**
C., Hodgson, J.L. & Mashaly,
M.M.   (1984)
Serum testosterone concentration during
two hours of moderate intensity treadmill
running in trained men and women
Endocr Res **10,** 27-38
Acute exercise, Adult, AEROBIC
CAPACITY, ANAEROBIC
CAPACITY, Androgens, Comparative,
Female, Male, Running

630/17   **Weiss, L.W., Cureton, K.J. &**
Thompson, F.N.   (1983)
Comparison of serum testosterone and
androstenedione responses to
weightlifting in men and women
Eur J Appl Physiol **50,** 413-419
Acute exercise, Adult, Androgens,
Comparative, Endocrine, Female, Male,
MUSCLE STRENGTH

610/18   **Wyshak, G., Frisch, R.E., Albright,**
N.L. & Schiff, I.   (1986)
Lower prevalence of benign diseases of
the breast and benign tumours of the
reproductive system among former
college athletes compared to non-athletes
Br J Cancer **54,** 841-845
Adult, Athlete, Cancer, Comparative,
Leisure activity, Vigorous

630/19   **Zonderland, M.L., Erich, W.B. &**
Peltenburg, A.L.   (1986)
Plasma lipoprotein profile in relation to
sex hormones in premenarcheal athletes
Int J Sports Med **7,** 241-245
Children, Comparative, LH, LIPIDS,
Menarche

KEYWORDS are listed in the appendix in addition the following specific keywords have been used in this section:

Bladder
Incontinence
Sexual function
Vagina

Summary of evidence: ameliorates stress incontinence in older women and cures or prevents stress incontinence following pregnancy or hysterectomy

THE PROBLEM

Urinary incontinence is a distressing problem which is common in elderly women. Does exercise of the pelvic floor muscles improve bladder control?

SCOPE

This section contains references on changes produced by pelvic floor exercises in stress incontinence in middle-aged and older women.

METHODOLOGICAL DIFFICULTIES

There are rather few well-controlled studies.

EVIDENCE

It is clear that improvements in bladder function can be obtained in some patients with exercise which strengthens the muscles of the pelvic floor. Such exercises may provide a prophylactic effect against the later development of incontinence especially for parous women or those who have had hysterectomies.

640/1   **Burgio, K.L., Robinson, J.C. & Engel, B.T.**   (1986)
The role of biofeedback in Kegel exercise training for stress urinary incontinence
Am J Obstet Gynecol **154**, 58-64
Adult, Bladder, Exercise programme, Female, Incontinence, Intervention, Vagina

640/2   **Castleden, C.M., Duffin, H.M. & Mitchell, E.P.**   (1984)
The effect of physiotherapy on stress incontinence
Age Ageing **13**, 235-237
Bladder, Elderly, Exercise programme, Female, Incontinence, Intervention

640/3   **Henderson, J.S.**   (1987)
Age as a variable in an exercise program for the treatment of simple urinary stress incontinence
J Obstet Gynecol Neonatal Nurs **16**, 266-272
Adult, Bladder, Exercise programme, Incontinence, Intervention

640/4   **Hendrickson, L.S.**   (1981)
The frequency of stress incontinence in women before and after the implementation of an exercise program
Issues Health Care Women **3**, 81-92
Adult, Bladder, Exercise programme, Female, Incontinence, Intervention

640/5   **Kujansuu, E.**   (1983)
The effect of pelvic floor exercise on urethral function in female stress urinary incontinence: an urodynamic study
Ann Chir Gynaecol **72**, 28-32
Adult, Bladder, Exercise programme, Female, Incontinence, Intervention

640/6   **Maly, B.J.**   (1980)
Rehabilitation principles in the care of
gynecologic and obstetric patients
Arch Phys Med Rehabil **61**, 78-81
Adult, Bladder, Exercise programme,
Female, Incontinence, PREGNANCY,
Vagina

640/7   **Mohr, J.A., Rogers, J. Jr., Brown,**
T.N. & Starkweather, G.   (1983)
Stress urinary incontinence: a simple and
practical approach to diagnosis and
treatment
J Am Geriatr Soc **31**, 476-478
Bladder, Elderly, Endocrine, Exercise
programme, Female, Incontinence,
Intervention, REPRODUCTIVE
HORMONES, Vagina

640/8   **Montgomery, E. & Shepherd,**
A.M.   (1983)
Electrical stimulation and graded pelvic
exercises for genuine stress incontinence
Physiotherapy **69**, 112
Adult, Bladder, Exercise programme,
Female, Incontinence, Intervention

640/9   **Schule, K.**   (1983)
The rank value of sports and movement
therapy in patients with breast or pelvic
cancer
Rehabilitation (Stuttg) **22**, 36-39
Adult, Cancer, Female, Review

640/10   **Stoddart, G.D.**   (1983)
Research project into the effect of pelvic
floor exercises on genuine stress
incontinence
Physiotherapy **69**, 148-149
Adult, Exercise programme, Female,
Incontinence, Intervention

640/11   **Trudel, G. & Saint-Laurent,**
S.   (1983)
A comparison between the effects of
Kegel's exercises and a combination of
sexual awareness relaxation and
breathing on insituational orgasmic
dysfunction in women
J Sex Marital Ther **9**, 204-209
Adult, Exercise programme, Female,
PERSONALITY, Sexual function,
Vagina

640/12   **Tweedale, P.G.**   (1973)
Gynecological hazards of water skiing
J Can Med Assoc **108**, 20-22
Adult, Bladder, Female, Hazards, Vagina

640/13   **Voigt, R.**   (1985)
Urodynamic results before and after
physiotherapy of women with stress
incontinence
Geburtshilfe Frauenheilkd **45**, 563-566
Adult, Bladder, Exercise programme,
Female, Incontinence, Intervention

640/14   **Williams, J.K., Lake, M. & Ingram,**
J.M.   (1985)
The bicycle seat stool in the treatment of
vaginal agenesis and stenosis
J Obstet Gynecol Neonatal Nurs **14**, 147-
150
Adult, Exercise programme, Female,
Intervention, Sexual function, Vagina

KEYWORDS are listed in the appendix in addition the following specific keywords have been used in this section:

Cognitive performance
Self-concept
Stress
Well-being

Summary of evidence: ameliorates, cures or prevents sub-optimal mental health in some subjects

THE PROBLEM

Does exercise improve mental health by increasing feelings of well-being or by reducing impairment such as anxiety and depression ?

SCOPE

This section contains mainly reviews which summarise often rather speculatively the changes attributed to exercise in various indices of mental health. There are few controlled studies.

METHODOLOGICAL DIFFICULTIES

Mental health is a concept not directly amenable to measurement. Its components are assessed using questionnaire data which is inevitably of low reliability. In addition the many factors other than exercise which affect mental health make controlled studies difficult.

EVIDENCE

Improvements in some indices of mental health have been reported and attributed to exercise, but the mechanism which would confirm a specific exercise effect is not yet clear (see following sections).

710/1　**Andersson, G. & Malmgren, S.**　(1986)
Changes in self-reported experienced health and psychosomatic symptoms in voluntary participants in a 1-year extensive newspaper exercise campaign
Scand J Soc Med **14**, 141-146
Adult, GENERAL HEALTH, Intervention, Leisure activity, SLEEP, Well-being

710/2　**Blumenthal, J.A., Schocken, D.D., Needels, T.L. & Hindle, P.**　(1982)
Psychological and physiological effects of physical conditioning on the elderly
J Psychosom Res **26**, 505-510
Adult, BLOOD PRESSURE, Elderly, Exercise programme, GENERAL HEALTH, Intervention, Self-concept

710/3　**Brown, R.S.**　(1982)
Exercise and mental health in the pediatric population
Clin Sports Med **1**, 515-527
Children, Review

710/4　**deCoverley Veale, D.M.W.**　(1987)
Exercise and mental health
Acta Psychiatr Scand **76**, 113-120
MOOD, PERSONALITY, Review

710/5　**Dishman, R.K., Ickes, W.J. & Morgan, W.P.**　(1980)
Self-motivation and adherence to habitual physical activity
J Appl Soc Psychol **10**, 115-131
Review

710/6　**Fasting, K.**　(1979)
Relationship between physical activity and health. Physical activity in leisuretime seen in relation to some health variables
NORA-rapport **60**,
Review

710/7   **Fasting, K.**   (1982)
Leisure time, physical activity and some
indices of mental health
Scand J Soc Med (Suppl) **29**, 113-119
Review

710/8   **Folkins, C.H. & Sime, W.E.**   (1981)
Physical fitness training and mental
health
Am Psychol **36**, 373-389
MOOD, PERSONALITY, Review

710/9   **Hayes, D. & Ross, C.E.**   (1986)
Body and mind: The effect of exercise,
overweight, and physical health on
psychological well-being
J Health Soc Behav **27**, 387-400
*Adult, CARBOHYDRATE
TOLERANCE, Comparative, Well-being*

710/10   **Howard, J.H., Cunningham, D.A. &
Rechnitzer, P.A.**   (1984)
Physical activity as a moderator of life
events and somatic complaints: a
longitudinal study
Can J Appl Sport Sci **9**, 194-200
*Adult, Male, GENERAL HEALTH,
Leisure activity, Longitudinal, Stress*

710/11   **Hughes, J.R.**   (1984)
Psychological effects of habitual aerobic
exercise: a critical review
Prev Med **13**, 66-78
*Cognitive performance, MOOD,
PERSONALITY, Review*

710/12   **Ingebretsen, R.**   (1982)
The relationship between physical
activity and mental factors in the elderly
Scand J Soc Med (Suppl) **29**, 153-159
*Cognitive performance, Elderly,
PERSONALITY, Review*

710/13   **Morgan, W.P.**   (1985)
Psychogenic factors and exercise
metabolism: A review
Med Sci Sports Exerc **17**, 309-316
Cognitive performance, MOOD, Review

710/14   **Mutrie, N.**   (1987)
The psychological effects of exercise for
women. In: Exercise: Benefits, Limits and
Adaptations. (Eds.) Macleod, D.,
Maughan, R., Nimmo, M., Reilly, T. &
Williams, C.
E. & F. Spon, London 270-288
Female, MOOD, Review

710/15   **Olson, J.M. & Zanna,
M.P.**   (1987)
Understanding and promoting exercise: a
social psychological perspective
Can J Public Health **78**, S1-7
Review

710/16   **Railo, W.S.**   (1982)
The relationship of sport in childhood
and adolescence to mental and social
health
Scand J Soc Med (Suppl) **29**, 135-145
Athlete, Children, Review

710/17   **Reid, R.M. & McGowan, I.**   (1986)
A longitudinal psycho-physiological
study of active and inactive men
Br J Sports Med **7**, 358-362
*Adult, Comparative, Leisure activity,
Male*

710/18   **Sachs, M. & Buffone, G.W.
(Eds.)**   (1984)
Running as Therapy
University of Nebraska Press
Review

710/19   **Shephard, R.J.**   (1983)
Physical activity and the healthy mind
Can Med Assoc J **128**, 525-530
MOOD, Review, Self-concept

710/20   **Szabadi, E.**   (1988)
Physical exercise and mental health
Br Med J **296**, 659-660
Review

710/21 **Taylor, C.B., Sallis, J.F. & Needle, R.** (1985)
The relation of physical activity to mental health
Public Health Reports **100,** 195-202
Review

710/22 **Tuckman, B.W.** (1986)
An experimental study of the physical and psychological effects of aerobic exercise on schoolchildren
Health Psychol **5,** 197-207
Children, Exercise programme, Intervention

KEYWORDS are listed in the appendix in addition the following specific keywords have been used in this section:

> Anxiety
> Body image
> Depression
> Endorphins
> Mental handicap
> Mental illness
> Self-concept
> Stress
> Well-being

Summary of evidence: exercise cures mild depression in some subjects

THE PROBLEM

Mood is a component of mental health which is labile and therefore potentially amenable to the effects of exercise. Does exercise improve mood or reduce depression?

SCOPE

This section contains references dealing with changes produced by exercise in anxiety and depression scales in patients and normal subjects. There are also studies of the effects of exercise on levels of endorphins, catecholamines and cortisol. There are studies of both men and women, all age groups and both active and sedentary groups.

METHODOLOGICAL DIFFICULTIES

Mood is assessed using questionnaire data which is inevitably of low reliability. In addition the many factors other than exercise which affect mood make controlled studies difficult. Methods for assessing low concentrations in plasma of stress hormones and opiate substances such as endorphins are now available but it is not clear how they relate to affective mood.

EVIDENCE

Exercise appears from controlled studies to have a beneficial effect by improving symptoms of depression in those who are slightly depressed. The mechanism is not yet clear; it may be due to the effects of endorphins or arise through the enhancement of feelings of mastery and control.

720/1   **Allen, M.**   (1983)
Activity-generated endorphins: a review of their role in sports science
Can J Appl Sport Sci **8**, 115-133
***Endocrine, Endorphins,
REPRODUCTIVE HORMONES,
Review***

720/2   **Bahrke, M.S.**   (1979)
Exercise, meditation and anxiety reduction: A review
Am Corr Ther J **33**, 41-44
Review

720/3   **Bahrke, M.S. & Morgan, W.P.**   (1978)
Anxiety reduction following exercise and meditation
Cog Ther Res **2**, 323-333
Acute exercise, Adult, Anxiety, Comparative, Inactivity,

720/4   **Bennett, J., Carmack, M.A. & Gardner, V.**   (1982)
The effect of a program of physical exercise on depression in older adults
Physical Educator **39**, 21-24
Depression, Elderly, Exercise programme, Intervention

720/5 **Berger, B.G. & Owen, D.R.** (1983)
Mood alterations with swimming:
swimmers really do 'feel better'
Psychomat Med **45**, 425-433
*Adult, Anxiety, Depression, Exercise
programme, Female, Intervention, Male,
Swimming*

720/6 **Birkui, P., Gianfrancesco, R. & di
Lesigne, C.L.** (1976)
Preliminary psychological survey in the
study of cardiac rehabilitation through
controlled physical activity
Sem Hop Paris **52**, 2291-2294
*Adult, Exercise programme, Intervention,
SECONDARY PREVENTION*

720/7 **Blumenthal, J.A., O'Toole, L.C. &
Chang, J.L.** (1984)
Is running an analogue of anorexia
nervosa? An empirical study of
obligatory running and anorexia nervosa
J Am Med Ass **252**, 520-523
*Adult, Anxiety, Depression, Hazards,
Mental illness, Running*

720/8 **Brown, J.D. & Lawton, M.** (1986)
Stress and well-being in adolescence: the
moderating role of physical exercise
J Human Stress **12**, 125-131
*Children, Depression, Female,
GENERAL HEALTH, Leisure activity,
Stress, Well-being*

720/9 **Bruning, N.S. & Frew, D.R.** (1987)
Effects of exercise, relaxation and
management skills training on
physiological stress: indicators: a field
experiment
J Appl Psychol **72**, 515-521
*Adult, Exercise programme, Intervention,
Stress*

720/10 **Cameron, O.G. & Hudson,
C.J.** (1986)
Influence of exercise on anxiety level in
patients with anxiety disorders
Psychosomatics **27**, 720-723
*Adult, Exercise programme, Intervention,
Mental illness*

720/11 **Carney, R.M.** (1987)
Exercise training reduces depression and
increases the performance of pleasant
activities in hemodialysis patients
Nephron **47**, 194-198
*Adult, Depression, Exercise programme,
Intervention, Kidney disease*

720/12 **Carney, R.M., McKevitt, P.M.,
Goldberg, A.P., Hagberg, J., Delmez,
J.A. & Harter, H.R.** (1983)
Psychological effects of exercise training
in hemodialysis patients
Nephron **33**, 179-181
*Adult, Exercise programme, Intervention,
Kidney disease*

720/13 **Carney, R.M., Wetzel, R.D.,
Hagberg, J. & Goldberg, A.P.** (1986)
The relationship between depression and
aerobic capacity in hemodialysis patients
Psychosom Med **48**, 143-147
*Adult, AEROBIC CAPACITY, Anxiety,
Depression, Kidney disease*

720/14 **Chastain, P.B. & Shapiro,
G.E.** (1987)
Physical fitness program for patients with
psychiatric disorders
Phys Ther **67**, 545-548
*Adult, Body image, Exercise programme,
Intervention, Mental illness, Self-concept*

720/15 **Cooper, K.H., Gallmon, J.S. &
McDonald, J.L.** (1986)
Role of aerobic exercise in reduction of
stress
Dent Clin North Am **30**, S133-S142
Review, Stress

720/16 **Crews, D.J. & Landers,
D.M.** (1987)
A meta-analytic review of aerobic fitness
and reactivity to psychosocial stressors
Med Sci Sports Exerc **19**, S114-S120
Review, Stress

720/17   de Meirleir, K., Naaktgeboren, N., Van Steirteghem, A., Gorus, F., Olbrecht, J. & Block, P.   (1986)
Beta-endorphin and ACTH levels in peripheral blood during and after aerobic and anaerobic exercise
Eur J Appl Physiol **55,** 5-8
Acute exercise, Adult, ANAEROBIC CAPACITY, Anxiety, Endocrine, Endorphins, Male

720/18   Dearman, J. & Francis, K.T.   (1983)
Plasma levels of catecholamines, cortisol, and beta-endorphins in male athletes after running 26.2, 6, and 2 miles
J Sports Med Phys Fitness **23,** 30-38
Acute exercise, Adult, Athlete, Endocrine, Endorphins, Leisure activity, Marathon, Running

720/19   Dorinsky, N.L.   (1984)
The effects of a regular aerobic exercise program on selected measures of the stress response
Health Care Women Int **5,** 459-462
Adult, Exercise programme, Female, Intervention, Stress

720/20   Doyne, E.J., Chambless, D.L. & Bentler, L.E.   (1983)
Aerobic exercise as a treatment for depression in women
Behav Ther **14,** 434-440
Adult, Depression, Exercise programme, Female, Intervention, Mental illness

720/21   Eide, R.   (1982)
The effect of physical activity on emotional reactions, stress reactions and related physiological reactions
Scand J Soc Med (Suppl) **29,** 103-107
Stress, Review

720/22   Elias, A.N., Iyer, K., Pandian, M.R., Weathersbee, P., Stone, S. & Tobis, J.   (1986)
Beta-endorphin/beta-lipotropin release and gonadotropin secretion after acute exercise in normal males
J Appl Physiol **61,** 2045-2049
Acute exercise, Adult, Endocrine, Endorphins, Male, REPRODUCTIVE HORMONES

720/23   Elliot, D.L., Goldberg, L., Watts, W.J. & Orwoll, E.   (1984)
Resistance exercise and plasma beta-endorphin/beta-lipotrophinimmunoreactivity
Life Sci **34,** 515-518
Adult, Endocrine, Endorphins, Exercise programme, Intervention, MUSCLE STRENGTH

720/24   Englund, C.E., Naitoh, P., Ryman, D. & Hodgdon, J.A.   (1983)
Moderate physical work effect on performance and mood during sustained operations
Naval Health Research Center Report, San Diego, CA 83-86
Acute exercise, Adult, Depression, Occupational activity

720/25   Farrell, P.A.   (1985)
Exercise and endorphins-male responses
Med Sci Sports Exerc **17,** 89-93
Endorphins, Male, PAIN, PERCEIVED EXERTION, Review

720/26   Farrell, P.A., Gates, W.K., Maksud, M.G. & Morgan, W.P.   (1982)
Increases in plasma beta-endorphin/beta-lipotropin immunoreactivity after treadmill running in humans
J. Appl Physiol **52,** 1245-1249
Acute exercise, Adult, AEROBIC CAPACITY, Anxiety, Depression, Endorphins, PERCEIVED EXERTION, Running

720/27 **Farrell, P.A., Gusttafson, A.B., Garthwaite, T.L., Kalkhoff, R.K., Cowley, A.W. Jr. & Morgan, W.P.** (1986)
Influence of endogenous opioids on the response of selected hormones to exercise in humans
J Appl Physiol **61**, 1051-1057
Acute exercise, Adult, Anxiety, Endocrine, Endorphins, Male

720/28 **Finocchiaro, M.S. & Schmitz, C.L.** (1984)
Exercise: a holistic approach for the treatment of the adolescent psychiatric patient
Issues Ment Health Nurs **6**, 237-243
Children, Depression, Exercise programme, Female, Intervention, Mental illness

720/29 **Folkins, C.** (1976)
Effects of physical training on mood
J Clin Psych **32**, 385-389
Adult, AEROBIC CAPACITY, Anxiety, Body image, Depression, Exercise programme, Intervention, Male, SECONDARY PREVENTION, Self-concept

720/30 **Folkins, C., Lynch, S. & Gardner, M.** (1972)
Psychological fitness as a function of physical fitness
Arch Phys Med Rehabil **53**, 503-508
Adult, Anxiety, Depression, Exercise programme, Female, Intervention, Male, Running, Self-concept

720/31 **Gentry, W.D. & Stewart, M.A.** (1985)
Psychologic effects of exercise training in coronary-prone individuals and in patients with symptomatic coronary heart disease. In: Exercise and the Heart, 2nd edition (Ed.) Brest, A.N
Cardiovascular Clinics, F.A.Davis Company, Philadelphia **15**, 255-260
Review, SECONDARY PREVENTION

720/32 **Goldwater, B.C. & Collis, M.L,** (1985)
Psychologic effects of cardiovascular conditioning: a controlled experiment
Psychosom Med **47**, 174-181
Adult, Anxiety, Exercise programme, Intervention, Male

720/33 **Gorbachenkov, A. A.** (1986)
Effect of a short course of physical training on the mental status of post-myocardial infarct patients
Kardiologiia **26**, 79-82
Adult, Depression, Exercise programme, Intervention SECONDARY PREVENTION

720/34 **Greist, J.H., Klein, M.H., Eischens, R.R., Faris, J., Gurman, A.S. & Morgan, W.P.** (1979)
Running as treatment for depression
Comp Psychiatry **20**, 41-54
Adult, Depression, Exercise programme, Intervention, Mental illness, Running

720/35 **Grossman, A., Bouloux, P., Price, P., Drury, P.L., Lam, K.S., Turner, T., Thomas, J., Besser, G.M. & Sutton, J.R.** (1984)
The role of opioid peptides in the hormonal responses to acute exercise in man
Clin Sci **67**, 483-491
Acute exercise, Adult, Endocrine, Endorphins, Male, PERCEIVED EXERTION, REPRODUCTIVE HORMONES, RESPIRATORY FUNCTION, Vigorous

720/36 **Grossman, A. & Sutton, J.R.** (1985)
Endorphins: what are they? How are they measured? What is their role in exercise?
Med Sci Sports Exerc **17**, 74-81
Endorphins, Review

720/37   Gurley, V., Neuringer, A. &
Massee, J.   (1984)
Dance and sports compared: effects on
psychological well-being
J Sports Med Phys Fitness **24**, 58-68
*Adult, Anxiety, Comparative, Depression,
Leisure activity, Self-concept*

720/38   Hales, R.E. & Travis, T.W.   (1987)
Exercise as a treatment option for anxiety
and depressive disorders
Milit Med **152**, 299-302
*Adult, Anxiety, Depression, Exercise
programme, Intervention, Mental illness*

720/39   Hartz, G.W., Wallace, W.L. &
Cayton, T.G.   (1982)
Effect of aerobic conditioning upon
mood in clinically depressed men and
women: a preliminary investigation
Percept Mot Skills **55**, 1217-1218
*Adult, Depression, Exercise programme,
Female, Intervention, Male, Mental illness*

720/40   Hatfield, B.D., Goldfarb, A.H.,
Sforzo, G.A. & Flynn, M.G.   (1987)
Serum beta-endorphin and affective
responses to graded exercise in young and
elderly men
J Gerontol **42**, 429-431
*Acute exercise, Adult, AEROBIC
CAPACITY, Anxiety, Comparative,
Depression, Elderly, Endorphins*

720/41   Hayden, R.M. & Allen,
G.J.   (1984)
Relationship between aerobic exercise,
anxiety, and depression: convergent
validation by knowledgeable informants
J Sports Med Phys Fitness **24**, 69-74
*Adult, Anxiety, Depression, Exercise
programme, Intervention, Running, Self-
concept*

720/42   Hayden, R.M., Allen, G.J. &
Camaione, D.N.   (1986)
Some psychological benefits resulting
from involvement in an aerobic fitness
from the perspectives of participants and
knowledgeable informants
J Sports Med Phys Fitness **26**, 67-76
*Adult, AEROBIC CAPACITY, Exercise
programme, Intervention*

720/43   Holmes, D.S. & Roth, D.L.   (1985)
Association of aerobic fitness with pulse
rate and subjective responses to
psychological stress
Psychophysiology **22**, 525-529
*Adult, AEROBIC CAPACITY,
Comparative, Female, Leisure activity,
Stress*

720/44   Howley, E.T.   (1976)
The effect of different intensities of
exercise on the excretion of epinephrine
and norepinephrine
Med Sci Sports **8**, 219-222
*Acute exercise, Adult, AEROBIC
CAPACITY, Endocrine, Male, Stress*

720/45   Hughes, J.R., Casal, D.C. & Leon,
A.S.   (1986)
Psychological effect of exercise: A
randomized cross-over trial
J Psychosom Res **30**, 355-360
*Adult, Depression, Exercise programme,
Intervention, Male*

720/46   Jamieson, J.L., Evans, J.F. & Cox,
J.P.   (1983)
Aerobic fitness and emotional arousal: a
further response to Zimmerman and
Fulton
Percept Mot Skills **56**, 250
Review

720/47   Kavanagh, T.   (1984)
Distance running and cardiac
rehabilitation: physiologic and
psychosocial considerations
Clin Sports Med **3**, 513-526
Review, SECONDARY PREVENTION

720/48   **Keller, S.**   (1980)
Physical fitness hastens recovery from
emotional stress
Med Sci Sports Exerc **12**, 118
Adult, Exercise programme, Intervention,
Stress

720/49   **Knuttgen, H.G., Vogel, J.A. &**
Portman, J. (Eds.)   (1983)
Biochemistry of exercise
Human Kinetics Publishers
Review

720/50   **Kowal, D.M., Patton, J.F. & Vogel,**
J.A.   (1978)
Psychological states and aerobic fitness
of male and female recruits before and
after basic training
Aviat Space Environ Med **49**, 603-606
Adult, Anxiety, Body composition,
Depression, Female, Male, Occupational
activity, Self-concept

720/51   **Kraemer, W.J., Noble, B., Culver,**
B. & Lewis, R.V.   (1985)
Changes in plasma proenkephalin
peptide F and catecholamine levels
during graded exercise in men
Proc Natl Acad Sci USA **82**, 6349-6351
Acute exercise, Adult, AEROBIC
CAPACITY, Comparative, Endocrine,
Endorphins, Leisure activity

720/52   **Lake, B.W., Suarez, E.C.,**
Schneiderman, N. & Tocci, N.   (1985)
The type A behavior pattern, physical
fitness, and psychophysiological
reactivity
Health Psychol **4**, 169-187
Adult, AEROBIC CAPACITY, Athlete,
BLOOD PRESSURE, Comparative,
Leisure activity, Male, PERSONALITY,
Stress

720/53   **Leste, A. & Rust, J.**   (1984)
Effects of dance on anxiety
Percept Mot Skills **58**, 767-772
Adult, Anxiety, Exercise programme,
Intervention

720/54   **Lobitz, W.C., Brammell, H.L. &**
Stoll, S.   (1983)
Physical exercise and anxiety
management training for cardiac stress
management in a nonpatient population
J Cardiac Rehabil **3**, 683-688
Adult, Anxiety, Exercise programme,
Intervention, PRIMARY
PREVENTION

720/55   **Lobstein, D.D., Mosbacher, B.J. &**
Ismail, A.H.   (1983)
Depression as a powerful discriminator
between physically active and sedentary
middle-aged men
J Psychosom Res **27**, 69-76
Adult, Comparative, Depression, Leisure
activity, Male

720/56   **MacDonald, M.R., Nielsen, W.R. &**
Cameron, M.G.P.   (1987)
Depression and activity patterns of spinal
cord injured persons living in the
community
Arch Phys Med Rehabil **68**, 339-343
Adult, Comparative, Customary activity,
Depression, Handicap

720/57   **Markoff, R.A., Ryan, P. & Young,**
T.   (1982)
Endorphins and moods changes in long
distance running
Med Sci Sports Exerc **14**, 11-15
Acute exercise, Adult, Anxiety,
Depression, Endorphins, Running

720/58   **Martinsen, E.W., Medhus, A. &**
Sandvik, L.   (1985)
Effects of aerobic exercise on depression:
a controlled study
Br Med J **291**, 109
Adult, AEROBIC CAPACITY,
Depression, Exercise programme,
Intervention, Mental illness

720/59   McCann, I.L. & Holmes, D.S.   (1984)
Influence of aerobic exercise on depression
J Pers Soc Psychol **46**, 1142-1147
Adult, Depression, Exercise programme, Intervention

720/60   McGlynn, G.H., Franklin, B., Lauro, G. & McGlynn, I.K.   (1983)
The effect of aerobic conditioning and induced stress on state-traitanxiety, blood pressure, and muscle tension
J Sports Med Phys Fitness **23**, 341-351
Adult, Anxiety, BLOOD PRESSURE, Comparative, Leisure activity, Stress

720/61   Mellion, M.B.   (1985)
Exercise therapy for anxiety and depression. 2. What are the specific considerations for clinical application?
Postgraduate Med **77**, 91-98
Anxiety, Depression, Endorphins, Review

720/62   Mobily, K.   (1982)
Using physical activity and recreation to cope with stress and anxiety: a review
Am Corr Ther J **36**, 77-81
Anxiety, Review, Stress

720/63   Morgan, W.P.   (1985)
Affective beneficence of vigorous physical activity
Med Sci Sports Exerc **17**, 94-100
Endorphins, Review

720/64   Mougin, C., Baulay, A., Henriet, M.T., Haton, D., Jacquiere, M.C., Tournill, D., Berthelay, S. & Gaillard, R.C.   (1987)
Assessment of plasma opiod peptides beta-endorphin and met-enkephalin at the end of an international nordic ski race
Eur J Appl Physiol **56**, 281-286
Acute exercise, Adult, Endocrine, Endorphins, Leisure activity, Male

720/65   Oltras, C.M., Mora, F. & Vives, F.   (1987)
Beta-endorphin and ACTH in plasma: Effects of physical and psychological stress
Life Sci **40**, 1683-1686
Acute exercise, Adult, Athlete, Endocrine, Endorphins, Male, Stress

720/66   Peronnet, F., Blier, P., Brisson, G., Diamond, P., Ledoux, M. & Volle, M.   (1986)
Plasma catecholamines at rest and exercise in subjects with high- and low-trait anxiety
Psychosom Med **48**, 52-58
Acute exercise, Adult, Anxiety, Comparative, Endocrine, Male

720/67   Raglin, J.S. & Morgan, W.P.   (1987)
Influence of exercise and quiet rest on state anxiety and blood pressure
Med Sci Sports Exerc **56**, 699-703
Acute exercise, Adult, Anxiety, BLOOD PRESSURE, Male

720/68   Rahkila, P., Hakala, E., Salminen, K. & Laatikainen, T.   (1987)
Response of plasma endorphins to running exercises in male and female endurance athletes
Med Sci Sports Exerc **19**, 451-455
Acute exercise, Adult, AEROBIC CAPACITY, Athlete, Endocrine, Endorphins, Female, Male

720/69   Ransford, C.P.   (1982)
A role for amines in the antidepressant effect of exercise: a review
Med Sci Sports Exer **14**, 1-10
Depression, Endocrine, Review

720/70   Ross, C.E. & Hayes, D.   (1988)
Exercise and psychologic well-being in the community
Am J Epidemiol **127**, 762-771
Adult, Anxiety, Depression, Female, GENERAL HEALTH, Leisure activity, Male

720/71   **Roth, D.L. & Holmes, D.S.**   (1985)
Influence of physical fitness in
determining the impact of stressful life
events on physical and psychologic health
Psychosom Med **47**, 164-173
Adult, AEROBIC CAPACITY,
Depression, GENERAL HEALTH,
Stress

720/72   **Roth, D.L. & Holmes, D.S.**   (1987)
Influence of aerobic training and
relaxation training on physical and
psychologic health following stressful life
events
Psychosom Med **49**, 355-365
Adult, Depression, Exercise programme,
Female, GENERAL HEALTH,
Inactivity, Intervention, Male, Stress

720/73   **Sanderson, F.H. & Reilly,**
T.   (1983)
Trait and state anxiety in male and female
cross-country runners
Br J Sports Med **17**, 24-26
Acute exercise, Adult, Anxiety, Athlete,
Female, Male, Running

720/74   **Schwartz, G.E., Davidson, R.J. &**
Goleman, D.J.   (1978)
Patterning of cognitive and somatic
processes in the self regulation of anxiety:
effects of meditation versus exercise
Psychosom Med **40**, 321-328
Adult, Anxiety, Comparative, Exercise
programme, Inactivity, Intervention

720/75   **Shephard, R.J., Kavanagh,T. &**
Klavora, P.   (1985)
Mood-state during post-coronary
cardiac rehabilitation
J Cardiac Rehabil **5**, 480-484
Adult, Anxiety, Depression, Exercise
programme, Intervention, SECONDARY
PREVENTION

720/76   **Shulhan, D., Scher, H. & Furedy,**
J.J.   (1986)
Phasic cardiac reactivity to psychological
stress as a function of aerobic fitness level
Psychophysiology **23**, 562-566
Adult, AEROBIC CAPACITY,
Comparative, HEART FUNCTION
TEST, Male, Stress

720/77   **Shyu, B.C.**   (1986)
Endorphin mechanisms and physical
exercise
University of Göteborg 1-66
Endorphins, Review

720/78   **Simons, C.W. & Birkimer,**
J.C.   (1988)
An exploration of factors predicting the
effects of aerobic conditioning on mood
state
J Psychosom Res **32**, 63-75
Adult, Anxiety, Depression, Exercise
programme, Intervention

720/79   **Sinyor, D., Golden, M., Steinert, Y.**
& Seraganian, P.   (1986)
Experimental manipulation of aerobic
fitness and the response to psychosocial
stress: heart rate and self-report measures
Psychosom Med **48**, 324-337
Adult, Exercise programme, Intervention,
Male, MUSCLE STRENGTH, Stress

720/80   **Sinyor, D., Schwartz, S.G.,**
Peronnet, F., Brisson, G. & Seraganian,
P.   (1983)
Aerobic fitness level and reactivity to
psychosocial stress: physiological,
biochemical, and subjective measures
Psychosom Med **45**, 205-217
Adult, AEROBIC CAPACITY, Anxiety,
Comparative, Endocrine, Male, Stress

720/81   **Sothmann, M.S. & Ismail, A.H.**   (1985)
Factor analytic derivation of the MHPG/ NM ratio: implications for studying the link between physical fitness and depression
Biol Psychiatry **20**, 579-583
Adult, AEROBIC CAPACITY, Comparative, Endocrine, Occupational activity

720/82   **Steinberg, H. & Sykes. E.A.**   (1985)
Introduction to symposium on endorphins and behavioural processes; review of literature on endorphins and exercise
Pharmacol Biochem Behav **23**, 857-862
Endorphins, Review

720/83   **Stern, M.J. & Cleary, P.**   (1982)
The national exercise and heart disease project. Long-term psychosocial outcome
Arch Intern Med **142**, 1093-1097
Adult, Anxiety, Depression, Exercise programme, Longitudinal, SECONDARY PREVENTION

720/84   **Stern, M.J., Gorman, P.A. & Kaslow, L.**   (1983)
The group counselling v exercise therapy study. A controlled intervention with subjects following myocardial infarction
Arch Intern Med **143**, 1719-1725
Adult, Depression, Exercise programme, Intervention, SECONDARY PREVENTION

720/85   **Taylor, C.B., Houston-Miller, N., Ahn, D.K., Haskell, W. & DeBusk, R.F.**   (1986)
The effects of exercise training programs on psychosocial improvement in uncomplicated myocardial infarction
J Psychosom Res **30**, 581-587
Adult, Anxiety, Depression, Exercise programme, Intervention, Male, SECONDARY PREVENTION

720/86   **Tucker, L.A., Cole, G.E. & Friedman, G.M.**   (1986)
Physical fitness: a buffer against stress
Percept Mot Skills **63**, 955-961
Adult, Comparative, Leisure activity, Male, MUSCLE STRENGTH, Stress

720/87   **Viswanathan, M., Van Dijk, J.P., Graham, T.E., Bonen, A. & George, J.C.**   (1987)
Exercise- and cold-induced changes in plasma beta-endorphin and beta-lipoprotein in men and women
J Appl Physiol **62**, 622-627
Acute exercise, Adult, AEROBIC CAPACITY, Endorphins, Female, Male, MENSTRUAL FUNCTION

720/88   **Weiss, C.R.**   (1987)
Affective aspects of an age-integrated water exercise program
Gerontologist **27**, 430-433
Depression, Elderly, Exercise programme, Intervention

720/89   **Wildmann, J., Kruger, A., Schmole, M., Niemann, J. & Matthaei, H.**   (1986)
Increase of circulating beta-endorphin-like immunoreactivity correlates with the change in feeling of pleasantness after running
Life Sci **38**, 997-1003
Acute exercise, Adult, Endocrine, Endorphins, Male, Running

720/90   **Williams, J.M. & Getty, D.**   (1986)
Effect of levels of exercise on psychological mood states, physical fitness, and plasma beta-endorphin
Percept Mot Skills **63**, 1099-1105
Adult, Depression, Endorphins, Exercise programme, Intervention, Mental illness

720/91   **Zaitsev, V.P., Aronov, D.M.,
Belaia, N.A., Alexseev, P.A. & Panina,
G.A.**   (1975)
Effect of intensive physical training on
the mental condition of patients after
myocardial infarct
Ter Arkh **47**, 59-64
*Adult, Depression, Exercise programme,
Intervention, SECONDARY
PREVENTION, Vigorous*

720/92   **Zimmerman, J.D. & Fulton,
M.**   (1982)
Aerobic fitness and emotional arousal: a
reply to Jamieson, Evans, and Cox
Percept Mot Skills **55**, 1301-1302
Review

730 PERSONALITY, BEHAVIOUR & COGNITIVE FUNCTION

KEYWORDS are listed in the appendix in addition the following specific keywords have been used in this section:

> Anxiety
> Behaviour
> Body image
> Cognitive performance
> Depression
> Learning
> Mental handicap
> Mental illness
> Personality (for personality tests)
> Self-concept
> Stress
> Well-being

Summary of evidence: exercise ameliorates low self-concept and poor cognitive function

THE PROBLEM

Does exercise have its alleged beneficial effects on mental health through improving self-concept or cognitive function ? Does it optimise the learning capabilities and mental development of handicapped children? Does it preserve mental function in old age ?

SCOPE

This section contains references dealing with changes produced by exercise in various aspects of personality, self-concept and cognitive functions such as learning and memory. There are studies of normal and mentally handicapped subjects, of males and females, all age groups and both sedentary and active groups.

METHODOLOGICAL DIFFICULTIES

These aspects of mental health are assessed using questionnaire data which is inevitably of low reliability. In addition the many factors other than exercise which affect them make it difficult to mount controlled studies in which a specific effect of exercise can be determined. The non-specific effects of attention from the observer or mental activity during the exercise may be causing the observed improvements.

EVIDENCE

Exercise is probably of benefit in optimising development in handicapped children who tend to have sedentary lifestyles. It appears to have a normalising effect on mental function in those who are very inactive because of various health problems. It also appears to improve personality factors such as self-concept in those with low initial values. In the elderly it has been shown to improve cognitive function including memory. The evidence is tentative as yet.

730/1 **Abood, D.A.** (1984)
The effects of acute physical exercise on the state anxiety and mental performance of college women
Am Corr Ther J **38**, 69-74
Acute exercise, Adult, Anxiety, Cognitive performance, Female

730/2 **Anderson, S.C. & Allen, L.R.** (1985)
Effects of a recreation therapy program on activity involvement and social interaction of mentally-retarded persons
Behav Res Ther **23**, 473-477
Adult, Behaviour, Exercise programme, Intervention, Mental handicap

730/3   **Balogun, J.A.**   (1986)
Muscular strength as a predictor of
personality in adult females
J Sports Med Phys Fitness **26**, 377-383
Adult, Female, MUSCLE STRENGTH,
Personality, Self-concept

730/4   **Bass, C.K.**   (1985)
Running can modify classroom behavior
J Learn Disabil **18**, 160-161
Children, Behaviour, Exercise
programme, Intervention, Learning,
Personality, Running

730/5   **Baumeister, A.A. & MacLean, W.E.**
Jr   (1984)
Deceleration of self-injurious and
stereotypic responding by exercise
Appl Res Ment Retard **5**, 385-393
Adult, Behaviour, Exercise programme,
Intervention, Male, Mental handicap

730/6   **Bennett, B.L., Schlichting, C.L. &**
Bondi, K.R.   (1985)
Cardiorespiratory fitness and cognitive
performance before and after
confinement in a nuclear submarine
Aviat Space Environ Med **56**, 1085-1091
Adult, AEROBIC CAPACITY,
ANAEROBIC CAPACITY, Cognitive
performance, Exercise programme,
Inactivity, Intervention, Male, Vigorous

730/7   **Blomquist, K.B. & Danner,**
F.   (1987)
Effect of physical conditioning on
information-processing efficiency
Percept Mot Skills **65**, 175-186
Adult, AEROBIC CAPACITY, Cognitive
performance, Exercise programme,
Intervention

730/8   **Buccola, V.A. & Stone,**
W.J.   (1975)
Effects of jogging and cycling programs
on physiological and personality
variables in aged men
Res Quart Am Assoc Health Phys Ed Rec
46, 134-139
AEROBIC CAPACITY, BLOOD
PRESSURE, Body composition,
Comparative, Cycling, Elderly, Exercise
programme, Intervention, JOINTS,
Male, Personality, Self-concept

730/9   **Chasey, W.C., Swartz, J.D. &**
Chasey, C.G.   (1974)
Effect of motor development on body
image scores for institutionalized
mentally retarded children
Am J Ment Deficiency **78**, 440-445
Body image, Children, Exercise
programme, Mental handicap

730/10   **Clark, B.A., Wade, M.G., Massey,**
B.H. & Van Dyke,R.   (1975)
Response of institutionalized geriatric
mental patients to a twelve-week
program of regular physical activity
J Gerontol **30**, 565-573
Cognitive performance, Elderly, Exercise
programme, Intervention, Mental illness

730/11   **Corder, W.O.**   (1966)
Effects of physical education on the
intellectual, physical and social
development of educable mentally
retarded boys
Exceptional Children **32**, 357-364
Behaviour, Children, Exercise
programme, Intervention, Learning,
Mental handicap

730/12   **Del Rey, P.**   (1982)
Effects of contextual interference on the
memory of older females differing in
levels of physical activity
Percept Mot Skills **55**, 171-180
Cognitive performance, Comparative,
Elderly, Female, Leisure activity

730/13 **Dickinson, J. & Perkins, D.** (1985)
Socialization into physical activity for disabled populations
C A H P E R J Nov-Dec, 4-12
Review, Self-concept

730/14 **Diem, L.** (1980)
Report of a longitudinal study of the effect of early motor stimulation on the personality development of children
Scottish J Phys Ed **8**, 16-19
Children, Cognitive performance, Exercise programme, Longitudinal, Personality, PSYCHOMOTOR PERFORMANCE, Swimming

730/15 **Diesfeldt, H.F.A. & Diesfeldt-Groenendijk, H.** (1977)
Improving cognitive performance in psycho-geriatric patients; the influence of physical exercise
Age and Ageing **6**, 58-64
Cognitive performance, Elderly, Exercise programme, Intervention, Mental illness

730/16 **Docherty, D. & Boyd, D.G.** (1982)
Relationship of disembedding ability to performance in volleyball, tennis, and badminton
Percept Mot Skills **54**, 1219-1224
Children, Cognitive performance, Comparative, Leisure activity

730/17 **Dresen, M.H.W.** (1985)
Effects of physical training program on aerobic energy expenditure, body composition and on class-room attention of handicapped children 8 to 14 years old. In: Proceedings of the workshop on disabled and sports (Eds) Hoeberigs, J.H. & Vorsteveld, H.
Velhoven, The Netherlands 37-43
Behaviour, Body composition, Children, Exercise programme, Intervention, Learning

730/18 **Eickhoff, J., Thorland, W. & Ansorge, C.** (1983)
Selected physiological and psychological effects of aerobic dancing among young adult women
J Sports Med Phys Fitness **23**, 273-278
Adult, Body composition, Exercise programme, Female, Intervention, Self-concept

730/19 **Eide, R.** (1982)
The relationship between body image, self-image and physical activity
Scand J Soc Med (Suppl) **29**, 109-112
Body image, Review, Self-concept

730/20 **Estok, P.J. & Rudy, E.B.** (1986)
Physical, psychosocial, menstrual changes/risks and addiction in the female marathon runner
Health Care Women Int **7**, 187-202
Adult, Anxiety, Female, Hazards, Leisure activity, Mental illness, MENSTRUAL FUNCTION, MOOD, Personality, Running, Self-concept, Vigorous

730/21 **Ewart, C.K., Stewart, K.J., Gillilan R.E. & Kelemen, M.H.** (1986)
Self-efficacy mediates strength gains during circuit weight training in men with coronary artery disease
Med Sci Sports Exerc **18**, 531-540
Adult, Intervention, Leisure activity, Male, MUSCLE STRENGTH, SECONDARY PREVENTION

730/22 **Fox, R., Burkhart, J.E. & Rotatori, A.F.** (1984)
Physical fitness and personality characteristics of obese and nonobese retarded adults
Int J Obes **8**, 61-67
Adult, Comparative, ENERGY BALANCE, Mental handicap, Personality, Self-concept

730/23   **Gary, V. & Guthrie, D.**   (1972)
The effect of jogging on physical fitness
and self-concept in hospitalized alcholics
Quart J Stud Alchol **33,** 1073-1078
*Adult, Body image, Intervention, Male,
Mental illness, Running, Self-concept*

730/24   **George, L.K.**   (1978)
The impact of personality and social
status factors upon levels of activity and
psychological well-being
J Gerontol **33,** 840-847
*Adult, Leisure activity, Personality, Well-
being*

730/25   **Godin, G. & Shephard,
R.J.**   (1985)
Gender differences in perceived physical
self-efficacy among older individuals
Percept Mot Skills **60,** 599-602
*Adult, Elderly, Female, Male, Self-
concept*

730/26   **Goldberg, G. & Shephard,
R.J.**   (1982)
Personality profiles of disabled
individuals in relation to physical activity
patterns
J Sports Med Phys Fitness **22,** 477-484
*Adult, Comparative, Handicap,
Personality*

730/27   **Goldfarb, L.A. & Plante,
T.G..**   (1984)
Fear of fat in runners: an examination of
the connection between anorexia nervosa
and distance running
Psychol Rep **55,** 296
*Adult, Hazards, Leisure activity, Mental
illness, Personality, Running*

730/28   **Gondola, J.C. & Tuckman,
B.W.**   (1985)
Effects of a systematic program of
exercise on selected measures of creativity
Percept Mot Skills **60,** 53-54
*Adult, Cognitive performance, Exercise
programme, Intervention, Running*

730/29   **Hatfield, B.D., Vaccaro, P. &
Benedict, G.J.**   (1985)
Self-concept responses of children to
participation in an eight-week precision
jump-rope program
Percept Mot Skills **61,** 1275-1279
*Body composition, Children, Exercise
programme, Intervention, Self-concept*

730/30   **Hendry, J. & Kerr, R.**   (1983)
Communication through physical
activity for learning disabled children
Percept Mot Skills **56,** 155-158
*Body image, Children, Cognitive
performance, Exercise programme,
Intervention, Learning, Mental handicap*

730/31   **Hilyer, J. & Mitchell, W.**   (1979)
Effect of systematic physical fitness
training combined with counselling on
the self concept of college students
J Counsel Psychol **26,** 427-436
*Adult, Exercise programme, Intervention,
Self-concept*

730/32   **Hilyer, J., Wilson, D., Dillon, C.,
Caro, L., Jenkins, C., Spencer, W.A.,
Meadows, M.E. & Brookes, W.**   (1982)
Physical fitness training and counselling
as treatment for youthful offenders
J Counsel Psychol **29,** 292-303
*Anxiety, Children, Depression, Exercise
programme, Intervention, Male, Self-
concept*

730/33   **Ismail, A.H. & El-Naggar,
A.M.**   (1981)
Effect of exercise on cognitive processing
in adult men
J Hum Ergol **10,** 83-91
Adult, Cognitive performance, Male

730/34   **Jasnoski, M.L. & Holmes,
D.S.**   (1981)
Influence of initial aerobic fitness,
aerobic training and changes in aerobic
fitness on personality functioning
J Psychosom Res **25,** 553-556
*Adult, Exercise programme, Female,
Intervention, Personality, Self-concept*

730/35   Johnson, S., Berg, K. & Latin,
R.   (1984)
The effect of training frequency of
aerobic dance on oxygen uptake, body
composition and personality
J Sports Med Phys Fitness **24**, 290-298
*Adult, AEROBIC CAPACITY, Body
composition. Exercise programme,
Female, Intervention, Personality,*

730/36   **Kagan, D.M. & Squires,
R.L.**   (1985)
Addictive aspects of physical exercise
J Sports Med Phys Fitness **25**, 227-237
*Adult, Hazards, Leisure activity,
Personality*

730/37   **Kern, L., Koegel, R.L., Dyer, K.,
Blew, P.A. & Fenton, L.R.**   (1982)
The effects of physical exercise on self-
stimulation and appropriate responding
in autistic children
J Autism Dev Disord **12**, 399-419
*Behaviour, Children, Exercise
programme, Intervention, Mental
handicap*

730/38   **Klein, S.A. & Deffenbacher,
J.L.**   (1977)
Relaxation and exercise for hyperactive
impulsive children
Percep Mot Skills **45**, 1159-1162
*Behaviour, Children, Exercise
programme, Intervention*

730/39   **Krementsov, Y.G.**   (1986)
Physical exercise among geriatric patients
in a psychiatric hospital. In: Physical
activity, sports and aging (Ed.) Harris, R.
Center for the Study of Aging, Albany
*Elderly, Exercise programme,
Intervention, Mental illness*

730/40   **Lagomarcino, A., Reid, D.H.,
Ivancic, M.T. & Faw, G.D.**   (1984)
Leisure-dance instruction for severely
and profoundly retarded
persons:teaching an intermediate
community-living skill
J Appl Behav Anal **17**, 71-84
*Adult, Exercise programme, Intervention,
Mental handicap*

730/41   **Leavitt, J.**   (1986)
Modifiability of cognitive functioning
because of physical activity: a review. In:
Physical activity, sports and aging (Ed.)
Harris, R.
Center for the Study of Aging, Albany
Cognitive performance, Review

730/42   **Lichtman, S. & Poser,
E.G.**   (1983)
The effects of exercise on mood and
cognitive functioning
J Psychosom Res **27**, 43-52
*Acute exercise, Adult, Anxiety, Cognitive
performance, MOOD*

730/43   **MacMahon, J.R.**   (1987)
Physical and psychological effects of
aerobic exercise in boys with learning
disabilities
J Dev Behav Pediatr **8**, 274-277
*Behaviour, Children, Exercise
programme, Intervention, Learning, Male*

730/44   **McGlynn, G.H., Laughlin, N.T. &
Rowe, V.**   (1979)
The effect of increasing levels of exercise
on mental performance
Ergonomics **22**, 407-414
*Acute exercise, Adult, Cognitive
performance, Female*

730/45   **McGowan, R.W., Jarman, B.O. &
Pedersen, D.M.**   (1974)
Effects of a competitive endurance
training program on self-concept and
peer approval
J Psychol **86**, 57-60
*Children, Exercise programme,
Intervention, Male, Self-concept*

730/46   **McLeavey, B.C., Corkery, M.B. & Cronin, T.E.** (1984)
The marathon runner: profile of health or vulnerable personality?
Ir Med J **77**, 37-39
Adult, Hazards, Leisure activity, Marathon, Running

730/47   **Milich, R., Loney, J. & Roberts, M.A.** (1986)
Playroom observations of activity level and sustained attention: two-year stability
J Consult Clin Psychol **54**, 272-274
Behaviour, Children, Customary activity, Male

730/48   **Molloy, D.W., Beerschoten, D.A., Borrie, M.J., Crilly, R.G. & Cape, R.D.T.** (1988)
Acute effects of exercise on neuropsychological function in elderly subjects
J Am Geriatr Soc **36**, 29-33
Acute exercise, Cognitive performance, Comparative, Elderly, Leisure activity

730/49   **Ohlsson, M.** (1977)
An experimental study on physical fitness related to information processing in elderly people. In: Physical Work and Effort. Proceedings of the First International Symposium (Ed.) Borg, G.
Pergamon Press, Stockholm 133-143
Cognitive performance, Comparative, Elderly, Leisure activity, Male

730/50   **Oliver, J.N.** (1958)
The effects of physical conditioning exercises and activities on the mental characteristics of educationally sub-normal boys
Br J Educ Psychol **28**, 155-165
Children, Exercise programme, Intervention, Learning, Male, Mental handicap, PSYCHOMOTOR PERFORMANCE

730/51   **Oliver, J.N.** (1972)
Physical activity and the psychological development of the handicapped. In: Psychological aspects of physical education and sport (Eds.) Kane, J.E.
Routledge & Kegan Paul, London
Mental handicap, Review

730/52   **Parízková, J., Mackova, E., Kabele, J., Mackova, J. & Skopova, M.** (1986)
Body composition, food intake, cardiorespiratory fitness, blood lipids and psychological development in highly active and inactive preschool children
Hum Biol **58**, 261-273
Body composition, Children, Cognitive performance, Comparative, ENERGY BALANCE, Learning, LIPIDS

730/53   **Perri, S. 2d. & Templer, D.I.** (1984)
The effects of an aerobic exercise program on psychological variables in older adults
Int J Aging Hum Dev **20**, 167-172
Anxiety, Cognitive performance, Depression, Elderly, Exercise programme, Intervention, Self-concept

730/54   **Powell, R.R.** (1974)
Psychological effects of exercise therapy upon institutionilized geriatric mental patients
J Gerontol **29**, 157-161
Cognitive performance, Elderly, Exercise programme, Intervention, Mental illness

730/55   **Rarick, G.L.** (1973)
Motor performance of mentally retarded children. In: Physical activity, human growth and development (Ed.) G.L.Rarick.
Academic Press
Review

730/56   **Salokun, S.O. & Toriola, A.L.**   (1985)
Personality characteristics of sprinters, basketball, soccer and field hockey players
J Sports Med Phys Fitness **25**, 222-226
Adult, Athlete, Male, Personality, Running, Self-concept, Vigorous

730/57   **Schurrer, R., Weltman, A. & Brammell, H.**   (1985)
Effects of physical training on cardiovascular fitness and behavior patterns of mentally retarded adults
Am J Ment Defic **90**, 167-170
Adult, AEROBIC CAPACITY, Behaviour, Exercise programme, Intervention, Mental handicap, Weight

730/58   **Segrave, J.O.**   (1983)
Sport and juvenile delinquency
Exerc Sport Sci Rev **11**, 181-209
Behaviour, Children, Review

730/59   **Short, M.A., DiCarlo, S., Steffee, W.P. & Pavlou, K.**   (1984)
Effects of physical conditioning on self-concept of adult obese males
Phys Ther **64**, 194-198
Adult, AEROBIC CAPACITY, ENERGY BALANCE, Exercise programme, Intervention, Male, Self-concept

730/60   **Sinyor, D., Brown, T., Rostant, L. & Seraganian, P.**   (1982)
The role of a physical fitness program in the treatment of alcoholism
J Stud Alcohol **43**, 380-386
Adult, Exercise programme, Intervention, Mental illness

730/61   **Sjöberg, H.**   (1980)
Physical fitness and mental performance during and after work
Ergonomics **23**, 977-985
Acute exercise, Adult, AEROBIC CAPACITY, Cognitive performance, Comparative, Leisure activity, Male

730/62   **Sonstroem, R.J.**   (1984)
Exercise and self-esteem
Exerc Sport Sci Rev **12**, 123-155
Review, Self-concept

730/63   **Sothmann, M.S. & Ismail, A.H.**   (1984)
Relationship between urinary catecholamine metabolites, particularly MHPG, and selected personality and physical fitness characteristics in normal subjects
Psychosom Med **46**, 523-533
Adult, Anxiety, Comparative, Depression, Endocrine, Male, Personality

730/64   **Sothmann, M.S., Ismail, A.H. & Chodepko-Zajiko, W.**   (1984)
Influence of catecholamine activity on the hierarchical relationships among physical fitness condition and selected personality characteristics
J Clin Psychol **40**, 1308-1317
Adult, Anxiety, Comparative, Depression, Endocrine, Male, MOOD, Personality

730/65   **Stamford, B.A., Hambacher, W. & Fallica, A.**   (1974)
The effects of daily physical exercise on the psychiatric state of institutionalized geriatric mental patients
Res Quart Am Assoc Health Phys Ed Rec **45**, 34-41
BLOOD PRESSURE, Body image, Cognitive performance, Elderly, Exercise programme, HEART FUNCTION TEST, Intervention, Male, Self-concept

730/66   **Stelmach, G.E. & Diewert, G.L.**   (1977)
Aging, information processing and fitness. In: Physical Work and Effort. Proceedings of the First International Symposium (Ed.) Borg, G.
Pergamon Press, Stockholm 122-130
Adult, Cognitive performance, Comparative, Elderly, Leisure activity

730/67 **Suominen-Troyer, S., Davis, K.J., Ismail, A.H. & Salvendy, G.** (1986)
Impact of physical fitness on strategy development in decision-making tasks
Percept Mot Skills **62,** 71-77
Adult, Cognitive performance, Comparative, Female, Leisure activity

730/68 **Svendsen, D.** (1982)
Physical activity in the treatment of mentally retarded persons
Scand J Soc Med (Suppl) **29,** 253-257
Mental handicap, Review

730/69 **Thoren, C.** (1971)
Physical training of handicapped schoolchildren
Scand J Rehab Med **3,** 26-30
Review

730/70 **Tomporowski, P.D. & Ellis, N.R.** (1984)
Effects of exercise on the physical fitness, intelligence, and adaptive behavior of institutionalized mentally retarded adults
Appl Res Ment Retard **5,** 329-337
Adult, Behaviour, Cognitive performance, Exercise programme, Mental handicap, Intervention, Vigorous

730/71 **Tomporowski, P.D. & Ellis, N.R.** (1985)
The effects of exercise on the health, intelligence, and adaptive behavior of institutionalized severely and profoundly mentally retarded adults: a systematic replication
Appl Res Ment Retard **6,** 465-473
Adult, Behaviour, Cognitive performance, Exercise programme, Mental handicap, Intervention, Vigorous

730/72 **Tomporowski, P.D., Ellis, N.R. & Stephens, R.** (1987)
The immediate effects of strenuous exercise on free-recall memory
Ergonomics **30,** 121-129
Acute exercise, Adult, Cognitive performance, Comparative

730/73 **Tucker, L.A.** (1983)
Muscular strength and mental health
J Person Soc Psychol **45,** 1355-1360
Adult, Anxiety, Male, MUSCLE STRENGTH, Personality, Self-concept

730/74 **Tucker, L.A.** (1983)
Muscular strength: a predictor of personality in males
J Sports Med Phys Fitness **23,** 213-220
Adult, Comparative, Male, MUSCLE STRENGTH, Personality

730/75 **Valliant, P.M. & Asu, M.E.** (1985)
Exercise and its effects on cognition and physiology in older adults
Percept Mot Skills **61,** 1031-1038
Body composition, Comparative, Depression, Elderly, Exercise programme, Intervention, Leisure activity, Personality, Self-concept

730/76 **Watters, R.G. & Watters, W.E.** (1980)
Decreasing self-stimulatory behavior with physical exercise in a group of autistic boys
J Autism Dev Disord **10,** 379-387
Behaviour, Children, Exercise programme

730/77 **Yates, A., Leehey, K. & Shisslak, C.M.** (1983)
Running–an analogue of anorexia?
N Engl J Med **308,** 251-255
Adult, Hazards, Leisure activity, Mental illness, Personality, Running

730/78 **Young, M.L.** (1985)
Estimation of fitness and physical ability, physical performance, and self-concept among adolescent females
J Sports Med Phys Fitness **25,** 144-150
Children, Comparative, Female, Leisure activity, Self-concept

740 PSYCHOMOTOR PERFORMANCE

KEYWORDS are listed in the appendix in addition the following specific keywords have been used in this section:

Cognitive performance
Self-concept

Summary of evidence: exercise improves skill through practice

THE PROBLEM

Exercise performance depends upon psychomotor skills as well as strength and aerobic capacity. Practice will improve these skills especially in children. Conversely, is there an improvement in psychomotor function to be obtained through physical exercise especially in the old and the handicapped of all ages?

SCOPE

This section contains references dealing primarily with changes produced by exercise in skill, coordination, reaction time and speed of movement in all age groups and both sexes.

METHODOLOGICAL DIFFICULTIES

The measurement of psychomotor performance is affected by many factors which affect both the state of arousal of the central nervous system and the effector muscles.

EVIDENCE

There is no evidence that physical exercise improves the function of the neural components of psychomotor function. However practice can greatly enhance performance.

740/1 **Halbert, J.A.** (1974)
The effects of physical exercise upon the performance of mentally handicapped in a rehabilitation setting: A preliminary report. In: Conference Proc of XXth World Congress in Sports Medicine 215-221
Adult, Exercise programme, Intervention, Mental Handicap

740/2 **Mauser, H-J. & Reynolds, R.P.** (1977)
Effects of a developmental physical activity program on children's body coordination and self-concept
Percep Mot Skills **44**, 1057-1058
Children, Exercise programme, Intervention, Self-concept

740/3 **Newell, K.M., Morris, L.R. & Scully, D.M.** (1985)
Augmented information and the acquisition of skill in physical activity
Exerc Sport Sci Rev **13**, 235-261
Review

740/4 **Reilly, T. & Smith, D.** (1986)
Effect of work intensity on performance in a psychomotor task during exercise
Ergonomics **29**, 601-606
Acute exercise, Adult, AEROBIC CAPACITY, Male

740/5 **Rutherford, O.M. & Jones, D.A.** (1986)
The role of learning and coordination in strength training
Eur J Appl Physiol **55**, 100-105
Adult, Exercise programme, Intervention, MUSCLE STRENGTH

740/6 **Sherwood, D.E. & Selder, D.J.** (1979)
Cardiorespiratory health, reaction time and aging
Med Sci Sports **11**, 186-189
Adult, Comparative, Leisure activity, Running

740/7   **Spirduso, W.W.**   (1975)
Reaction and movement time as a
function of age and physical activity level
J Gerontol **30,** 435-440
***Adult, Comparative, Elderly, Leisure
activity***

740/8   **Spirduso, W.W.**   (1980)
Physical fitness, Aging, and psychomotor
speed: A review
J Gerontol **35,** 850-865
Elderly, Review

740/9   **Williams, L.R., Pottinger, P.R. &
Shapcott, D.G.**   (1985)
Effects of exercise on choice reaction
latency and movement speed
Percept Mot Skills **60,** 67-71
***Acute exercise, Cognitive performance,
Male***

750 NEUROLOGICAL FUNCTION

KEYWORDS are listed in the appendix .

Summary of evidence: exercise such as boxing is a hazard for the brain

THE PROBLEM

Does exercise have a tranquillising effect on the nervous system as has been suggested or cause any changes in neuronal function within the CNS?

SCOPE

This section contains references dealing primarily with changes produced by exercise in brain function manifest as motor neurone activity, seizure discharges in epilepsy and vision. It also includes the hazards of boxing.

METHODOLOGICAL DIFFICULTIES

Measurement of neuronal function in man is indirect and crude at the present time.

EVIDENCE

Boxing can produce significant and permanent brain damage. The significance of changes in the level of arousal or other more specific effects of exercise on higher mental function are as yet obscure.

750/1   **Casson, I.R., Siegel, O., Sham, R., Campbell, E.A., Tarlau, M. & DiDomenico, A.** (1984)
Brain damage in modern boxers
J Am Med Ass **251,** 2663-2667
Adult, Hazards, Male

750/2   **DeVries, H.A., Wiswell, R.A., Bulbulian, R. & Moritani, T.** (1981)
Tranquilizer effect of exercise
Am J Phys Med **60,** 57-66
Acute exercise, Elderly

750/3   **Eickelberg, W., Kaylor, P., Less, M., Baruch, I. & Megarr, J.** (1983)
Effects of passive physical exercise on peripheral vision in muscular dystrophic children
Percept Mot Skills **56,** 167-170
Children, Exercise programme, Handicap, Intervention

750/4   **Enoka, R.M. & Stuart, D.G.** (1985)
The contribution of neuroscience to exercise studies
Fed Proc **44,** 2279-2285
Review

750/5   **Gandevia, S.C. & Burke, D.** (1985)
Effect of training on voluntary activation of human fusimotor neurons
J Neurophysiol **54,** 1422-1429
Adult, MUSCLE METABOLISM

750/6   **Horyd, W., Gryziak, J., Niedzielska, K. & Zielinski, J.** (1981)
Effect of physical exertion on seizure discharges in the EEG of epilepsy patients
J Neurol Neurochir Pol **15,** 545-552
Acute exercise, Adult, Handicap

750/7   **Morrison, R.G.** (1986)
Medical and public health aspects of boxing
J Am Med Ass **255,** 2475-2480
Hazards, Review

750/8   **Rossi, B. & Zani, A.** (1986)
Differences in hemispheric functional asymmetry between athletes and nonathletes: evidence from a Unilateral Tactile Matching Task
Percept Mot Skills **62,** 295-300
Adult, Athlete, Comparative, Male, Leisure activity

KEYWORDS are listed in the appendix in addition the following specific keywords have been used in this section:

Endorphins

Summary of evidence: exercise ameliorates pain during the exercise

THE PROBLEM

Does exercise have an effect which mimics that of the natural brain opiates which reduce affective pain, or reduce pain sensitivity in any other way?

SCOPE

This section contains references dealing primarily with changes produced by exercise in pain perception and opiate levels in plasma.

METHODOLOGICAL DIFFICULTIES

Studies of pain are difficult to justify ethically. Plasma levels of opiates have an uncertain relation to the levels in specific target areas of the brain.

EVIDENCE

Studies using naloxone which blocks opiate receptors suggest that exercise has no effect on this system in the brain. There may be other non-specific reasons such as gating mechanisms which explain a reduction in pain sensitivity during exercise, but there is no evidence that habitual exercise lowers pain sensitivity in the long term.

760/1   **Campbell, J.F., Stenstrom, R.J. & Bertrand, D.**   (1985)
Systematic changes in perceptual reactance induced by physical fitness training
Percept Mot Skills **61**, 279-284
Adult, Exercise programme, Inactivity, Intervention

760/2   **Carmody, J. & Cooper, K.**   (1987)
Swim stress reduces chronic pain in mice through opiod mechanisms
Neuroci Lett **74**, 358-363
Acute exercise, Animal, Endorphins

760/3   **De Meirleir, K., Arentz, T., Hollmann, W. & Vanhaelst, L.**   (1985)
The role of endogenous opiates in thermal regulation of the body during exercise
Br Med J **290**, 739-740
Acute exercise, Adult, Endorphins, Male

760/4   **Doleys, D.M., Crocker, M. & Patton, D.**   (1982)
Response of patients with chronic pain to exercise quotas
Phys Ther **62**, 1111-1114
Adult, Exercise programme, Intervention

760/5   **Haier, R.J., Quaid, K. & Mills, J.S.C.**   (1981)
Naloxone alters pain perception after jogging
Psychiatr Res **5**, 231-232
Acute exercise, Adult, Endorphins, MOOD, Leisure activity, Running

760/6   **Janal, M.N., Colt, E.W., Clark, W.C. & Glusman, M.**   (1984)
Pain sensitivity, mood and plasma endocrine levels in man following long-distance running: Effects of naloxone
Pain **19**, 13-25
Acute exercise, Adult, Endocrine, Endorphins, Male, MOOD, REPRODUCTIVE HORMONES, Running, Vigorous,

760/7   Kemppainen, P., Pertovaara, A.,
Huopaniemi, T., Johansson, G. &
Karonen, S.L.   (1985)
Modification of dental pain and
cutaneous thermal sensitivity by physical
exercise in man
Brain Res **360**, 33-40
Acute exercise, Adult, Endocrine, Male

760/8   Olausson, B., Eriksson, E.,
Ellmarker, L., Rydenhag, B., Shyu, B.C.
& Andersson, S.A.   (1986)
Effects of naloxone on dental pain
threshold following muscle exercise and
low frequency transcutaneous nerve
stimulation: a comparative study in man
Acta Physiol Scand **126**, 299-305
Acute exercise, Adult, Endorphins

760/9   Pertovaara, A., Huopaniemi, T.,
Virtanen, A. & Johansson, G.   (1984)
The influence of exercise on dental pain
thresholds and the release of stress
hormones
Physiol Behav **33**, 923-926
Acute exercise, Adult, Endocrine, Male,
REPRODUCTIVE HORMONES

760/10   Surbey, G.D., Andrew, G.M.,
Cervenko, F.W. & Hamilton,
P.P.   (1984)
Effects of naloxone on exercise
performance
J Appl Physiol **57**, 674-679
Acute exercise, Adult, Athlete,
Endorphins, Leisure activity, Male,
PERCEIVED EXERTION, Running

760/11   Vecchiet, L., Marini, I., Colozzi, A.
& Feroldi, P.   (1984)
Effects of aerobic exercise on muscular
pain sensitivity
Clin Ther **6**, 354-363
Acute exercise, Adult

770 SLEEP

KEYWORDS are listed in the appendix.

Summary of evidence: exercise does not ameliorate insomnia

THE PROBLEM

Does exercise improve sleep or cure insomnia?

SCOPE

This section contains references dealing primarily with changes produced by exercise on quality and quantity of sleep.

METHODOLOGICAL DIFFICULTIES

The study of sleep requires monitoring with EEG electrodes in order to obtain reliable information. This in itself perturbs the natural situation unless the recordings are made in the home and habituation to the technique is adequate.

EVIDENCE

There is no good evidence that exercise enhances sleep or cures insomnia. It may have a non-specific arousing effect in sedentary subjects which tends to disturb sleep. Athletes and those with active lifestyles have different sleep patterns from those who are sedentary, for reasons which are not yet clear, and their sleep is not perturbed by further strenuous exercise.

770/1　**Bunnell, D.E., Bevier, W.C. & Horvath, S.M.** (1985)
Effects of exhaustive submaximal exercise on cardiovascular function during sleep
J Appl Physiol **58**, 1909-1913
Acute exercise, Adult, CARDIAC PERFORMANCE, Endocrine, Vigorous

770/2　**Bunnell, D.E., Bevier, W. & Horvath, S.M.** (1983)
Effects of exhaustive exercise on the sleep of men and women
Psychophysiology **20**, 50-58
Acute exercise, Adult, Female, Male, Vigorous

770/3　**Griffin, S.J. & Trinder, J.** (1978)
Physical fitness, exercise, and human sleep
Psychophysiology **15**, 447-450
Acute exercise, Adult, Comparative, Leisure activity

770/4　**Kupfer, D.J., Sewitch, D.E., Epstein, L.H., Bulik, C., McGowen, C.R. & Robertson, R.J.** (1985)
Exercise and subsequent sleep in male runners: failure to support the slow wave sleep-mood-exercise hypothesis
Neuropsychobiology **4**, 5-12
Adult, Comparative, Leisure activity, Male, MOOD, PSYCHOMOTOR PERFORMANCE, Running

770/5　**Matsumoto, K., Saito, Y., Abe, M. & Furumi, K.** (1984)
The effects of daytime exercise on night sleep
J Hum Ergol **13**, 31-36
Acute exercise, Adult, Male

770/6　**Montgomery, I., Trinder, J. & Paxton, S.J.** (1982)
Energy expenditure and total sleep time: Effect of physical exercise
Sleep **5**, 159-168
Adult, Exercise programme, Intervention

770/7   Paxton, S.J., Trinder, J. &
Montgomery, I.   (1983)
Does aerobic fitness affect sleep?
Psychophysiology **20**, 320-324
Adult, AEROBIC CAPACITY,
Comparative, Exercise programme,
Intervention, Male

770/8   Paxton, S.J., Trinder, J., Shapiro,
C.M., Adam, K., Oswald, I. & Graf,
K.J.   (1984)
Effect of physical fitness and body
composition on sleep and sleep-related
hormone concentrations
Sleep **7**, 339-346
Adult, Athlete, Body composition,
Comparative, Endocrine, GROWTH,
Male, REPRODUCTIVE HORMONES

770/9   Roussel, B. & Buguet, A.   (1982)
Changes in human heart rate during sleep
following daily physical exercise
Eur J Appl Physiol **49**, 409-416
Acute exercise, Adult, Male

770/10   Shapiro, C.M., Warren, P.M.,
Trinder, J., Paxton, S.J., Oswald, I.,
Flenley, D.C. & Catterall, J.R.   (1984)
Fitness facilitates sleep
Eur J Appl Physiol **53**, 1-4
Acute exercise, Adult, AEROBIC
CAPACITY, ANAEROBIC
CAPACITY, Intervention, Male,
Occupational activity, Vigorous

770/11   Torsvall, L.   (1981)
Sleep after exercise: A literature review
J Sports Med Phys Fitness **21**, 218-225
Review

770/12   Torsvall, L., Akerstedt, T. &
Lindbeck, G.   (1984)
Effects on sleep stages and EEG power
density of different degrees of exercise in
fit subjects
Electroencephalogr Clin Neurophysiol **57**,
347-355
Acute exercise, Adult, Comparative,
Leisure activity

770/13   Trinder, J., Paxton, S.J.,
Montgomery, I. & Fraser, G.   (1985)
Endurance as opposed to power training:
the effect on sleep
Psychophysiology **22**, 668-673
Adult, Athlete, Comparative, Leisure
activity, Male, MUSCLE STRENGTH,
Running

770/14   Walker, J.M., Floyd. T.C., Fein, G.,
Cavness, C., Lualhati, R. & Feinberg,
I.   (1978)
Effects of exercise on sleep
J Appl Physiol **44**, 945-951
Acute exercise, Adult, Comparative,
Leisure activity, Male, MOOD,
PERSONALITY, Running

KEYWORDS are listed in the appendix in addition the following specific keywords have been used in this section:

Anxiety
Depression
Endorphins

Summary of evidence: exercise ameliorates fatigue during rhythmic exercise

THE PROBLEM

Does perceived exertion during a standard task decrease as exercise improves performance capacity such that the standard task requires a smaller proportion of that capacity ?

SCOPE

This section contains references dealing primarily with changes produced by exercise in perceived exertion recorded using validated rating scales.

METHODOLOGICAL DIFFICULTIES

The original scale for perceived exertion was developed for cycling, the transfer of the scale to other situations has not been so well validated, moreover it is a subjective scale easily perturbed by the subject's interpretation of the purpose of the study and his self-image.

EVIDENCE

It is clear that improvements in perceived exertion occur, roughly in proportion to the magnitude of the improvements in stamina. This is a major benefit of exercise available to anyone and of consequence for the quality of life especially in those with poor initial capacity.

780/1   **Birk, T.J. & Birk, C.A.**   (1987)
Use of ratings of perceived exertion for exercise prescription
Sports Med **4**, 1-8
Exercise programme, Review

780/2   **Borg, G.A.**   (1982)
Ratings of perceived exertion and heart rates during short-term cycle exercise and their use in a new cycling strength test
Int J Sports Med **3**, 153-158
Acute exercise, Adult, Cycling

780/3   **Borg, G.A.**   (1982)
Psychophysical bases of perceived exertion
Med Sci Sports Exerc **14**, 377-381
Review

780/4   **Borg, G.A., Hassmen, P. & Lagerstrom, M.**   (1987)
Perceived exertion related to heart rate and blood lactate during arm and leg exercise
Eur J Appl Physiol **56**, 679-685
Acute exercise, Adult, Comparative, Male

780/5   **Borg, G.A., Ljunggren, G. & Ceci, R.**   (1985)
The increase in perceived exertion, aches and pain in the legs, heart rate and blood lactate during exercise on a bicycle ergometer
Eur J Appl Physiol **54**, 343-349
Acute exercise, Adult, Male, PAIN

780/6   **Cabanac, M.**   (1986)
Performance and perception at various combinations of treadmill speed and slope
Physiol Behav **38**, 839-843
Acute exercise, Adult, Comparative

780/7   **Cafarelli, E.**   (1982)
Peripheral contributions to the perception of effort
Med Sci Sports Exerc **14**, 382-389
Review

780/8   Carton, R.L. & Rhodes,
E.C. (1985)
A critical review of the literature on
ratings scales for perceived exertion
Sports Med **2**, 198-222
Review

780/9   Demello, J.J., Cureton, K.J., Boineu,
R.E. & Singh, M.M. (1987)
Ratings of perceived exertion at the
lactate threshold in trained and untrained
men and women
Med Sci Sports Exerc **19**, 354-362
Acute exercise, Adult, Body composition,
Comparative, AEROBIC CAPACITY,
ANAEROBIC CAPACITY, Female,
Leisure activity, Male, RESPIRATORY
FUNCTION

780/10   Dishman, R.K. (1987)
Using perceived exertion to prescribe and
monitor exercise training heart rate
Int J Sports Med **8**, 208-213
Adult, Exercise programme

780/11   Ekblom, B. & Goldbarg,
A.N. (1971)
The influence of physical training and
other factors on the subjective rating of
perceived exertion
Acta Physiol Scand **83**, 399-406
Adult, AEROBIC CAPACITY, Exercise
programme, Intervention, Male

780/12   Gamberale, F. (1985)
The perception of exertion
Ergonomics **28**, 299-308
Review

780/13   Higgs, S.L. & Robertson,
L.A. (1981)
Cyclic variations in perceived exertion
and physical work capacity in females
Can J Appl Sport Sci **6**, 191-196
Adult, AEROBIC CAPACITY,
ANAEROBIC CAPACITY, Female,
MENSTRUAL FUNCTION, MUSCLE
STRENGTH

780/14   Hughes, J.R., Crow, R.S., Jacobs,
D.R. Jr., Mittelmark, M.B. & Leon,
A.S. (1984)
Physical activity, smoking, and exercise-
induced fatigue
J Behav Med **7**, 217-230
Acute exercise, Adult, BLOOD
PRESSURE, Comparative, Inactivity,
Leisure activity, LIPIDS, Male,
PRIMARY PREVENTION

780/15   Jones, L.A. & Hunter, I.W. (1983)
Perceived force in fatiguing isometric
contractions
Percept Psychophys **33**, 369-374
Adult, MUSCLE STRENGTH

780/16   Kraemer, W., Noble, B.J.,
Robertson, K. & Lewis, R.V. (1985)
Response of plasma proenkephalin
peptide F to exercise
Peptides (Suppl) **6**, 167-169
Acute exercise, Adult, Comparative,
Endorphins, Leisure activity, Male,
Running

780/17   Löllgen, H., Graham, T. &
Sjorgaard, G. (1980)
Muscle metabolites, force, and perceived
exertion bicycling at varying pedal rates
Med Sci Sports Exerc **12**, 345-351
Acute exercise, Adult, AEROBIC
CAPACITY, MUSCLE
METABOLISM

780/18   Marks, L.E., Borg, G.A. &
Ljunggren, G. (1983)
Individual differences in perceived
exertion assessed by two new methods
Percept Psychophys **34**, 280-288
Acute exercise, Adult, Comparative, Male

780/19   McCloskey, D.I., Gandevia, S.,
Potter, E.K. & Colebatch, J.G. (1983)
Muscle sense and effort: Motor
commands and judgments about
muscular contractions
Adv Neurol **39**, 169-211
Acute exercise, Adult, MUSCLE
STRENGTH

780/20 **Mihevic, P.M.** (1981)
Sensory cues for perceived exertion: A review
Med Sci Sports Exerc **13**, 150-163
Review

780/21 **Mihevic, P.M.** (1983)
Cardiovascular fitness and the psychophysics of perceived exertion
Res Q Exerc Sport **54**, 239-246
Review

780/22 **Morgan, A.D, Peck, D.F., Buchanan, D.R. & McHardy, G.J.** (1983)
Effect of attitudes and beliefs on exercise tolerance in chronic bronchitis
Br Med J **286**, 171-173
Acute exercise, Adult, Anxiety, Depression, MOOD, RESPIRATORY FUNCTION

780/23 **Muza, S.R. & Zechman, F.W.** (1984)
Scaling of added loads to breathing: Magnitude estimation vs. handgrip matching
J Appl Physiol **57**, 888-891
Acute exercise, Adult, Comparative, Male, MUSCLE STRENGTH, RESPIRATORY FUNCTION

780/24 **Myles, W.S. & Maclean, D.** (1986)
A comparasion of response and production protocols for assessing perceived exertion
Eur J Appl Physiol **55**, 585-587
Acute exercise, Adult, Comparative

780/25 **Noble, B.J.** (1982)
Clinical applications of perceived exertion
Med Sci Sports Exerc **14**, 406-411
Review

780/26 **Noble, B.J., Borg, G.A., Jacobs, I., Ceci, R. & Kaiser, P.** (1983)
A category-ratio perceived exertion scale: relationship to blood and muscle lactates and heart rate
Med Sci Sports Exerc **15**, 523-528
Acute exercise, Adult, Male

780/27 **O'Sullivan, S.B.** (1984)
Perceived exertion. A review
Phys Ther **64**, 343-346
Review

780/28 **Pandolf, K.B.** (1982)
Differentiated ratings of perceived exertion during physical exercise
Med Sci Sports Exerc **14**, 397-405
Review

780/29 **Pandolf, K.B.** (1983)
Advances in the study and application of perceived exertion
Exerc Sport Sci Rev **11**, 118-158
Review

780/30 **Pandolf, K.B., Billings, D.S., Drolet, L.L., Pimental, N.A. & Sawka, M.N.** (1984)
Differential ratings of perceived exertion and various physiological responses during prolonged upper and lower body exercise
Eur J Appl Physiol **53**, 5-11
Acute exercise, Adult, Male, MUSCLE STRENGTH

780/31 **Pandolf, K.B., Burse, R.L. & Goldman, R.F.** (1975)
Differentiated ratings of perceived exertion during physical conditioning of older individuals using leg-weight loading
Percep Mot Skills **40**, 563-574
Acute exercise, Adult, Male, MUSCLE STRENGTH

780/32 **Rejeski, W.J.** (1985)
Perceived exertion: An active or passive process?
J Sports Psychol **7**, 371-378
Exercise programme, Review

780/33   **Robertson, R.J.**   (1982)
Central signals of perceived exertion
during dynamic exercise
Med Sci Sports Exerc **14**, 390-396
Review

780/34   **Robertson, R.J., Caspersen, C.J.,
Allison, T.G., Skrinar, G.S., Abbott, R.A.
& Metz, K.F.**   (1982)
Differentiated perceptions of exertion
and energy cost of young women while
carrying loads
Eur J Appl Physiol **49**, 69-78
Acute exercise, Adult, Female

780/35   **Robertson, R.J., Falkel, J.E.,
Drash, A.L., Swank, A.M., Metz, K.F.,
Spungen, S.A. & LeBoeuf, J.R.**   (1986)
Effect of blood pH on peripheral and
central signals of perceived exertion
Med Sci Sports Exerc **18**, 114-122
*Acute exercise, Adult, AEROBIC
CAPACITY, ANAEROBIC
CAPACITY, Male*

780/36   **Sidney, K.H. & Shephard,
R.J.**   (1977)
Perception of exertion in the elderly,
effects of aging, mode of exercise and
physical training
Percep Mot Skills **44**, 999-1010
*Acute exercise, AEROBIC CAPACITY,
BLOOD PRESSURE, Body composition,
Comparative, Elderly, Exercise
programme, Female, Intervention, Male,
MUSCLE STRENGTH,*

780/37   **Skrinar, G.S., Ingram, S.P. &
Pandolf, K.B.**   (1983)
Effect of endurance training on perceived
exertion and stress hormones in women
Percep Mot Skills **57**, 1239-1250
*Adult, AEROBIC CAPACITY, Body
composition, Endocrine, Female,
Intervention, Leisure activity, Running*

780/38   **Smutok, M.A., Skrinar, G.S. &
Pandolf, K.B.**   (1980)
Exercise intensity: Subjective regulation
by perceived exertion
Arch Phys Med Rehabil **61**, 569-574
*Acute exercise, Adult, Exercise
programme, Male*

KEYWORDS are listed in the appendix in addition the following specific keywords have been used in this section:

Immune response
Longevity
Lymphocyte
Vitamins

Summary of evidence: exercise does not increase longevity, reduce the incidence of cancer, nor affect the immune response nor constipation

SCOPE

The references in this section deal with some of the questions which do not fit into other sections. They deal with matters which are indicated to some extent by the keywords above.

EVIDENCE

There is no good evidence that exercise affects longevity apart from its effects on chronic diseases such as coronary heart disease. There are references which show changes of various kinds in the immune response during and soon after strenuous exercise. It is not yet clear whether they amount to an increase or a decrease in the body's defence mechanisms. It has been suggested that an active lifestyle is associated with an increased bowel transit time and a reduced risk of colonic cancer, however the number of studies is few and the evidence somewhat conflicting.

800/1 **Anderson, R.A., Bryden, N.A., Polansky, M.M. & Deuster, P.A.** (1988)
Exercise effects on chromium excretion of trained and untrained men consuming a constant diet
J Appl Physiol **64**, 249-252
Acute exercise, Adult, Comparative, Leisure activity, Male

800/2 **Belko, A.Z.** (1987)
Vitamins and exercise – an update
Med Sci Sports Exerc (Suppl 5) **19**, S191-196
Review

800/3 **Berk, L.S., Nieman, D., Tan, S.A., Nehlsen-Cannarella, S., Kramer, J., Eby, W.C. & Owens, M.** (1986)
Lymphocyte subset changes during acute maximal exercise
Med Sci Sports Exerc **18**, 706
Acute exercise, Adult, Immune response, Lymphocyte, Male, PERCEIVED EXERTION, Vigorous

800/4 **Borisova, A.I.** (1976)
Role of therapeutic physical training and its methods in different periods of burns
Klin Khir **6**, 20-22
Adult, Exercise programme, Intervention

800/5 **Branch, L.G. & Jette, A.M.** (1984)
Personal health practices and mortality among the elderly
Am J Public Health **74**, 1126-1129
Cohort, Customary activity, Elderly, Female, Longevity, Male

800/6 **Campbell, W.W. & Anderson, R.A.** (1987)
Effects of aerobic exercise and training on the trace minerals chromium, zinc and copper
Sports Med **4**, 9-18
Adult, Exercise programme, Intervention

800/7   **Cordain, L., Latin, R.W. & Behnke, J.J.**   (1986)
The effects of an aerobic running program on bowel transit time
J Sports Med **26**, 101-104
Adult, AEROBIC CAPACITY, Exercise programme, Intervention, Male, Running, Vigorous

800/8   **D'Alessio, D.J., Minor, T.E., Allen, C.I., Tsiatis, A.A. & Nelson, D.B.**   (1981)
Study of the proportions of swimmers among well controls and children with enterovirus-like illness shedding or not shedding an enterovirus
Am J Epidiol **113**, 533-541
Children, Comparative, Hazards, Leisure activity, Swimming

800/9   **Dreon, D.M.**   (1986)
Vitamin B6 utilization in active and inactive young men
Am J Clin Nutr **43**, 816-824
Adult, Exercise programme, Intervention, Male, Running, Vitamins

800/10   **Eskola, J., Ruuskanen, O., Soppi, E., Viljanen, M.K., Jarvinen, M., Toivonene, H. & Kouvalainen, K.**   (1978)
Effect of sport stress on lymphocyte transformation and antibody formation
Clin Exp Immunol **32**, 339-345
Acute exercise, Adult, Comparative, Immune response, Leisure activity, Lymphocyte, Male, Marathon, Running, Vigorous

800/11   **Fernandes, G., Rozek, M. & Troyer, D.**   (1986)
Reduction of blood pressure and restoration of T-cell immune function in spontaneously hypertensive rats by food restriction and/or by treadmill exercise
J Hypertens (Suppl 3) **4**, S469-74
Animal, BLOOD PRESSURE, Exercise programme, Immune response, Intervention

800/12   **Garabrant, D.H., Peters, J.M., Mack, T.M. & Bernstein, L.**   (1984)
Job activity and colon cancer risk
Am J Epidemiol **119**, 1005-1014
Adult, Cancer, Case-control. Male, Occupational activity

800/13   **Gleeson, M.**   (1987)
Influence of exercise on ascorbic acid status in man
Clin Sci **73**, 519-523
Adult, Vitamins

800/14   **Gohiul, K., Rothfuss, L., Lang, J. & Packer, L.**   (1987)
Effect of exercise training on tissue vitamin E and ubiquinone content
J Appl Physiol **63**, 1638-1641
Animal, Exercise programme, Intervention, Vitamins

800/15   **Heikkinen, H., Parkatti, T., Forsbergh, S, & Kisskinen,K.**
Effects of 'lifelong' physical training on functional aging in men
Proc. of III Nordic Congress of Gerontology, Turku.
Elderly, Leisure activity, Longevity

800/16   **Holloszy, J.O. & Smith, E.K.**   (1987
Effects of exercise on longevity of rats
Fed Proc. **46**, 1850-1853
Longevity, Review

800/17   **Houston, H., Hoffman-Goetz, L., Houston, M.E. & Keir, R.**   (1987)
Immunological response to exercise training in man
Fed Proc **46**, 681
Adult, AEROBIC CAPACITY, Exercise programme, Immune response, Intervention, Male

800/18   **Hunter, K.E. & Turkki, P.R.**   (1987)
Effect of exercise on riboflavin status of rats
J Nutr **117**, 298-304
Animal, Exercise programme, Intervention, Muscle metabolism, Vitamins

800/19   **Jensen, G.D. & Bellecci, P.**   (1987)
The physical and mental health of
nonagenarians
Age and Ageing **16**, 19-24
Elderly, Leisure activity, Longevity, Male

800/20   **Kaplan, G.A., Seeman, T.E., Cohen,
R.D., Knudsen, L.P. & Guralnik,
J.**   (1987)
Mortality among the elderly in the
Alameda county study: behavioural and
demographic risk factors
Am J Public Health **77**, 307-312
***Cohort, Elderly, Female, Leisure activity,
Longevity, Male***

800/21   **Karpova, J.I., Mokhov, E.N. &
Volkov, N.I.**   (1987)
The effect of mitochondrial energetics
inhibitors on spontaneous rosette
formation of lymphocytes from athletes
J Sports Med Phys Fitness **27**, 165-171
***Acute exercise, Adult, Athlete, Female,
Immune response, Leisure activity,
Lymphocytes, Male***

800/22   **Keeling, W.F. & Martin,
B.J.**   (1987)
Gastrointestinal transit during mild
exercise
J Appl Physiol **63**, 978-981
Acute exercise, Adult, Male

800/23   **Kottke, T.E., Caspersen, C.J. &
Hill, C.S.**   (1984)
Exercise in the managment and
rehabilitation of selected chronic diseases
Prev Med **13**, 47-65
***JOINTS, RESPIRATORY
FUNCTION, Review, SECONDARY
PREVENTION***

800/24   **Larson, E.B. & Bruce,
R.A.**   (1986)
Exercise and aging
Ann Intern Med **105**, 783-785
Elderly, Longevity, Review

800/25   **Larsson, B., Renstrom, P.,
Svardsudd, K., Welin, L., Grimby, G.,
Eriksson, H., Ohlson, L.-O., Wilhelmson,
L. & Bjorntorp, P.**   (1984)
Health and ageing characteristics of
highly physically active 65-year-old men
Eur Heart J (Suppl E) **5**, 31-35
***Body compostion, Comparative,
CARBOHYDRATE TOLERANCE,
Elderly, Leisure activity, Longevity***

800/26   **Lewicki, R.**   (1987)
Effect of physical exercise on some
parameters of immunity in conditioned
sportsmen
Int J Sports Med **8**, 309-314
***Acute exercise, Adult, Athlete, Immune
response, Leisure activity***

800/27   **McCarthy, D. A., Perry, J.D.,
Melson, R.D. & Dale, M.M.**   (1987)
Leucocytosis induced by exercise
Br Med J **295**, 636
***Acute exercise, Adult, Immune response,
Leisure activity, Male***

800/28   **Molinaro, J.**   (1986)
Physical therapy and dance in the surgical
management of breast cancer. A clinical
report
Phys Ther **66**, 967-969
***Adult, Cancer, Exercise programme,
Intervention***

800/29   **Ohno, H., Sato, Y., Yamashita, K.,
Doi, R., Arai, K., Kondo, T. & Taniguchi,
N.**   (1986)
The effect of brief physical exercise on
free radical scavenging enzyme systems in
human red blood cells
Can J Physiol Pharmacol **64**, 1263-1265
***Acute exercise, Adult, Immune response,
Male***

800/30   **Paffenbarger, R.S.Jr., Hyde, R.T.
& Wing, A.L.**   (1987)
Physical activity and incidence of cancer
in diverse populations: a preliminary
report
Am J Clin Nutr **45**, 312-317
*Adult, Cancer, Leisure activity,
Longitudinal, Male*

800/31   **Schaefer, R., Kokot, K., Heidland,
A. & Plass, R.**   (1987)
Jogger's leukocytes (letter)
N Engl J Med **316**, 223-224
Acute exercise, Adult, Immune response

800/32   **Stotts, K.M.**   (1986)
Health maintenance: Paraplegic athletes
and non-athletes
Arch Phys Med Rehabil **67**, 109-114
*Adult, Comparative, Handicap, Leisure
activity*

800/33   **Vena, J.E., Graham, S., Zielezny,
M. & Brasure, J.**   (1987)
Occupational exercise and risk of cancer
Am J Clin Nutr **45**, 318-327
*Adult, Cancer, Case-control, Male,
Occupational activity*

800/34   **Wiley, J.A. & Camacho,
T.C.**   (1980)
Life-style and future health: Evidence
from the Alameda county study
Prev Med **9**, 1-21
Adult, Female, Leisure activity, Male

800/35   **Wu, A.H., Paganini, A., Ross, R.K.
& Henderson, B.E.**   (1987)'
Alcohol, physical activity and other risk
factors for colorectal cancer: a
prospective study
Br J Cancer **55**, 687-694
*Cancer, Cohort, Elderly, Female, Leisure
activity, Male*

Index of keywords

All the keywords which have been used are listed together here. Keywords listed in capital letters are also subsection headings (apart from abbreviations such as COPD) and can be identified on the contents page.

   Some keywords are restricted to subsections. They are followed by the appropriate subsection code numbers (see contents page). They are defined where necessary at the beginning of the subsection in the body of the bibliography. The other keywords are global, that is they are used throughout the bibliography and so are not followed by subsection code numbers. They are defined in a separate 'Grouped Index of Global Keywords'.

Index of global keywords

These keywords have been used throughout the bibliography. Where necessary definitions are given in brackets; these are not exhaustive but provide guidelines. Where sub-section headings have been used as keywords they are listed in capital letters.

Subject

Adult
Animal
Athlete (professional athletes, or as designated by author)
Children (less than 18 yrs)
Elderly (greater than 70 yrs)
Female (only if results differentiated by sex)
Male (only if results differentiated by sex)

Type of study

Acute exercise (single exercise session, from a marathon to an exercise test, in which the acute response has been measured)
Autopsy
Case-control
Comparative (two or more different protocols or groups, comparison of sedentary and active, but not a control group of an intervention study)
Cohort (large group of individuals sharing a common characteristic studied over a number of years)
Intervention (contrived change usually in exercise levels lasting some weeks)
Longitudinal (group of individuals studied for at least two years)

Type of exercise

Customary activity (activities of daily living, domestic activity)
Cycling (not bicycle egometer test)
Exercise programme (intervention where exercise is prescribed and monitored, exercise prescription, see Leisure activity)
Inactivity (immobilization, bedrest, spaceflight, reduction in activity levels)
Leisure activity (games, sports, athletic activity)
Marathon (full or half)
Occupational activity (not professional athletes)
Running
Swimming
Vigorous (activity requiring more than 75% of individuals' maximal oxygen uptake)

Physiological function

AEROBIC CAPACITY (maximal oxygen uptake- measured or predicted)
ANAEROBIC CAPACITY (short term power output, ventilatory, lactate or anaerobic threshold)
ARTERIES
BLOOD PRESSURE
Body composition (%bodyfat, skinfold thickness)

BONES
CARBOHYDRATE TOLERANCE
(diabetes, glucose sensitivity)
CARDIAC PERFORMANCE (stroke
volume, cardiac output)
COAGULATION (factors affecting
coagulation of the blood)
COLLATERALS (development of
coronary blood vessels)
Endocrine (cortisol, epinephrine, etc.)
ENERGY BALANCE (obesity, weight
control or metabolism)
GROWTH (growth hormone, growth and
development in children)
HEART FUNCTION TEST (screening for
ECG abnormalities)
JOINTS (arthritis, stiffness, collagen, range
of movement)
LIPIDS (blood lipids, cholesterol, HDL,
LDL, triglycerides)
MENSTRUAL FUNCTION
MENTAL HEALTH
METABOLIC FUNCTION
MOOD
MUSCLE METABOLISM (enzyme
concentration, capillary density)
MUSCLE STRENGTH (fibre type, weight
training, body building)

Neurological function
PAIN
PERCEIVED EXERTION
PERSONALITY (behavioural changes,
learning, cognitive performance, self-
concept)
PREGNANCY
PSYCHOMOTOR PERFORMANCE
REPRODUCTIVE HORMONES
RESPIRATORY FUNCTION (cystic
fibrosis, asthma, etc.)
SLEEP
URO-GENITAL TRACT
VEINS
Weight (weight change as main focus)

Diseases and disorders
(other than those specified in the appropriate
subsection)

Cancer
EPIDEMIOLOGY-CHD (studies of
incidence or prevalence of coronary heart
disease)
Handicap (physical, mental)
Hazards (risks and injuries other than
cardiovascular)
HAZARDS-CVS (cardiovascular hazards
other than in section 233)
Kidney disease
PRIMARY PREVENTION (risk factors
for coronary heart disease, see also LIPIDS
and BLOOD PRESSURE)
SECONDARY PREVENTION (studies of
established coronary heart disease)

Other

GENERAL HEALTH
Review (books, reviews, editorials,
supplements)

Author index

Hoffman-Goetz, L. — 800/17
Hofman, A. — 220/35
Hofmann, V. — 231.3/52
Hohimer, A.R. — 620/40, 78
Hoiberg, A. — 232/68
Holdich, T.A.H. — 240/21
Hodgson, D.R. — 120/13
Hodgson, J.L. — 110/30, 231.4/43, 510/43, 45, 116, 630/16
Hodgson, S.F. — 420/87
Hodsman, G.F. — 220/13
Hoe, S. — 231.4/81
Hoepfel-Harris, J. — 231.2/28
Hofer, V. — 234/11
Hoffman, A. — 232/67, 69, 231.4/69, 164
Hoffman, D.I. — 610/101
Hoffman, M.D. — 110/83